Suicides in prison

The suicide rate in prisons in England and Wales is 40 per 100,000 – four times that of the general population. How can this rate be explained? Recent prison suicides have aroused much public concern and media attention, yet there has been very little research examining their true cause or nature. Previous studies have tended to rely exclusively on official statistics and prison records, and have had little effect on formulating policy and practice.

Suicides in Prison is the first major study in this area to draw directly on the experiences of both prisoners and staff. The interviews conducted by the author help to cast new light on the circumstances which can lead to suicide or attempted suicide. The book provides further evidence to support the growing recognition that suicide is not an exclusively psychiatric problem. The coping mechanisms and social support given to the people involved can play a crucial role.

Alison Liebling also shows how serious difficulties in the management of prisoners at risk of suicide may be exacerbated by problems of communication between departments, and that prison officers may lack the necessary training to play a potentially major role in suicide prevention. Most importantly, if staff perceptions and attitudes are not addressed, any attempt to improve procedures may well be ineffective.

Suicides in Prison will be of interest to probation officers, social workers and prison staff and governors as well as those studying penology. It traces the recent history of the problem and provides the first major theoretical discussion of the nature and causes of suicide in prison.

Alison Liebling is Research Associate at the Institute of Criminology in Cambridge.

Also available from Routledge:

Prisoners' Children: What are the Issues?
Edited by Roger Shaw

Children Inside: Rhetoric and Practice in a Locked Institution for Children
Barbara Kelly

The State of the Prisons – 200 Years On
Edited by Dick Whitfield for the Howard League

Racism and Anti-Racism in Probation
David Denney

Suicides in prison

Alison Liebling

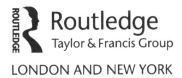

Routledge
Taylor & Francis Group

LONDON AND NEW YORK

First published in 1992 by
Routledge
2 Park Square, Milton Park, Abingdon, Oxfordshire OX14 4RN

Simultaneously published in the USA and Canada by
Routledge
a division of Routledge, Taylor & Francis.
711 Third Avenue, New York, NY 10017

First issued in paperback 2014

Routledge is an imprint of the Taylor and Francis Group,
an informa business

British Library Cataloguing in Publication Data
A catalogue record for this book is available from the British Library.

Library of Congress Cataloging in Publication Data
Liebling, Alison, 1963–
    Suicides in prison / Alison Liebling.
    p.   cm.
    Includes bibliographical references and index.
    1. Prisoners—Great Britain—Suicidal behavior.   I. Title.
    HV6545.6.L54   1992
    365'.6–dc20   92–4230
                                                                          CIP
ISBN 13: 978-0-415-07559-6 (hbk)
ISBN 13: 978-1-138-88141-9 (pbk)

Typeset by Michael Mepham, Frome, Somerset

Social death begins when the institution ... loses its interest or concern for the individual as a human being and treats him as a body – that is, as if he were already dead.

(Schneidman, 1973:159)

For my brother Jonathan, and my sister Helen

Contents

Tables and figures

FIGURE

Acknowledgements

The research on which this book is based was supported by a grant from the Economic and Social Research Council. I am indebted to them for their award. A research fellowship from Trinity Hall supported me in all ways once that research was complete and enabled this book to be written.

I would like to thank all those people who gave their time and interest so generously in the early stages of the research carried out during the course of writing this book. In particular, Mark Williams, Enda Dooley, Simon Backett, Keith Hawton, Derek Chiswick and Brian Burtch. I have to thank friends and colleagues at the Institute of Criminology in Cambridge for support and inspiration, particularly my fellow PhD students. Thanks to Ania Wilczynski, also to Richard Sparks and Will Hay, for guidance and example. I would also like to thank Tony Bottoms, Nigel Walker and Brenda McWilliams for their advice, and Adrian Grounds, my supervisor, for his. I am indebted to Jean Kenworthy and particularly to Thelma Norman and Pam Paige for sympathetic rescue in administrative crises, and to all the library staff at the Institute, particularly Jean Taylor and Betty Arnold for tolerating increasing demands on their resources, desk space and coffee. I also thank Helen Krarup for her time, and interest, and for joining the new team.

I have to thank staff at the Home Office Prison Department and the Research and Planning Unit for allowing this research to begin and for making the necessary arrangements. To John Ditchfield in particular, I am grateful for his interest and his time. Thanks to Martin Steer for suggesting that I should attend the Prison Chaplaincy Conference, and to the Prison Service Chaplaincy for being such enthusiastic hosts. My thanks go to the staff and prisoners who made this research possible and enjoyable, despite its nature. I hope the book makes some contribution to their needs.

To Trinity Hall, especially David Thomas, I owe my sanity. A special 'thank you' to informers and listeners, and to Geoff Parks, for the CD-player, the car and the table-tennis. To a few special friends: Fran, Judith and Andrew, thanks for everything. To Alastair MacDonald, up the road, thank you for your encouragement and for placing some important signposts. To my family, thank you for being there. Finally, for his continuing interest, and for inspiration, I thank Professor Keith Bottomley.

Abbreviations

ADP	Average daily population
AG	Assistant governor
BGO	Basic grade officer
BOV	Board of Visitors
CG	Comparison group
CI	Circular Instruction
CIES	Correctional Institutions Environment Scale
CNA	Certified Normal Accommodation
CSC	Correctional Service of Canada
DC	Detention centre
DPS	Directorate of Psychological Services
DRSMU	Directorate of Regimes and Services Management Unit
EDR	Earliest date of release
ESA	Education, Science and Arts Committee
ETL	Essential task list
HORPU	Home Office Research and Planning Unit
LDR	Latest date of release
(S)MO	(Senior) medical officer
MSC	Massachusetts Special Commission
NEPO	New entrant prison officer
OPCS	Office of Population Censuses and Surveys
PED	Parole eligibility date
PGO	Personal group officer
PO	Principal officer
POA	Prison Officers' Association
SER/SIR	Social E(I)nquiry Report
SG	Subject group
SHHD	Scottish Home and Health Department
SO	Senior officer
SSO	Strict suicide observation
VO	Visiting order
YCC	Youth custody centre
YOI	Young offenders' institution

Introduction

In 1981, a series of self-inflicted deaths and suicides began in the Glenochil complex for young offenders, in Scotland. There had been no deaths at the establishment until this time. The suicide rate for Scotland as a whole had been increasing over many years and this increase had been quite marked amongst young men in the 15–24 age group. The annual rate of suicide per 100,000 had increased from 7.2 in 1971 to 11.6 in 1981 (Scottish Home and Health Department (SHHD) 1985:15). However, as the authors of a Working Group Report reviewing suicide precautions at Glenochil pointed out, there was:

> no remarkable change in the national trend in 1981 that would help to explain the deaths at Glenochil over the past few years. In any case, it is clear that the rates within the complex are much higher than in the general population.
>
> (SHHD, 1985:15)

Since the Glenochil suicides occurred in the early 1980s, similar deaths amongst young offenders in custody occurred in England and Wales, sometimes in series, and increasingly, in apparently disproportionate numbers to those occurring either in the community or in prison. The relative neglect of the prison suicide problem in research, yet its attraction for media and campaigning organisations left an absence of reliable or helpful information from which policy and practice could be advised. The gap was filled by myth, cliché and fear on the one hand, and innovation on the other. Inside prisons, a wealth of information and experience existed and examples of good practice in averting suicide attempts could be found. Importantly, staff and prisoners could provide many clues as to the possible causes of suicides in prison. They had never been asked for their account of the problem; where they had spoken, their voices had seldom been heard.

These events and the official and public responses to them provide an important context in which the material to follow in the rest of this book might be understood. This Introduction will trace the rise in young prisoner suicides throughout the 1980s and attempts made by the Prison Department to reduce these and other prison suicides. The increasing prominence of the young prisoner suicide issue in the media, and the distress caused to prison staff expected to manage and prevent such attempts precipitated many important initiatives intended to tackle the problem in several different ways. New Circular Instructions on suicide prevention were issued, new training programmes for staff were designed and a review of suicide prevention procedures was carried out by the Chief Inspector of Prisons in 1990. A long-term research project was commissioned into suicide attempts in male prisons to be carried out by the Cambridge Institute of Criminology.

It is in this context, of the increasing incidence of young prisoner suicides and of growing Prison Department concern that the research upon which this book is based was initially carried out. It is presented here in the knowledge that more remains to be said and discovered about the nature and extent of the prison suicide problem and that yet it demands to be understood. The available literature has been gathered together from many disciplines in order to assess the current state of the art. It has been found wanting. What it lacks is coherence, theoretical reflection, balance and co-ordination. Whilst no one book can fulfil these requirements, nor one author possess all the necessary skills to perform such a task alone, what follows is an attempt to redress the balance. If the reader can stay to the end and feel a greater concern for and understanding of the young prisoners who have taken their own lives, for the many who have tried, and for those who have felt or who continue to feel tempted, this book will have achieved much of its aim. If the reader can also appreciate the task facing those who are charged with the care and containment of these and other such prisoners and if he or she feels moved to continue the struggle to understand and improve, it will have accomplished a greater goal.

At the time when the Scottish Working Group was set up there had been a total of five deaths at the Glenochil complex within a period of three years. Two more deaths occurred in 1985, during the time of the review. At this stage, the Report noted: 'Not only has the heightened anxiety extended to both establishments, but parasuicidal activity[1] had also developed. At the time of our review, we found both features to be predominant aspects of the complex' (SHHD, 1985:31). The Secretary of State for Scotland, Mr George Younger, told the Commons that there was no evidence to suggest a 'common link' between the deaths. Members of the Working Group on suicide precautions at Glenochil included Dr Derek Chiswick (Chairman), a Senior Lecturer in Forensic Psychiatry at the University of Edinburgh. Their report included a description of the regimes in operation, the sort of offenders received and the typical problems facing inmates and staff. A certain level of bullying and harassment of the more vulnerable young offenders, including, on occasion, incitement of the inmate to hang himself, was a feature of the 'inmate sub-culture'. The Working Group described the outbreak of suicidal behaviour within a closed institution as a familiar phenomenon:

> They tend to follow a pattern: after the first one or two incidents, both staff and inmates become very sensitive to the possibility of suicidal behaviour; staff anxiety rises and leads to increased surveillance and security, which may be counter-productive; among inmates, the initial shock gives way to an acceptance

of self-injury and suicide, so that at times of stress it becomes a more likely reaction.

(SHHD, 1985:16)

A Circular Instruction (CI 1/83) was issued by the Scottish Home and Health Department (SHHD) to all penal establishments in Scotland, in January 1983, giving guidelines on identifying inmates who may be suicidal, and information on the procedures to be followed when a risk was identified. In the next two years, however, four more deaths were to follow.

Increased staff sensitivity towards all acts of self-injury arising as a result of the first few deaths, and a conscientious adherence to stringent guidelines in the recent Circular, gave rise to an unprecedented number of inmates who declared themselves to be suicidal, or who injured themselves superficially in order to remove themselves from difficulties they were experiencing in the mainstream of the young offenders institution.

The Working Party interviewed 24 inmates being kept under suicide observation during the time of their review (21 of these were under strict suicide observation (SSO), which involves the removal of all potentially dangerous items from the cell). They fell into three main groups:

1 those who were mentally disturbed, either as a result of mental illness or a temporary emotional upset;
2 those seeking protection because they were being bullied owing to the nature of their offence, or because they could not cope in the mainstream, e.g. due to mental handicap, or weakness (this was the largest group).
3 those seeking a way out of the (DC) regime in which they found themselves.

It appeared, therefore, that many inmates were willing to endure long periods in conditions of severe deprivation on SSO rather than return to life in the mainstream wings. It should be noted at this stage that not one of the seven young men to take his own life was being kept under strict suicide observation at the time of his death (although one had been taken off special watch a few weeks before he hanged himself). In 1984, 164 inmates were placed on SSO for periods ranging from two to 365 days (SHHD, 1985:33).

According to the Working Party Report, prolonged use of SSO was found to be a feature peculiar to Glenochil. In England, at Aylesbury, Feltham and Glen Parva, for example, 'sanctuary', where it was necessary, was provided by accommodation in the prison hospital or in a separate wing, so that association could take place; and shared cells were encouraged. The Working Party seemed to feel that arrangements in England were better:

In the three youth custody centres in England of comparable size to Glenochil ... there are extensive prison hospital facilities either on site or close at hand. In addition there is a range of different programmes designed to cater for groups of young offenders with different needs. For example there was separate accommodation for those serving long sentences, those in need of a more structured regime, those in need of closer supervision and those who are emotionally vulnerable.

(SHHD, 1985:38)

Current suicide prevention procedures in Glenochil were thought to be unsatisfactory, not least because the regime, originally intended for those at risk of suicide, had become: 'contaminated by its use for those who seek a refuge and those who find the conditions preferable to the mainstream' (SHHD, 1985:40). Dr Chiswick felt that 'this is not a psychiatric problem, it is a management problem' (Chiswick, 1988, pers. comm.), troubling words from a psychiatrist. Since this Report has been published, Glenochil has been closed as a young offenders establishment. The members of the Working Group felt that the prime causes of suicide were in fact largely situational, and that this was a feature particularly salient to young offender establishments. The establishment's approach to the prevention and management of suicide attempts had been to 'batten down the hatches', and attempt to make Glenochil 'suicide-proof'. Instead, there was a need to address issues of staff confidence, inmate bullying and other non-medical aspects of suicide management.

In England and Wales, throughout the corresponding period (1981–5), there had been three hangings within 12 months, in HMYCC Swansea. Elsewhere, in 1982, a young prisoner suicide at Ashford Remand Centre led to a verdict of 'lack of care' by the inquest jury (Home Office, 1984:vii). This verdict spurred considerable concern amongst Home Office personnel, sufficient to lead to the first 'thematic review' to be carried out by the Inspectorate of Prisons: 'Suicides in Prison', in 1983 (Home Office, 1984). This report marked a new departure for the Prison Inspectorate. It was the first of the Chief Inspector's reports to focus on a theme, rather than an individual prison, and was undertaken as a result of both public and official concern over the number of suicides in prison.

No mention of the Glenochil suicides was made in this report, published on 3 September 1984. (However, detention centres for young offenders were abolished by the Criminal Justice Act, 1988 in England and Wales.) Instead, the focus was on current suicide prevention procedures in the prison system as whole. The report included some limited statistical and case-history data on suicides that had been collected by the Prison Department.

The report pointed out, perhaps unhelpfully at the time, that the suicide rate in prisons overall was 40 per 100,000, about four times that of the general population. Calculations of suicide rates in prison are complex and misleading (see Chapter 1). More cautious estimates suggest that given the particular demographic characteristics of the prison population, a fair comparison would have been with equivalent groups in the general community. It should also take account of the number of receptions arriving at each prison annually: a figure which far exceeds the average daily population (ADP), on which most figures are based. Underestimations of the total number of suicides per annum are likely. Suicide verdicts are not always brought: at least a fifth of all prison suicides are likely to receive other verdicts, such as 'open' or 'misadventure' (Dooley, 1990b). Verdicts outstanding on inquests also affect the annual figures, as deaths are not registered as suicides until the cause of death has been established by an inquest, to be held with a jury (see Chapter 4). After the sudden rise in 1987, the prison suicide figures reached a 'plateau' (Dooley, 1990c). From 29 self-inflicted deaths in prisons in England and Wales in 1985 and 21 in 1986, the figures leapt by over 100 per cent to 46 in 1987, 37 in 1988 and 48 in 1989 (Home Office, 1990a:8).[2] The figure for 1990 reached 50. In line with both official and popular assumptions about prisoners, which present them as a particularly 'suicide-prone' group, the Prison Department Report commented: 'Given their background and circumstances, it is perhaps not surprising that prisoners should be particularly prone to kill themselves' (Home Office, 1984:1.12.). 'High-risk' groups included remand prisoners, the mentally ill and lifers, according to evidence summarised in the Chief Inspectors' Report (Home Office, 1984). Suicides were most likely to occur early in the period of custody. Between 1972 and 1982, in England and Wales, there were 169 suicides in prisons; 45 per cent of these were remand prisoners, even though they made up only 10–15 per cent of the prison population at that time (Home Office, 1984). This over-representation of remand prisoners is the most consistent finding of prison suicide research.

A Working Group was to follow, and their recommendations culminated in a new Circular Instruction (3/1987) issued to all Prison Department establishments to come into effect on 1 March of that year. In its introduction, the Circular refers to the 'substantial task' of suicide prevention in custody:

> The rate of suicide in prison may be as much as four times that in the community; and suicide accounts for over a quarter of all deaths of inmates. And for every inmate who kills him or herself there are many more who injure themselves with apparent suicidal intent; and even larger numbers seriously consider killing themselves. So at any one time there is a small but significant part of the prison population which is at risk.
>
> (CI 3/1987:3)

The Working Group, the Instruction continues, defined the task of the Prison Service in preventing suicide as follows: 'to take all reasonable steps to identify prisoners who are developing suicidal feelings; to treat and manage them in ways that are humane and are most likely to prevent suicide; and to promote recovery from suicidal crisis' (CI 3/1987:3).

A SUICIDE CRISIS?

Ironically, the year following the implementation of the new Circular was the worst in the Prison Service's history for suicides. The numbers doubled. Media interest, questions in Parliament and local campaigns raised the profile of an issue which was automatically linked to the 'other prison crisis': overcrowding. 'Epidemics' in particular prisons (and on particular wings) raised questions about situational factors – the problem of suicides in prison became a media and campaign issue (R. Smith, 1985; Smith, 1986).

Risley remand centre, in Cheshire, was the first English establishment to suffer from a rash of suicides. Risley had in fact been the subject of a public campaign a decade earlier for the same reason (Walker, 1991, pers. comm.). Twelve prisoners had hanged themselves there within five years of its opening (1964 to 1969) (*The Observer*, 20 July 1980). A total of 20 prison suicides in 1979 had attracted the attention of the media. Brixton, Oxford, Dartmoor and Leeds had all suffered suicides in 1980, bringing the total in that year to 21. By 1987 this figure had more than doubled. Eight verdicts of suicide at Risley were recorded in a period of 18 months between 1988 and 1989 following the deaths of six men and two women. Risley was severely overcrowded and understaffed. A Chief Inspector's Report by the new Inspector of Prisons, Judge Tumim, announced that inmates lived in 'barbarous and squalid conditions', a comment for which he was immortalised in the press. He found a 'shocking disregard' for the Circular Instructions intended to manage and prevent suicide attempts. Risley became the subject of severe criticisms: it provided profoundly depressing conditions for unconvicted prisoners; inadequacies of design had laid the foundation of 'hopelessness and apathy'; 'grave omissions' had occurred. In respect to the report, Governor grades were removed, and a six-year redevelopment plan was announced, which was to transform Risley from a remand centre into a local prison. One immediate change was that all offenders under the age of 21 were to be transferred out.

As the problem continued to attract attention and concern in the media, the link between 'suicides and overcrowding' became more refined. In May of 1989, *The Independent* linked suicides in prison to four basic problems, all with practical solutions: the problem of remands in custody; the number of mentally ill offenders on remand; the unaccountable operation of the prison medical service; and the inadequate implementation of a Circular on suicide prevention (*The Independent*, 5 April 1989). Sympathy for the 'overstressed' officers expected to deal with 'the types of disturbed and vulnerable people who are sent there by the court' began to appear for the first time: 'Conditions in the jail had been exacerbated by the high percentage of psychotic and drug-addicted prisoners, combined with overcrowding and an absence of any proper training for officers to deal with vulnerable inmates' (*The Independent*, 5 April 1989). Mr Harry Fletcher, general secretary of the National Association of Probation Officers, was reported to say that the Prison Department needed 'to look beyond the squalor and the food before things can change' (*The Independent*, 5 April 1989), suggesting that physical conditions alone were not a sufficient explanation for prison suicides. The situation was to deteriorate further. In January of 1989 the Home Secretary was urged to launch an inquiry into a series of suicides at Armley prison in Leeds. There was something particularly distressing about these deaths: they were all young offenders and they were all awaiting trial. At that time there had been four deaths within six months. The Home Secretary agreed to an internal inquiry. The confidential inquiry concluded that there was no connection between the deaths, and that conditions in the prison were not to blame. Domestic problems were the major trigger. Some recommen-dations such as more sophisticated lighting, the establishment of a suicide-prevention management group, staff training and improvements to the reception areas were made, and swiftly implemented.

The Home Secretary declined to bring an Inspection of Leeds prison forward from December of that year. The following month there was another suicide. Again, this occurred on the young-offender remand wing. The Howard League for Penal Reform began their own inquiry into the deaths. Evidence was submitted from many quarters, but they were not allowed access to the prison (Grindrod and Black, 1989). Evidence of incitement to suicide by cell-mates hoping to be treated sympathetically by the courts, and of systematic bullying appeared in coroners' inquests. It was rumoured that inmates sometimes injured themselves before a court appearance, hoping that this would mitigate a sentence (*The Independent*, 12 April 1989).

In April, 1989, Mr Barry Sheerman, the Labour Home Affairs spokesman said: 'There has been a very profound leap in the suicide figures. I believe this is a fundamental symptom of the problems in our prison system – the overcrowding and the unacceptably high number of prisoners on remand' (*The Guardian*, 5 April 1989). Leeds prison launched its own campaign against suicides, training its staff and improving its recording and management approach to self-injury. In 1989, 106 cases of deliberate self-injury occurred: 47 were considered to be possible suicide attempts; 36 were attempted hangings; 28 were amongst people aged 19 and under (Home Office, 1990a:33). In July of 1991, the young offenders were removed from Leeds. They were transferred to a new prison (Moorlands) near Doncaster.

In May of 1989 the Home Office issued a shorter and clearer Circular on Suicide Prevention (CI 20/1989), replacing the thorough but unwieldy 3/1987. This restated and modified their suicide prevention procedures in several ways. A certain amount of the form-filling on reception was trimmed in busy remand centres, to allow more time for interviewing those inmates who were thought to be at risk. The Circular represented a sensitive response to problems establishments were having in follow-ing the previous procedures, and led to improved operations by restricting reception screening in this way. But problems continued. A 'lack of care' verdict was brought in the case of a prisoner who hanged himself in Winson Green prison in Birming-ham, after a failure of communication regarding his risk category resulted in his being left unsupervised in an ordinary cell. The Home Office contested the case (R v. Birmingham and Solihull Coroner, Ex-parte Secretary of State for the Home Department, July 1990); the Divisional Court quashed the verdict and ordered a fresh inquest. The second inquest jury returned a verdict of 'suicide in circum-stances aggravated by lack of care'. This case raised several fundamental questions about suicides in prison: could the failure to prevent a suicide in custody constitute 'lack of care' on the part of the prison authorities?[3] Only three such verdicts had ever been brought in cases of prison deaths before 1989, and only one of these was a suicide. Was 'failing to prevent' suicide an act of commission, or one of omission – and how substantial an omission?

At Brixton prison in the first months of 1989 there were eight suicides of mentally disturbed remand prisoners. An official inquiry was launched into the professional conduct of one of the doctors. Three members of staff also committed suicide during the year. It was not just the inmates who were being exposed to 'unacceptable levels of stress' (*The Sunday Correspondent*, 29 October 1989). In 1989, Hull prison also suffered from an 'epidemic' of self-injury on its 'B-Wing' – a remand unit for young offenders. The wing was severely overcrowded and 15-year-old boys were held amongst the 200 young remand prisoners:

> Each cell, built for one inmate, held two and they were confined for some 18 hours a day or more. The wing was extensively vandalised both inside and out. Many windows were broken and the exterior wall surface was dirty from inmates throwing fouled clothing, food, the contents of slop pails and packets of faeces from their cell windows.
>
> (Home Office, 1988c:10)

An entire preface in the Chief Inspector's Annual Report of 1989 was devoted to the plight of these young remand prisoners:

> On wet days, when the normal one hour's exercise is not available, many do not leave their cells at all save for a few minutes to collect meals on trays, and to slop out. Education classes are limited for those who attend to about two hours a day. There are no evening classes. The 'midday' meal is served so that the inmates can all be locked back in their cells by midday ... B wing inmates do not have access to the prison library, but only to a wholly inadequate cupboard of paperbacks on the wing.
>
> There is much self-mutilation. More than one inmate a week on average cuts his wrist or arms and needs medical treatment. Whether this is done to attract attention, or out of sheer boredom, or in pursuance of a belief that it will facilitate bail, or bring about longer family visits, we do not know.
>
> (Home Office, 1990a:1)

Hull's Board of Visitors published their annual report, condemning conditions on the wing, and they also contacted the Home Secretary about 'the appalling and deteriorating situation' (*The Times*, 4 April 1989; Hull BOV, 1989). In 1990 a young man facing a murder charge committed suicide at Hull. By August 1991 arrangements had been made for the young prisoners to be transferred to Moorlands. The move was delayed as a result of damage to one wing by young prisoners from Leeds and Everthorpe arriving at Moorlands during early August.

On 1 February 1990, the Chief Inspector of Prisons, Judge Tumim, was asked to undertake a review of the policies and procedures intended to manage and prevent suicides in custody, taking particular account of the problems presented by mentally disturbed inmates. His terms of reference were:

> To review the effectiveness of the current policy and procedures for the prevention of suicide and self-harm in Prison Service establishments in England

and Wales, with particular reference to the risks posed by mentally disturbed prisoners; and to make recommendations.

(Home Office, 1990d:1)

Judge Tumim reported in December 1990. He called for evidence to be submitted from many quarters, including Inquest, the Prison Reform Trust and informally, from the Institute of Criminology; he visited many establishments and sent letters to all Prison Department establishments asking for co-operation and advice. He suggested that possible explanations for the drastic increase in prison suicides were the closure of long-stay mental hospitals, resulting in an increase in mentally disordered prisoners, the introduction of new screening procedures, which had focused the minds of both inmates and staff on the problem, and the rapid changes in the working arrangements and management of establishments brought about by Fresh Start.[4] He commented that it was unfortunate that the increase in the number of prison suicides was occurring 'at a time when the Home Office has re-affirmed its commitment to improving conditions and the treatment of inmates' (Home Office, 1990d:3).

His Inspectorate Report of 1990 included for the first time a separate chapter on prison medical services, including suicide prevention procedures. He argued that attempts at suicide were inadequately recorded. Thirty-three verdicts of suicide had been brought during 1989. The Annual Report suggested that 'the destabilising effect of sensory deprivation produced by harsh regimes and containment in a cell, with or without others, for over 20 hours a day' created a depressing life for inmates (Home Office, 1990a:34). This situation was compounded by inadequate sanitation, difficulties of direct access to medical officers, and the use of unfurnished cells for the potentially suicidal. Poor and uneven hospital provision made the observation and treatment of suicide risks difficult and dangerous (Home Office, 1990a: *passim*; Bluglass, 1990). There was no doubt that conditions and facilities in many prisons were poor. In July 1990 the UK received its first visit from a committee established by the Council of Europe: The European Convention for the Prevention of Torture and Inhuman or Degrading Treatment or Punishment, as prohibited by article 3 of the European Convention of Human Rights. The team visited prisons and police cells. The Council intended to report at the end of the year. They expressed 'curiosity about England's regressive and vengeful prison system' (*The Independent*, 9 August 1990). Their visit came 7 months after the Prison Department had issued a new mission statement:

Her Majesty's Prison Service serves the public by keeping in custody those committed by the Courts.
Our duty is to look after them with humanity and to help them lead law-abiding and useful lives in custody and after release.

In May of 1990 the Samaritans published a report showing that suicide amongst young males in the general population had increased by over 50 per cent over the last 10 years, from 10 per 100,000 to 15 per 100,000 (Samaritans, 1990). Mortality

Statistics for England and Wales showed that the suicide rate for all males aged between 16 and 44 had increased from 26 per 100,000 in 1986 to 28 per 100,000 in 1988 (OPCS, 1990). For women there was a decline from 14 per 100,000 in 1985 to 11 per 100,000 in 1988 (OPCS, 1990). At least 600 young men between 15 and 24 killed themselves in 1989 (BBC 2: 'Public Eye' – Suicide: Young Men at Risk). Unemployment, frustrated ambition, consumerism and advertising, confusing role models and lack of social ties were suggested as possible causes. These factors were not sufficient to account for the increasing number of young prisoner suicides. It was possible that the 50 per cent increase in young suicides could be accounted for largely by young men in social-class five: the marginally employed, the unemployed, those with homelessness, drug and alcohol problems, those with poor educational histories and even poorer prospects (Kreitman *et al.*, 1991). This argument supplies at least the beginning of an explanation for the increasing incidence of young prisoner suicides. A group of young people who are especially at risk of suicide in the community are a group who share a particularly high risk of imprisonment. Increasingly, our prisons are full of vulnerable people. As alternatives to custody such as community service, intermediate treatment and curfews are found for those with the remotest chance of succeeding in the community, it is arguable that the prison population has become more concentrated with the recidivist, the high-tariff offender and the 'failure'.

In July 1990, another cluster of suicides and attempted suicides occurred. A 15-year-old boy hanged himself in Swansea prison, within hours of being convicted of theft. The court had deemed him too unruly for local authority care, and no other secure accommodation was available for juveniles in Wales. He had slashed his wrists whilst in Swansea on remand, and was placed in the hospital on his return, where special watch procedures were ordered. Six suicides had occurred at Swansea since 1984. Three of them had occurred during 1990. A Working Party was set up at Swansea to review the suicide problem and suggest improvements. Recommendations made included a review of the practice of isolating inmates at risk, increased use of the Samaritans, improved reception procedures, better training for staff, greater input from Education and other staff, and the voluntary use of personal officers[5] (Davies, 1990). Earlier in July, two 17-year-old boys in adjacent cells had hanged themselves at Hindley Young Offenders Institution. The following weekend, six serious attempts occurred in the same establishment:

> Between Friday and Sunday, two 17-year-olds were resuscitated after being found hanging in their cells. Another two 17-year-olds were taken to the prison hospital with slashed wrists or arms. A 15-year-old and a 20-year-old were found together with sheets knotted around their necks attempting to hang themselves in their cell.
>
> (*The Guardian*, 17 July 1990)

On Monday 6 August 1990, a 17-year-old remand prisoner hanged himself in Leeds prison: the sixth teenage remand prisoner to die by his own hand at Leeds since 1989. He was taken to a local hospital and put on a life-support machine, but he died shortly afterwards. The governor began a second inquiry. A Home Office spokesman was reported in the *The Independent*, saying: 'If the inquiry indicates that something needs to be changed to ensure that it doesn't happen again it will be done' (*The Independent*, 13 August 1990).

Five prison suicides in one month in August 1990 preceded the completion of Judge Tumim's inquiry into suicide prevention procedures. Three of the five occurred at Brixton, and involved mentally ill prisoners. Could the increasing presence of mentally ill prisoners in the prison population account for the increasing suicide rate? The campaigning organisation Inquest were providing expert legal advice to families of prisoners who committed suicide in prison. They also communicated their concern about these deaths to the extensively interested press. The number of 'lack of care' verdicts brought at inquests increased. Still, no satisfactory understanding of the problem emerged.

It was becoming clear that not every 'suicide attempt' was related to suicide. Nor was every suicide related to psychiatric illness. Some young offenders in custody saw the opportunity to influence their current situation, either within the prison, or in the courts by appearing to be suicidal. Some hoped they could secure their own release, or obtain a transfer to another prison. Many attempts, however, were clearly real – and many succeeded. Others came dangerously close. Half occurred amongst sentenced young prisoners. It was thought by many that several suicides were the result of 'staged attempts which went wrong'. Prison staff were faced with a problem of preventing suicides, in restricted conditions, minimising the contagion of the problem, and trying to distinguish between those who were 'genuine' and those who were, in their view, manipulating or 'attention-seeking'. Very little helpful information was available; not only was there very little research on the topic, but what little there was remained unpublished, and ventured no further than the records of the suicides concerned. No-one had ever asked the inmates, or indeed the staff, 'what was going on', and why? In practice, a concern with procedures often diverted attention away from possible reasons for suicides or suicide attempts.

It is this gap that the research on which this book is based set out to fill. Its aim was to bring together the scattered strands of research and literature already existing, to consider explanations already put forward, and to gain information directly from prisoners and staff involved in such incidents, rather than from the retrospective analysis of official records, which formed the basis of much of the material currently available on suicides in prison.

The aim of this book is to assess our current understanding of the nature and causes of suicides in prison, to explore the validity of previous research and to show how research methods which move beyond recorded information alone may contribute to our understanding of the problem. It presents the results of an extensive fieldwork project based on detailed and semi-structured interviews with young inmates treated in prison hospitals for self-inflicted injuries, suicide attempts and threats. Their experiences of the prison world, their histories and their views about the causes of suicides in prison are compared with those of a comparison group drawn randomly from the general population of the four centres in which the research was carried out. Prison staff are also interviewed in order to elicit their own views about suicide and suicide attempts in custody, and to understand some of the problems they face in its management and prevention. By concentrating on a particular group of inmates – young sentenced prisoners – some of the generalisations and contradictions inherent in previous research may be avoided.

The book is divided into three parts. The first part deals with current literature and research in the field, bringing together for the first time a disparate body of material on suicides, suicide attempts and self-injury in prison, and showing how previous research has been limited in several fundamental respects. Research in other areas of prison life suggests that record-based research must be supplemented by interviews with staff and inmates involved in suicide attempts in custody. Chapter 1 discusses early and contemporary international studies of suicides in prison. It shows the limitations of our current calculations of prison suicide rates and presents alternative methods. Much of the existing information on suicides in prison is based on a flawed understanding of prison suicide rates. Chapter 2 brings together current (post-1980) research and evidence relating to 'the prison suicide profile'. Individual and situational factors thought to be associated with suicide risk in prison are considered and some comparisons are drawn with the results of studies of suicide in the community. The validity of a single 'prisoner suicide profile' is brought into question as a result of this review. Chapter 3 reviews the literature and presents current data on young prisoner suicides, showing that they may be distinct from adults in significant respects. Young prisoner suicides are less likely to resemble suicides in the community and are less likely than other prison suicides to show evidence of psychiatric illness, suggesting that prison-related factors may play a significant and distinct part in their causation. Chapter 4 presents a critique of previous research methods and theory, exposing serious gaps in our understanding of the problems of both suicides in prison, and young prisoner suicides in particular. Statistics and recorded information on suicides and suicide attempts in prison are unreliable and a preoccupation with prediction has limited research: few studies discuss the possible reasons for suicide or suicide attempts in prison. Research on prison coping behaviour offers significant insights into the notion of vulnerability to suicide, and suggests a new route for research for our theoretical understanding.

Part II presents the methodological approach developed as a result of the limitations found in existing research and outlines the results of an intensive investigation of young prisoner suicide attempts. Chapter 5 relates precisely how the research was carried out, arguing that the subjective experiences of the individual must be understood in order for his or her actions to be interpreted. The chapter ends with a discussion of matters of ethics and gender in prison suicide research, and other important reflections on the research experience. Chapter 6 comprises a statistical presentation of the results of the interviews, with quotations from selected examples illustrating differences between the subject and comparison groups in their histories and their perceptions of the sentence. Previous research has omitted to investigate whether the experience of imprisonment may be different for the potentially suicidal. What emerges is that the experience of prison is not uniform: inmates' own resources and opportunities vary. These aspects of the prison experience appear to be related to suicidal behaviour. It is also possible to gain a valuable understanding of 'the pains of imprisonment' for all inmates from these interviews: most of these pains are hidden, and yet they are accessible to the interested interviewer. This chapter then presents inmates' views about suicide attempts in prison, and illustrates how and why these attempts occur: their method, timing, location and motivation, illustrating 'the onset of a suicidal crisis' in the inmates' own words. A profile of the 'vulnerable inmate' is drawn up based on the material presented in this chapter. Chapter 7 shows that important differences emerged between the male and female young prisoners, particularly in relation to their deliberate self-harm. Young female prisoners are for many reasons more difficult to differentiate according to factors relating to coping ability and the expression of suicidal feelings.

Chapter 8 presents the results of interviews carried out with 80 prison staff, illustrating their understanding of the problem of suicide and self-injury in prison. An outline of current suicide prevention procedures is included, and staff attitudes towards both these procedures, their appropriateness and the possible causes of suicide and suicide attempts in prison are discussed. Serious problems encountered by prison officers interfere with the successful operation of prevention procedures.

Part III draws together the main arguments and conclusions to emerge from the rest of the book and discusses the theoretical, methodological and practical implications of the research results, suggesting a course for future reflection and research.

Part I

The literature

Chapter 1

Suicides in prison

Rates and explanations

For prisoners ... the death rate from suicide ... is over four times as great ... Is this increased incidence of suicide also a direct effect of the prison environment; or is it due to the fact that persons with marked suicidal tendency are more liable to be imprisoned for crime? This question cannot be definitely answered from the statistical evidence before us, although, in the circumstances of the case, there can be little doubt as to what the correct answer should be. We know that the suicidal act does require a certain conjunction of favourable conditions for its successful accomplishment; and that these conditions would be least likely found in the prison environment, which, with its constant supervision of, and restrictions upon, a prisoner's actions, operates in every direction against his committing suicide easily. Consequently, we should assume that the greater the intensity of the suicidal tendency, the less would be the likelihood of the suicidal act deferred until a time particularly unfavourable for its consummation; but on the other hand, we would conjecture that, amongst persons possessing an *equal* tendency to commit suicide, the additional strain of imprisonment would inevitably lead to an increased desire of death amongst suicides.

(Goring, *The English Convict*, 1913:152)

SECTION I: EARLY PRISON SUICIDE STUDIES

The first UK-published survey of suicides in prison was commissioned by Dr R. M. Gover, the first Medical Inspector to be appointed by the newly established Board of Prison Commissioners in 1878. It appeared in the Third Report of the Commissioners of Prisons (1880). The figures covered the five and a half years preceding the study (1873–31 March 1879). The study was carried out in response to growing concern over the apparently large number of suicides in English prisons at that time (Prison Commission, 1880). Dr Gover concluded from his survey of 81 suicides in local prisons (the ten that occurred in convict prisons were excluded from his study) that suicides occurred most frequently during the first week in custody. He observed that those most vulnerable to suicide were first-time prisoners (42 per cent of the suicides had no previous convictions recorded against them) and those on remand. Of all prison suicides during this period, 34 per cent occurred amongst prisoners on remand or awaiting trial (Gover, 1880:58). Suspense and anxiety relating to the trial were possible explanations for these excesses. Other groups particularly prone to suicide were violent prisoners (that is, those prisoners convicted of violent offences), those anticipating penal servitude and those awaiting transfer to a convict prison, having already received a sentence of penal servitude. An analysis of the occupations of those ending their lives in this way showed that most were mechanics and labourers. Fear – of penal servitude – but also of other fates, was the most influential of the motives for suicide. He noted that prison staff's lack of knowledge about individual prisoners was a relevant factor. Those prisons least able to assign a motive to the suicides were those with the largest numbers of suicides occurring in them.

Gover concluded that in prison, the operation of 'a principle analogous to that of the survival of the fittest' could be detected, 'the most hardened criminals being those who are best able to endure imprisonment' (Gover, 1880:59): the most-often imprisoned were not the most at risk.

Dr Smalley, Gover's successor, analysed those prison suicides occurring between 1902 and 1911 (Prison Commission, 1911). He found that there was an average of 9.5 suicides per annum (range 4–14). The total number for the whole period was 95 (86 males and nine females). The most striking differences between suicides in prison and ordinary suicides was in respect of their age: the incidence of suicide in prison was much higher in the younger age groups. Outside, it was known that suicides occurred more frequently amongst the older age groups: at least 55 per cent of male suicides were aged over 45 (Smalley, 1911:41). Of the 86 male prison suicides in his study,[1] six were under 20 years old, 19 were aged between 20 and 24, 22 were aged 25–34, 18 were aged 35–44 and only 21 (24.4 per cent) were aged 45 or over. This difference in age distribution between suicides in and outside of prison could not be accounted for by the uneven age distribution of the prison population alone. Smalley concluded: 'It is probable, therefore, that some other influences are operative either in the special character of persons going to prison or in the special conditions that attach to imprisonment' (Smalley, 1911:41).

Three of his 86 male suicides had been imprisoned for the offence of attempted suicide,[2] 43 (50 per cent) had been imprisoned for acquisitive crimes, 12 (14 per cent) for homicide (murder, manslaughter and wounding with intent), four for assault and threats, seven for sexual offences (carnal knowledge, rape and sodomy), three for indecent exposure, four for arson, four for vagrancy, four for drunkenness, one for wilful damage and one for brothel-keeping. Those convicted of crimes of impulsive violence or crimes against morality (sexual offences) were found to be most 'prone to suicide': for example, 14 per cent of prison suicides were imprisoned for homicide offences, yet persons charged with such offences accounted for only 2.4 per cent of the prison population (Smalley, 1911:41). Crimes of arson were also over-represented amongst prison suicides.

Smalley commented that suicidal tendency appeared in most cases to be related to the nature of the offence and not the effects of the anticipated severity of the punishment facing the prisoner, except perhaps in offences of exceptional gravity. He argued that although insanity is frequently associated with impulsive and violent crimes:

> It is not, however, to be assumed from this that suicide in such cases is necessarily the result of insanity. It is quite probable that in many instances an impulsive suicide, like the impulsive crime which preceded it, may be an initial symptom of mental disease, but in the absence of other evidence it is at least as likely that the emotional instability shown in the crime and in the suicide may be due to conditions within the limits of mental health.
>
> (Smalley, 1911:41)

He continued:

> This is notably the case, for instance, in children and adolescents; and the earlier age incidence in prison suicides ... may perhaps be taken to point to the influence of the physiological instability of youth as shown by impulsive reaction to the shock of detection or of imprisonment.
>
> (Ibid. :41).

Charles Goring noted in his study of 'The English Convict' that the suicide rate amongst prisoners was over four times as great as that for the general population (73 and 17 per 1,000 deaths, respectively) (Goring, 1913:152).[3] He remarked that these and other death rates were directly modified by the special environmental conditions of English prisons.[4]

No other systematic study of prison suicides was carried out until D. O. Topp, Regional Principal Medical Officer for the South East Regional Office of the Prison Department, carried out his study of suicides in British prisons, published in 1979. Topp analysed the records of 186 prisoners who committed suicide between 1958 and 1971. This figure – the total number of officially recorded prison suicides for that period, with an unusual additional group of deaths receiving open verdicts but thought to be suicides – represents a mean of 13.3 deaths per annum, a suicide rate of 42 per 100,000 daily average population and 14 suicides per 100,000 receptions into custody (Topp, 1979:25).

Topp obtained the official figures for suicides in prison from Prison Department Annual Reports published between 1880 and 1971. The 775 suicides found were divided into seven-year periods, and related to the average daily population of these time intervals, in order to establish trends over time. Topp found that between 1880 and 1971, the suicide rate declined from about 60 to about 40 per 100,000. There were significant variations, with a peak between 1916 and 1922, and a trough (of 28 per 100,000) between 1937 and 1950. No explanation was offered for these variations.

Of the 189 suicides and probable suicides studied by Topp, 69 (37 per cent) were carried out by unsentenced prisoners, or those being held on remand. Of the 117 (63 per cent) sentenced prisoners 66 (35 per cent of the total) were serving sentences of 18 months or more, and 51 (27 per cent of the total) were serving sentences of less than 18 months, or were young people serving borstal/detention orders. Topp's figures showed that a sentence of more than 18 months' duration, whether antici- pated or actually received, was associated with a greater risk of suicide. Not surprisingly, according to Topp, 'life sentenced inmates, the vast majority of whom were murderers, showed the highest individual rate of suicide, with seven deaths for 1,018 receptions' (Topp, 1979: 26; see also West, 1965 and Danto, 1978 on murder followed by suicide). The suicide rate for lifers is about four times higher than for the prison population as a whole (Topp, 1979; see also Dooley, 1990a).

Seventy-seven (41 per cent) inmates committed suicide during their first month in custody; 23 (12 per cent) in their second, 12 in their third, eight in their fourth, and thereafter less than one per month by the end of the first year. Topp concluded that suicide is most likely to be committed during the first few weeks in custody. This finding has been confirmed by virtually all studies, which agree that the period following reception, whether on remand or under sentence, is a time of very high risk.

Almost half (47 per cent) of the suicides were imprisoned for theft or 'acquisi- tive' crimes, and just over a quarter (28 per cent) for violent crime, in contrast to Gover's findings. Also in contradiction to Gover, Topp found that 90 per cent of his suicides had previous convictions, and of these, 64 per cent had previous experience of custody. Topp omits to relate these figures to those for the general prison population, which makes his findings difficult to interpret. No particular patterns were established in relation to the timing of these suicides, but as to method, 168 (90 per cent) died from hanging. Six inmates died as a result of self-cutting, five from falling from a height and four from self-poisoning.

Just over a third (38 per cent) of his subjects had received psychiatric treatment in the past, 56 (30 per cent) as in-patients. Gunn and his colleagues indicated that a history of some form of psychiatric treatment outside prison is about twice as common among prisoner suicides as among the general prison population (Gunn et al., 1978); a history of in-patient psychiatric treatment outside prison is two and a half times more common (Home Office, 1986a:94).

Almost half (42 per cent) of the suicides were said to have shown some tendency to depression in the past, a quarter (19) of these (10 per cent of the total) amounting to a definite depressive illness. Half (51 per cent) had made previous suicide attempts or threats, and these had been multiple in 38 subjects (20 per cent of the total). This is much higher than the 16 per cent of all sentenced men found by Gunn to have attempted suicide (Gunn et al., 1978). A history of previous suicide attempts is one of the more reliable indicators of future risk, especially during the six months following an attempt. As reported in Topp, 5–10 per cent of suicide attempters eventually take their own lives, illustrating that their suicide rate is many times that of the general population. In 65 per cent of those who had attempted or threatened suicide before, the interval between their latest threat or attempt and their actual suicide was less than six months.

Almost a quarter (22 per cent, or 40) of the suicides were under 21, 63 (34 per cent) were between 25 and 34. Information regarding proportions of the prison population of these age groups is not reported, but Topp suggests that the 25–34 group is probably the peak age group of the prison population. Most (79 per cent) of his subjects were single or separated; 54 per cent (100) had been living alone, or were homeless, prior to their arrest. Almost half (45 per cent) had no known contact with relatives or friends, and 62 per cent had a history of 'social mobility'. This evidence of 'anomie' or lack of social integration amongst prison suicides is one characteristic they share with non-prisoner suicides – a finding which Durkheim would have predicted. It suggests that social isolation is a contributory factor amongst suicides in general, though its implications for prisoners are particularly significant.

Over a third (38 per cent) had a history of parental deprivation before the age of 16. No comparative data is given for the general prison population, so the significance of these findings cannot be assessed. Fifty-two per cent had shown some degree of aggression in their lifestyle; 30 per cent had had a drink problem and 11 per cent a drug problem. Gunn *et al.* found that 15 per cent of sentenced adult males had a 'drink problem' and 32 per cent a history of drug abuse. This indicates that alcohol abuse may be more prevalent among suicides than the general prison population, though drug abuse did not appear to be so.

In half of the cases, it appeared that the fatal event was performed on impulse, although Topp claims that in 59 per cent of cases there could have been some expectation of being saved. Despite this judgement, and the fact that over a third (39 per cent) of subjects were under medical/psychiatric treatment at the time of their suicide, only 15 per cent had been recognised as presenting a potential suicide risk. Sixty-nine per cent had seen doctors for complaints with a psychiatric content whilst in custody; 9 per cent had either demonstrated manipulative, attention-seeking behaviour (undefined in this study) or presented problems of control; 30 per cent of the subjects were located in the prison hospital at the time of their suicide.

Topp concluded with a reminder that the prison population is clearly not representative of the population at large, differing both in age distribution and social composition. It is hardly surprising, he argued, that the prison population has 'a higher incidence of depressive episodes and of suicides than exists in the general population' (Topp, 1979:26), a statement repeated in many subsequent studies (Home Office, 1984; Winfree, 1985). Successful suicides were often committed by those with previous criminal records and previous institutional experience, especially when facing a long sentence, or early in custody, before they become 'integrated into the prison inmate culture' (Topp, 1979:26). Topp warned that generalisations risk masking the unique features of each case so that, for example, fear of release may provide sufficient motivation to some prisoners, where the prospect of long periods of confinement is a more common factor in the decision to commit suicide. He ascribed attention-seeking behaviour to many of the suicides, and suggested that altruistic motives concerned with shame about the offence were rarely significant (however, again see West, 1965 and Danto, 1973 on murder followed by suicide). Anxiety about the disruption of already tenuous relationships may have contributed, especially amongst those anticipating long sentences.

Topp's comparison of prison suicide rates with those of in-patient suicides in psychiatric hospitals showed the latter to be significantly higher (by a factor of ten). This does not detract from the main findings of his study: that prisoners are at least three times more likely to commit suicide than the population at large, and many of these suicides could have been predicted or prevented, especially as so many come to the attention of doctors or other staff during the course of their sentence. Topp did not comment on the significant number (40 – 22 per cent) of young offenders in his sample, but ended instead with the comment that his results 'emphasise the deviance of the prison population, and suggest(ed) that it will give rise to a disproportionate number of suicides' (Topp, 1979:27).

Two further key studies of suicides in prison were published in the 1970s, one in Canada and one in the US (Burtch and Ericson, 1979; Danto, 1973). Both were concerned with the search for the prisoner suicide profile. As both studies have been reviewed elsewhere (Lloyd, 1990; Correctional Service of Canada, 1981) only the details of importance to the arguments in this book will be summarised here. Danto edited a collection of studies based mainly on small samples (e.g. 10, 6, 13, 26 inmates) in single institutions. He pointed out that we know little of the 'inside narrative' of being a prisoner. Together the studies confirm that prison suicides may be distinguished from the community suicide by their younger age, the increased isolation and their relatively high association with drugs and alcohol. Prison suicides occurred early in the sentence, especially during the remand period and by hanging. Different 'types' of suicidal inmate can be identified in Danto's study: the disgraced serious offender and the persistent but isolated recidivist (Danto, 1973:17–26). Both of these suicidal types may be distinguished from the attempted suicide, who may be manipulative, and who injure themselves to live, not to die. Some limited descriptive data about the prison environment is included in many of the studies, which is used to illustrate the part played by imprisonment (a 'social death') in the suicide rates. Only one of the studies (Johnson, 1973) gives clear evidence of the contribution made by the prison environment to the various types of self-injury encountered in custody.

The most comprehensive study to be carried out on suicides in prison before 1980 was Burtch's and Ericson's official document analysis (1979) of 96 suicides in four maximum security prisons (1959–1975) in Canada. They found that the young and unmarried were over-represented amongst the suicides, and that those serving both very short and very long sentences were particularly at risk. Suicides were most likely early in the sentence and in 'protective' areas of the prison (hospital, punishment and segregation areas). Offence-type did not seem to deter-mine risk. They argued that control and containment are given a higher priority by prison staff than suicide prevention and that our notion of the prison as a system of 'social defence' leads to the neglect of inmate welfare. The 'silent system' – the secrecy within prisons and the inadequate inquest system – interferes with a proper understanding of prisoner suicides. They suggest that the prisoner population may be 'suicide-prone'.

Summary

Prison suicide research began in the wake of concern about its increasing incidence, and about its possible causes. Early studies recognised both that prisoner suicides may differ from those in the general community, and that they differed less than might be expected from the general prison population. The young, those on remand, those serving long sentences and those facing pressure from other inmates were particularly at risk. Efforts to assess motivation were grounded in the wish to develop appropriate prevention strategies. In prison, with its special environmental features, 'suicide may be due to conditions within the limits of mental health' (Smalley, 1911:41). This early notion that psychiatric history may not be responsible for the high numbers of suicides in prison was an important feature of these two studies, but it was lost in the path of subsequent research.[5]

By 1979, studies were more detailed, but they had become dominated by the search for the suicidal inmate profile. Individual factors were analysed intensely, whilst vague references were made to the prison environment. The 'deviance of the prisoner population' was thought to account for the high incidence of suicide in prison. Particular features of prisoner populations: their social, behavioural and clinical characteristics, provided an adequate explanation for the rates (Topp, 1979). This approach continues to dominate prison suicide research to date.

In the decade since Topp's study, some important advances have been made in our understanding of suicides in prison. Many of the features of prisoner suicide identified in earlier studies have been confirmed (such as the disproportionate frequency of suicide amongst remand prisoners and lifers, and the importance of the early stages of custody). Others have been introduced: the role of social and outside contacts, the process of socialisation within the prison, the importance of timing and particular stages of risk and so on. Still others (for example, the possible contribution made by the experience of imprisonment, the role of psychiatric illness and the validity of prison suicide figures) remain poorly understood.

The following review will present a survey of the most recent and significant studies from the UK, Europe, Australia, North America and Canada, in order to illustrate the most important features of recent prison suicide studies. At the outset, it is important to outline and explore recent evidence relating to prison suicide rates. This will be the task of the next section.

SECTION II: PRISON SUICIDE RATES: CONTEMPORARY STUDIES

The general topic of dying in jail, which itself occurs with admitted regularity, has been largely overlooked by social scientists. Most of the extant suicide research remains either (1) highly speculative with little 'hard facts' to corroborate the author's conclusions or (2), if available data are used, the findings are suspect due to questionable analytical techniques or problems with conceptualization and/or operationalization processes.

(Winfree, 1985:2)

The prison suicide rate in England and Wales is, at the most recent available count (up to 1987), at least 40–50 per 100,000 inmates in the average daily population (ADP) of prisons in England and Wales, or about four times the rate of suicides in the community (Home Office, 1984; McClure, 1987; Backett, 1987; Dooley, 1990a). US figures are much higher: the most comprehensive US studies find the prison suicide rate to be about 200 prisoners per 100,000 ADP, or between five and 15 times greater than the suicide rate in the general population (Flaherty, 1983; Hayes, 1983; Winfree, 1985). In Europe and Australia, the prison suicide rates are between three and 11 times the rate in the general community (Bernheim, 1987; Hatty and Walker, 1986; Biles, 1990). Suicide has been said to be the leading cause of death in prison (Tuskan and Thase, 1983; Danto, 1973; Burtch and Ericson, 1979). Suicides occur between ten and 20 times as often as homicides in prison (Winfree, 1985; Dooley, 1990b). There were 23–24 homicides reported in all US jails in 1977, and ten in 1982. There were 297 and 294 suicides, respectively (Winfree, 1985). Dooley reports an average of one homicide per year in prisons in England and Wales (Dooley, 1990b).

Before seeking to explain these rates, it is an important task of the present review to explore their meaning and validity. Are suicide rates in prison excessively high, or are they simply demographically representative of the population they contain? There are few satisfactory answers to this question in the current literature, as we shall see.

Prison suicide: a preliminary survey of international rates

Studies of prison suicide invariably begin by presenting rates of suicide in custody. Most compare their rates to those for the general community. Most studies base their prison suicide rates on the average daily population in prison: that is, the average number of inmates in the population on any one day. This rate is without exception found to be several times higher than the suicide rate in the general community. An outline of the most recent available international figures will be presented here (see Table 1.1).

UK

In the UK, Backett found the suicide rate in Scottish prisons between 1970 and 1982 to be 51.8 per 100,000 prisoners per year. This rate is calculated on the basis of 33 prison deaths recorded as suicides over 12 years, using the mean average daily population during this time. Backett does not compare this rate with any suicide rate in the community, but other studies estimate that the suicide rate in Scotland at this time lies between 11 and 13 per 100,000 (McCloone and Crombie, 1987).

Dooley found the prison suicide rate in English and Welsh prisons between 1972 and 1987 to have increased from 31 per 100,000 prisoners in the average daily population per year in 1972–5, to 56 per 100,000 in 1984–7, an increase of 81 per

Table 1.1   International prison suicide rates (based on average daily population)

Country	Prison suicide rate		Rate as multiple of general population suicide rate
England and Wales[1]	56	per 100,000	4+
Scotland[2]	52	per 100,000	4[a]
Austria[3]	56–106	per 100,000	2.5–5
Belgium[3]	60	per 100,000	3
Italy[3]	80	per 100,000	10
Switzerland[3]	465	per 100,000	14
France[3]	43–169	per 100,000	1.8–7.4
Australia[4]	90–180	per 100,000	5–11
USA[5]	200	per 100,000	11–16
Canada[3]	120	per 100,000	5–6

Notes: 1 Dooley, 1990a; 2 Backett, 1987; 3 Bernheim, 1987; 4 Hatty and Walker, 1986; New South Wales Bureau of Crime Statistics and Research, 1990; 5 Winfree, 1985; Hayes, 1983; a Calculated from McCloone and Crombie (1987) who show that the suicide rate in Scotland increased from 11 per 100,000 in 1974 to 13 per 100,000 in 1984.

cent (Dooley, 1990a; see Table 1.2). The prison suicide rates based on reception figures will be discussed below. In the community, the suicide rate for males aged 15–44 has risen from 10 per 100,000 to 15 per 100,000 in the last decade (Samaritans, 1990; OPCS, 1990).

In a thematic review carried out in response to increasing concern about the apparently increasing problem of suicides in prison, the Chief Inspector of Prisons compared prison suicide rates with those in the community and found the prison suicide rate to have been between 30 and 50 prisoners per 100,000 ADP between 1958 and 1982 (Home Office, 1984:49). This rate is likely to be 'true', according

Table 1.2   Prison suicides 1972–1987

	1972–75	1976–79	1980–83	1984–87	Increase(%) 1972–75 to 1984–87
Total receptions	544,760	572,277	642,826	671,170	(23)
Average daily pop. (ADP)	37,947	41,757	43,185	46,181	(22)
Suicides	47	69	80	104	(121)
Suicides per 100,000 receptions	8.6	12.1	12.4	15.5	(80)
Suicides per 100,000 ADP	31	41	46	56	(81)

Source: Dooley, 1990a:41

to the report, 'since suicides occurring in prison are unlikely to resemble, and thus be confused with, deaths from other causes' (Home Office, 1984:5). The report calculates that the suicide rate in prison is 'therefore roughly four times that for the general population of males aged 17 and over' (Ibid.). The Chief Inspector comments that it would be much more informative to explore suicide rates for different sub-groups within the prison population (males and females, those on remand and those under sentence and so on) to see whether they show disparate rates (Home Office, 1984:5).

Europe [6]

In Austria the prison suicide rate is between 56 and 106 per 100,000 ADP, or 2.45 times higher than the rate in the general community (Bernheim, 1987:56). In Belgium the rate is 60 per 100,000 ADP, or three times the rate for the general community. In 1979–1984 this ratio increased to 163 per 100,000 ADP, or five times the community rate (Bernheim, 1987:62).

In Italy the prison suicide rate has risen from an average of 31 per 100,000 ADP in 1960–1969, to 80 per 100,000 ADP in the 1970s, an increase from four to ten times the community rate (Bernheim, 1987:103). In Switzerland, the three years for which information is available (1975–1977) show a rather high rate of prison suicides, at 465 per 100,000 (845 per 100,000 for remand prisoners only). This rate is 14 times higher than the rate of 33 per 100,000 for the free community (Bernheim, 1987:109). It is based on a total of 51 suicides, however (an average of 17 per year), in a population of 3,655 prisoners.

In France, for which the most complete and comprehensive figures are available, since 1955 (until 1985) the suicide rate has varied between 43 and 169 per 100,000 ADP, moving higher and lower sporadically, but reaching one of its many peaks between 1980 and 1985 at 139 per 100,000 ADP. The ratio between prison and community suicides has varied between 1.8 and 7.4, the prison suicide rate always reaching higher than the community rate (Bernheim, 1987:93).

Australia

In Australia, the suicide rate is given in only one of the available studies: it lies between 90 and 180 per 100,000 prisoners per year (Hatty and Walker, 1986). Confirming figures can be calculated from the available information in two studies by Biles in his investigation of Australian Deaths (1989b; 1990b).[7] Biles' figures give a prison suicide rate of 138 per 100,000 ADP. The suicide rate in the community in New South Wales in 1988 was 11.7 per 100,000 pop. (New South Wales Bureau of Crime Statistics and Research, 1990:1).

USA

In the US, Flaherty found the suicide rate amongst children in adult jails to be 12.3

per 100,000 ADP – four times the rate amongst children in the general population[8] (Flaherty, 1983). Hayes finds the jail suicide rate in county jails and police lock-ups to be 16 times greater than the rate in the community in his national study (Hayes, 1983). US jail figures are significantly higher than the rates for sentenced prisoners alone; Tuskan and Thase estimate that the rate for US jails and prisons is at least three times the national average (Tuskan and Thase, 1983). Based on figures available in US Department of Justice Criminal Statistics, it is possible to calculate that the jail suicide rate was 180 per 100,000 (401 suicides) in 1987. For sentenced inmates, the rate was 18 per 100,000 (97 suicides), based on average daily population (US Department of Justice, 1988:606–662).

Canada

Bernheim found that suicide rates in Canadian prisons during the early 1980s varied considerably according to region. The ratio of prison suicides to those in the community varied from 2.5 times higher in Alberta to 12.75 times higher in Manitoba. Overall, the prison suicide rate was five times higher than those in the community (Bernheim, 1987:83). The Correctional Service of Canada found the suicide rate in maximum security institutions to be 160 per 100,000 inmate-years, and 90 per 100,000 inmate-years in both maximum and medium security establishments (Correctional Service of Canada, 1981:50–51).

These average figures (see Table 1.1) mask large differences between regions, types of facility and particular years. In particular prisons (for example, many remand centres and local prisons in the UK and elsewhere) suicide rates are much higher, whatever the base from which the figures are calculated.

Accounting for differences

It is consistently found that prison suicide rates calculated on the basis of ADP are several times higher than those rates for the general community. Most of the studies looking at rates over time show both an increase in the rate of prison suicides over and above any rate of increase in the ADP (Dooley, 1990a; Bernheim, 1987; Correctional Service of Canada, 1981) and many show an increase, of varying degrees, in the ratio of suicides in prison to those in the community (Bernheim, 1987; Dooley, 1990a; OPCS, 1990). The differences in prison suicide rates may be accounted for by differences in the relative size and nature of each country's prison population, the proportion of prisoners held on remand and the length of time they stay there. The criteria for bringing suicide verdicts in each country may vary, as may the particular requirements involved in the certification of prison deaths (for example, in the UK and in Australia, a full inquest with jury is to be held; see Chapter 4). In Scandinavia, proof of intent is not a requirement for a verdict of suicide; their rates both in and out of prison are significantly higher than most other countries' (Bernheim, 1987). These comparative rates therefore have certain limitations.

Such comparisons between suicide rates in the community and suicide rates in prison inform most of the research and current opinion on suicides in prison, however. There are some fundamental flaws in these rates. Despite being the most widely used base from which to calculate prison suicide rates, the average daily population is not an appropriate base from which to make comparisons with the general community.

The limitations of prison suicide rates based on average daily population

Whilst the ADP of a local UK prison may vary between 90 and 1500 inmates, over 25,000 inmates may pass through its gates each year (Prison Statistics, 1988; Home Office, 1988a). The same is true of prisons in all countries, some of which (for example, the USA) will have much larger numbers passing through their gates each year. The number of inmates 'exposed to risk' for varying periods of time is therefore much higher than most prisons' ADP. It is recognised that inmates are most at risk of suicide early in custody (Topp, 1979; Backett, 1987; Dooley, 1990a) and during the remand period. During reception high (ultimately unknown) numbers of inmates pass through the gates at a time of maximum risk. There are also serious problems relating to demographic differences between the prison population and the general community, these will be discussed below.

Rates using annual reception figures

Some studies have used annual reception figures as the base rate from which to calculate the rate of suicides in prison. In Bernheim's study in Canadian prisons, if annual reception figures are used, the prison suicide rate is still 1.5 times higher than those in the community, or three times higher amongst remand prisoners (Bernheim, 1987:83).

Using annual reception figures, Scott-Denoon showed that Correctional suicide rates in Canada have fluctuated erratically between 10 and 20 per 100,000 admissions per year during the 1970s. For seven years between 1970 and 1980 the prison suicide rates exceeded community suicide rates, and for three years they were lower than the community rates in Canada, for four years lower than the rates in British Columbia. The author points out, however, that British Columbia has the highest rate of suicide in the country (Scott-Denoon, 1984:4).

Dooley also uses reception figures as an alternative to rates based on the ADP (see Table 1.2). He finds that the prison suicide rate is still 15.5 inmate suicides per 100,000 annual receptions (in 1984–1987), and that this rate has increased by 80 per cent since 1972–1975. This figure will be lower than the equivalent community rate, as most prisoners do not remain 'exposed to risk' (in custody) for a whole year (Prison Statistics, 1988).

The limitations of prison suicide rates based on annual reception figures

These figures are also flawed. They may underestimate the annual rate of suicides in prison, as the average length of time spent in custody by inmates is less than one year. The number of inmates exposed to risk during a one-year period is higher than the average population of prisoners on any one day of that year. For inmates on remand the average length of time spent in custody was 56 days during 1985–1988; for sentenced prisoners the average length of sentence was 24.5 months for adult males (Home Office Statistical Bulletin, 1990). The amount of time spent in custody will be between a half and a third less than this, with remission (or two-thirds less with parole, for some). Most prisoners are at the 'short end' of the sentence scale, those serving long sentences contributing disproportionately to the average length of sentence received. The average length of sentence will be even shorter for young offenders. Some measure of 'exposure to risk' is required.

Reception figures are also flawed demographically, just as the ADP will be: receptions into custody are not representative of the general community. Prisons overwhelmingly contain adult males, whose average age is younger than that of the general population. Any meaningful comparisons between the two populations would have to take these demographic differences into account. Suicidal activity is not an equal-risk behaviour amongst the general community; children under 14 rarely commit suicide, for example (Winfree, 1985; Hawton, 1986). Particular sections of the community are more 'at risk' than others. In other words the suicide rate for 'at risk' people in the community will be considerably higher than the average suicide rate per 100,000 population (Winfree, 1985). Prisons specialise in the 'at risk' population (Bowker, 1982; Hayes, 1983): the homeless, the unemployed, the poorly educated, the alcohol- and drug-dependent, offending males from homes broken by separation, divorce and violence. Despite this, certain sections of the prison population may present a greater risk of suicide than the prison population as a whole (such as lifers, for example, Topp, 1979; West, 1965; Dooley, 1990a). Certain segments of the prison population may contain more individuals who fit the profile of the suicide risk (Winfree, 1985; Hayes, 1983). The 'at risk' in prison should perhaps be compared with the 'at risk' in the community. Young prisoners are amongst those least likely to fit the profile of the suicide risk as we think of this profile in the community.

Only one study calculates comparative suicide rates by taking account of the differences between the prison population and the general community with which it is compared (Winfree, 1985). Two less-detailed studies make some effort to improve on previous methods of calculation, using 'inmate-years' as the base rate from which to calculate prison suicide figures (Correctional Service of Canada, 1981; Harding-Pink, 1990).

Winfree found that when the adjusted general population death rate is employed, the death rates for certain causes (natural causes and homicide) are lower and have decreased in jails (Winfree, 1985). This is not the case for suicides, which are between five and fifteen times higher than the rate for the general community.

These ratios can only be interpreted in terms of the base that is used to create the figures, Winfree argues, and he dismisses the ADP as an insufficient base from which to begin any comparison. Winfree argues that we should develop national equivalent (adjusted or standardised) population rates against which we can compare jail suicide rates in order to reflect the unique character of jail population. His study is carried out in the US, and the appropriate weighted adjustments he carries out are on gender, race and age. The appropriate annual base figure lies between the ADP and the annual reception rate, using an average time of exposure or average length of time spent in custody (the 'exposure to risk factor', or 'person-years-at-risk'). Still this average may mask large and important differences between individuals and groups within the prison population.

In Winfree's US census study, the suicide rate in the general population is 12–13 per 100,000 individuals. The general population *equivalent* (adjusted by age, gender and race) rate is 69–85 per cent higher. The unadjusted jail rate is 11 times higher, the sex-adjusted rate fifteen times higher than the general population rates and 6–8 times higher than the general population equivalent rates. Taking the person-years-at-risk rate produces an annual prison suicide rate of 112–120 suicides per 100,000 person-years-at-risk, a rate five times higher than the general population equivalent rate. It is surprising that Winfree does not consider the possibility that suicide rates in the community may be a serious underestimation of the 'actual suicide rate' for the general population, equivalent or otherwise. Some authors suggest that the underestimation of suicides (the proportion of self-inflicted deaths receiving 'open', 'accidental' or other verdicts) could be as high as 90 per cent of all unnatural deaths receiving verdicts other than suicide (Barraclough and Hughes, 1987; see also Chapter 4).

Winfree concludes that the suicide rate in jails is substantially higher than that in the equivalent group within the general community. He suggests that we should divide ratios calculated on the basis of ADPs by three, giving a figure of a third of that suggested by most authors. If this is done to the studies summarised in Table 1.1, all but two countries would have a prison suicide rate higher than that for the general community. Given that US prisons have a higher ratio of receptions to ADP (US Department of Justice, 1988[9]), these adjusted figures will be a serious underestimation of the relative frequency of prison suicides when applied to many countries other than the US. Winfree also notes that the base population is by definition uniquely disposed towards acts of self-destruction (Winfree, 1985:17). This is a most important aspect of prisoner suicide and should be explored: the proposition will be considered in Chapter 2. If prisons collect the 'suicide prone', this fact should be considered and the reasons for it understood. If they do not, then the high rate of suicides in prison requires an alternative explanation. The two possibilities are not mutually exclusive: high rates of suicides in prison may be explained by *both* the collection of vulnerable individuals and the subjection of many inmates to unacceptable levels of stress.

In Winfree's study of US prisons, person-years-at-risk are highly associated with individual establishment's suicide figures, suggesting that suicides occur where the largest number of prisoners are exposed to risk – that is – where they are most expected. Comparing the suicide rates of prisons like Birmingham (Winson Green) and Durham (whose average annual receptions figure is 50,000 and 25,000, respectively) with those of Littlehey or Sudbury (long-term, Category C and D prisons whose annual reception figures are considerably lower, at as little as 250 per annum) illustrates this point. What is not clear from his study is whether those inmates who do commit suicide are those one might describe as vulnerable. Winfree expresses some reservations about the use of census data, but maintains that his report 'remains our only best picture of death and dying in American Jails' (Winfree, 1985:33).

A study of suicides and self-inflicted injuries in Canadian prisons between 1974 and 1983 calculates rates on the basis of inmate-years served (= ADP $\times 6\frac{7}{12}$ (i.e. 6 years 7 months); Correctional Service Canada, 1981:49). The rate of suicides per 100,000 inmate years served based on these figures is 90 per 100,000 (ranging from 60 in medium security establishments to 160 in maximum security conditions. (N.B. Minimum security establishments are not included in this study, the rates will therefore be an over-estimate of the total prison rate.) These figures will, however (for the reasons given above), be several times lower than those calculated on the basis of ADP alone. This conservative method of calculation still leaves the prison suicide rate at about five times the rate in the general community (Correctional Service of Canada, 1981; Bernheim, 1987). In Geneva, the sudden-death rate[10] per 1,000 inmate years was found to be 8.7 deaths per 1,000 person years. The equivalent death rate, age- and sex-adjusted, for the Geneva population was 1.2 deaths per 1,000 person years (Harding-Pink, 1990).

Reported increases

As few studies have employed such a detailed analysis of suicide rates, little other evidence of the disproportionately high levels of suicides in prison is available. A final method of assessment of prison suicide rates is to compare rates over time, taking changes in the size of the population into account. Dooley (1990a) found that when the increasing numbers of annual receptions were used as the basis of prison suicide rate calculations, it still appeared that the rate had increased over 15 years by 80 per cent (see Table 1.2).

Of those few studies that look at suicide rates over time, most report an increase in prison suicide rates over recent years (Hammerlin and Bodal, 1988; Biles, 1991; Bernheim, 1987; Correctional Service of Canada, 1981; Massachusetts Special Commission, 1984; Hatty and Walker, 1986; Dooley, 1990a). Few studies look in detail at changes in the prison population besides ADP. Public interest in prison suicides has also increased, resulting in a more fastidious reporting of such deaths, particularly recently in the UK, amongst young prisoners.

As we shall see in Chapter 4, there are other important problems concerning suicide and prison suicide figures, but at this stage it is appropriate to conclude that prison suicides are more frequent than might be expected from the age and other demographic characteristics of the prison population and taking into account the 'through-put' of receptions. In addition, prison suicide rates appear to have been increasing over time. A more careful analysis of suicide rates both in and out of prison, and of the notion of equivalent populations, should be a prerequisite for future research. Clearly what is needed is a population base or denominator which is modified to take account of both the through-put factor (which is essentially what 'person-years' attempts to do) and the demographic characteristics of the two populations. It remains to consider whether prison suicides differ in other respects from suicides in the general community. This may be a more instructive approach to prison suicides than the contemplation of suicide rates alone.

Chapter 2

The prison suicide profile

Suicidal fatalities in the prisoner population present a profile which is distinct from the population of suicides generally, but little different from that of the general prison population.

(Hankoff, 1980:166)

SECTION I: PRISON SUICIDES – A SPECIAL CASE?

Prison suicides rates have been shown to be higher than those in the community, even for equivalent population groups, as far as we can tell from available information. Prison suicides also differ in qualitative respects from suicides in the community: their profiles are different. Of most significance is the finding that a history of psychiatric treatment may be less likely amongst prison suicides than amongst those in the community (Backett, 1987; 1988; Barraclough and Hughes, 1987) despite the high levels of psychiatric treatment in the prison population (Coid, 1984; Gunn *et al.*, 1978). On the other hand, prison suicides differ less than might be expected from the general prison population in most respects.

This chapter will look in detail at what we know of prisoner suicides, using recent research and reports to present the available evidence describing those inmates thought to be most at risk. Section II will look at attempted suicide and self-injury, addressing the question of the traditional distinction between these activities and the populations engaging in them. Section III will draw together the two often separate bodies of literature, showing that suicidal behaviour may be conceptualised as a continuum, along which the vulnerable may quickly move.

The prison suicide profile: identification of high-risk groups

Most prison suicide studies are still concerned with the identification of a profile of the high-risk prisoner: what are the common features of prison suicides, and what do they tell us about possible factors associated with risk? This profile, once accomplished, is typically aimed at the prediction (and therefore prevention) of future prison suicides.

This section will summarise the most salient findings of research carried out in the last decade, to explore the notion that prison populations are an especially at-risk group (Home Office, 1984; Winfree, 1985), and to discover which features of prisoner suicides are associated with maximum risk. As most of these studies are either unpublished or not yet reviewed, a detailed examination of their findings on all variables is presented.

Prison suicide studies: descriptive features

Descriptive studies based on the demographic, social and psychiatric charac-teristics of prison suicides have been explored in order to find the common features of those inmates most likely to take their own lives in custody. They are features which are easy to discover, the details are recorded for many other purposes, and they provide a guideline (if valid) to staff, who are expected to be alert to potential suicide risk. These descriptive characteristics are 'facts' about the individual or his or her situation whose possible association with suicide does not necessarily imply or require an explanation – the association alone is a sufficient indication of risk.

Individual characteristics

There is some confusion about the strict division of factors into 'individual' and 'situational'. Many factors (such as penal status and sentence length, family contacts and so on) are assumed to be individual factors as they can be seen as characteristics relating to the individual, rather than features of his or her situation. Some situational variables may only be unbearably stressful because of the par-ticular characteristics of the individual, as we shall see in Chapter 4. For clarity of presentation, this review has attempted to deal with each variable according to its place in the 'individual v. situational' debate. Some do not have a definitive place in such a scheme, and so have been placed according to the author's choice.

Demographic characteristics

Age

Most studies find the average age of the prison suicide to be lower than that for suicide in the general community (Bernheim, 1987; Hayes, 1983; Kennedy, 1984). Prison suicides are reported by at least three studies as being concentrated in the younger age groups (Hatty and Walker, 1986; Kennedy, 1984; Bernheim, 1987). Kennedy found, for example, that 84 per cent of his sample of suicides were under 35, with the mid-20s to early-30s constituting a particularly high-risk age group (Kennedy, 1984:193). As we saw in the previous section, this is in part because the average age of the prison population is relatively low. However, many studies also report that suicides (and particularly suicide attempts) are younger than the average age of the prison population (Correctional Service of Canada, 1981; Hatty and Walker, 1986). Hatty and Walker found that 34 per cent of 77 suicides occurring in Australian prisons between 1980 and 1985 were aged 20–24 (there were 24 per cent of 20–24-year-olds in the prison population during this period); 30 per cent were aged 25–29 (there were 24 per cent of 25–29-year-olds in the prison population). The only other age group to be over-represented were the 50–69 age groups (Hatty and Walker, 1986:16). The particular case of young adults (aged 17–21) will be discussed in more detail in Chapter 3. Backett found the mean age of suicides in Scottish prisons during a similar period to be low, at 28.6 years. He makes no comparisons with the general prison population. As Lloyd points out in his literature review, the lack of any control group for the prison population and/or the general population makes many of these studies of little use in the exploration of the profiles of prison suicides (Lloyd, 1990:4).

Dooley found the mean age of 295 recorded suicides in England and Wales in 1972–1987 to be 32.9 years (Dooley, 1990a). This was significantly *higher* than the mean age for the prison population. Dooley reports that 56 per cent of his suicides were over 30 compared with 33 per cent of the sentenced prison population (Dooley, 1990a:43). Dooley suggests that the unexpectedly high mean age of prison suicides may be linked to the disproportionate presence of those suicides showing some mental illness, which tends to be associated with older age groups. It may be that life-sentence prisoners (who are disproportionately represented in prison suicide figures) are older than their shorter-sentence colleagues. As we will see in Chapter 3, in Dooley's study the figures for young offenders are still disproportionately high, and they are increasing slightly faster than other age groups. Scott-Denoon concludes: 'The early "twenties" appear across the board to show the heaviest suicide rates' (Scott-Denoon, 1984:9). He identifies several groups of particularly 'at risk' inmates, who may be masked by the overall figures, such as the 'very young, noncommunicative inmate with little or no community resources' (Scott-Denoon, 1984:11).

It appears from the available studies that the young are at least as prone to suicide in prison (if not more) as any other age group. This trend remains largely unexplored. In the community, the rate of suicide is consistently found to increase with age, reaching a peak at age 70–80 for men and 60–70 for women (McCloone and Crombie, 1987; Seager and Flood, 1965). The suicide rate has increased amongst young people, but is still lower in the community than for other age groups, at 13 per 100,000 (OPCS, 1990; Samaritans, 1990). The suicide rate for people in the community aged 15–44 has increased in the last decade by 50 per cent (Samaritans, 1990). In prison, during the same period, the figures suggest that the suicide rate for the under-21s has increased by over 100 per cent (see Chapter 3).

Gender

Men have consistently been found to commit suicide two and a half to four times as often as women in the general population (Rich *et al.*, 1988; McClure, 1987; Barraclough *et al.*, 1974).[1] Women make more suicide attempts, but use less lethal methods, such as overdoses as opposed to firearms and strangulation. The use of lethal methods by women has increased in recent years (Rich *et al*., 1988), and the ratio of male to female suicides is thought to be decreasing (McClure, 1987), although recent studies show that the suicide rate for women in the UK is now increasing more slowly than for men (OPCS, 1990). Depressive disorders are more likely to be attributed to females who commit suicide, and economic problems and substance abuse to male suicides (Rich *et al*., 1988).[2]

In prison suicide studies, few female suicides are found (see Chapter 7). This is largely due to the small number of female prisoners in the population (between 3 and 4 per cent, in most countries; Bernheim, 1987), but it is also due to the fact that most studies use all-male samples. Only six of the 13 studies reviewed by Lloyd (1990) provided any specific information on female inmate suicides, and the samples were usually too small to allow any meaningful comparisons to be made. Bernheim demonstrates that in all studies included in his survey, none include more than four female suicides. Table 2.1 summarises the available evidence showing the relative rarity of female suicides appearing either in prison suicide studies, or in the suicide figures on which the studies are based.

Dooley found that the five females in his prison suicide study did not differ from the males; they were therefore not analysed separately (Dooley, 1990a). Only Hatty and Walker find both the death rate and the suicide rate to be higher for women prisoners than for men, but as the numbers are only eight and four, respectively, they do not draw any conclusions from these findings (Hatty and Walker, 1986:14).

Table 2.1   Females in prison suicide research

Country	Author	Dates in study	No. suicides	No. female suicides	% Females in prison pop.
UK	HMCIP	1972–1983	169 (28)	3 (0)	3–4
UK	Backett	1970–1982	33	0	3–4
UK	Dooley	1972–1987	295 (51)	5 (4)	3
France	Fully	1955–1964	183	2	3.2
France	Tournier & Chemithe	1975–1978	173	0	3.2
Belgium	Cosym & Wilmotte	1958–1965	46	5	nk
Italy	Italie	1960–1969	100	4	nk
Switzerland	Suisse	1975–1977	51	0	<3
Canada	Scott-Denoon	1970–1980	35	2	6
Canada	Bernheim	1960–1985	200+	3	2–3
Quebec	Bernheim	1964–1985			
USA	Hayes	1979	419	12	7
Australia	Hatty & Walker	1980–1985	77	4	nk

Note: Compiled from Bernheim (1987); Lloyd (1990); Dooley (1990a; 1990b); Backett (1987); Hayes (1983), Scott-Denoon (1984) and US Department of Justice (1988) (av. no. suicides = 159; av. no. female suicides = 3, 1.8%). Probable suicides not receiving suicide verdicts appear in brackets.

As a result of these small numbers and the tendency of prison suicide studies not to consider women separately, there is no available profile of the female prison suicide.[3] Scott-Denoon concludes: 'The incidence of females in our Correctional Centres appears closely related to their proportion of total inmate population and thus sex cannot be considered a significant factor in predicting suicidal behaviour or assessing suicide risk' (Scott-Denoon, 1984:14).

Ethnicity

Ethnic minorities are over-represented in custody in many countries, including the UK (NACRO, 1985; Casale, 1989; Genders and Player, 1989; Walker et al. 1990). They are not over-represented in the suicide statistics if the rate of suicide is compared with their proportions in the general prison population.

In the UK, no ethnic minority group is over-represented in the suicide figures. In Dooley's study, 83.7 per cent of suicides were UK white or Irish, 6.1 per cent were Afro-Caribbean and 10.2 per cent were Asian or other. The proportions in the general prison population were 83 per cent, 9 per cent and 8 per cent, respectively (Dooley, 1990a:41). These very small differences were not statistically significant. No information about ethnicity is given in Backett's study.

In the US, and in Australia, the significance of ethnic origin is more apparent. Hankoff found that most of his (seven) prison suicides were black or Hispanic, as do many of the US studies taking very small samples (Hankoff, 1980; Gaston, 1979; Esparza, 1973; Heilig, 1973). Larger studies seem to contradict this pattern, finding that the rate for white, single males far exceeds that for other ethnic groups (Hayes, 1983; MSC, 1984; see also Johnson, 1976). The racial mix in particular establishments clearly affects findings in small studies. Scott-Denoon concluded that:

> Clearly the factors of race and ethnic background of our suicide victims are of little value in providing an indicator of suicidal potential ... It appears from our BC Corrections data that as far as native offenders are concerned, that there are not a disproportionate number of their group suiciding in our institutions.
>
> (Scott-Denoon, 1984:28)

It is in Australia that the significance of ethnic origin is most pertinent. Aboriginal deaths in custody became the subject of a Royal Commission in 1988 due to the large and disproportionate numbers of Aborigines dying in Australian prisons. Aborigines comprise less than 1.2 per cent of the Australian population (aged 15 years or more). They die in prison at a rate about 13 times that of non-Aborigines (Biles, 1989a). In police cells this ratio is 20 times higher than that for non-Aborigines (Biles, 1989a). Hatty and Walker found that Aboriginals appeared to be at no greater risk of suicide than non-Aboriginals, considering their numbers in the prison population. However, they found that their prison death rates from all causes was around 50 per cent higher, and that their average age at death was lower than for non-Aboriginals. They make up 13.6 per cent of the prison population (a proportion ten times higher than would be expected from their numbers in the general population, see Biles, 1989a). They constitute 10.9 per cent of all prison suicides (Hatty and Walker, 1986:18). Broadhurst and Maller show that the assumption that Aboriginals' over-representation in prison suicide rates can be accounted for by their over-representation in custody omits to consider their additional disproportionate 'exposure-to-risk' over time. Aborigines are between three and four times more likely than non-Aborigines to return to custody after release, thus increasing the likelihood that any individual Aborigine will die in custody during their lifetime (Broadhurst and Maller, 1990).

No explanations for the high rates of Aboriginal deaths and suicides are offered in either Biles' study or that by Hatty and Walker. A Royal Commission Interim Report suggests that factors contributing to the excess of Aboriginal deaths include their disproportionate representation in the prison population, social and legal discrimination and deprivation, a lack of adequate drug and alcohol facilities for Aborigines and the impact of programmes of separation of Aboriginal families, forced relocation and institutionalisation (Royal Commission Interim Report, 1988:12). Increased exposure to custody over time may also account for the disproportionate number of Aboriginal suicides.

Scott-Denoon concludes from his Canadian study that inmates on immigration detention are slightly more vulnerable to suicide than the general inmate population[4] (Scott-Denoon, 1984:21). He argues that:

> Depending on the seriousness of the charges awaiting a foreign national facing deportation and/or depending on his feelings of anxiety concerning the severing of current Canadian ties or disruption of life, we may have a potential suicide candidate.
>
> (Scott-Denoon, 1984:xvi).

Of Canadian suicides, 8.5 per cent (3/35) were carried out by foreign nationals facing deportation. They constitute between 1 and 3 per cent of the Canadian prison population (Scott-Denoon, 1984:21).

Factors of ethnic background (alone) do not provide an indication of suicide potential in Canada (Scott-Denoon, 1984:27), despite the fact that ethnic minorities are grossly over-represented in the prison population (17–19 per cent, compared to 2.5 per cent of the general community).

Social characteristics

Marital status

Most studies show that inmates who commit suicide are likely to be single (Scott-Denoon, 1984; Backett, 1987; Dooley, 1990a; Hatty and Walker, 1986; Correctional Service of Canada, 1981). The same is true of most prisoners, however. As few of the studies have any control group either for the general prison population or the community, descriptive studies of marital status are seriously flawed. Cohabitation is often unrecorded, and the status of relationships outside may not be static. Dooley found that 21 per cent of his sample of prison suicides were married; 54 per cent had never been married, 20 per cent were separated, divorced or widowed (although 13 (4.4 per cent) had killed their spouse). In three cases (1 per cent) marital status was not recorded. Information relating to the general population was not available for comparison (Dooley, 1990a).

In Backett's sample, 18 (55 per cent) of his suicides were single, a further six (18 per cent) were divorced or separated and nine (27 per cent) were married. Lloyd compares the figures for Backett's and Dooley's study of 73 per cent and 79 per cent of single, separated or divorced inmates, respectively with a figure for a sample of the South-East prison population (Home Office, 1978). He shows that the figure of 71 per cent of single, separated, divorced or widowed inmates is remarkably similar to the figures shown for prison suicides in the two studies (Lloyd, 1990:9). Lloyd adds in a footnote that the Home Office sample consisted of adult inmates only, and may be even higher for the total population.

Phillips also reported in her study of suicides at Brixton that there was a high proportion of widowers amongst the suicide group, which was accounted for by the fact that three of the four were charged with the murder of their spouse. This was the only significant difference relating to marital status between suicides, attempted suicides and the general population (Phillips, 1986:4.5).

In a Canadian study, Scott-Denoon found that 66 per cent of prison suicides were single, separated, divorced or widowed. He concludes that: 'Single, separated, divorced or widowed prisoners ... have a two-thirds greater risk of suicide than married prisoners (common law included)' (Scott-Dennon, 1984:31–33). However, he also argues:

> Certainly the key issue is not the mere designation of marital status but the quality of the interpersonal relationships behind these labels ... negative relationships in a marriage or common-law arrangement can in fact be a crucial factor in an inmate's decision to commit suicide.
>
> (Scott-Denoon, 1984:33)

A spouse refusing to bail out her husband, declining to write or disclosing an affair could well be a sufficient trigger to an impulsive suicidal act. Marriage is not an insulator from suicide. It may be that single, divorced or separated status indicates another social state. Scott-Denoon suggested that: 'While marital status alone is by no means a factor which indicates potential for suicide, it can be indicative of important community relationship support or lack thereof' (Scott-Denoon, 1984:xvii). Similarly, Jenkins argues that: 'there is considerable evidence that even when out of prison, many of those who eventually kill themselves are likely to be less socially integrated' (Jenkins et al., 1982:8). Many of their deaths arise from the 'anomic' nature of their lives, according to Jenkins. Topp had shown, as we saw in the previous chapter, that: '79 per cent. (of prison suicides) were single or separated, 100 (54 per cent.) had been living in lodgings, alone, or were vagrant, prior to their arrest; 83 (45 per cent.) had no known contact with relatives or friends' (Topp, 1979:26).

The most detailed evidence on marital status comes from the Correctional Service of Canada, whose report shows that although there are no significant differences between prison suicides and the general penitentiary population in relation to marital (including common-law) status, it is amongst the single, separated and common-law groups that the highest prison suicide rates are found (Correctional Service of Canada, 1981:56). The report concludes that married inmates are somewhat less likely to commit suicide, but this does not mean that they never do: 11 per cent of their 46 suicides were amongst married inmates.

In Australia, Hatty and Walker found a similar pattern, showing 'that an existing marital relationship is negatively related to the probability of suicide', although 23 per cent (16) of their suicides were married at the time of death. They also show that no differences exist in relation to marital status between the prison suicide group and the overall prison population (Hatty and Walker, 1986:19).

In the community, marital status has a 'marked effect' upon suicide rates, the divorced, single and widowed having the highest rates (Kreitman, 1977). It appears that in prison, marital status itself is not a reliable indicator of suicide risk, and it certainly cannot discriminate between the general prison population and those at risk of suicide. It does seem that the lack of stable and supportive relationships, or the disruption of such relationships may be a precipitating factor, particularly if this isolation extends beyond the most significant relationships. Social isolation is an important factor in community studies of suicide (Sainsbury, 1988; Barraclough and Hughes, 1987) and is of great significance in the study of prison suicide (Scott-Denoon, 1984; Topp, 1979).

Family background

Since the discovery by Topp in 1979 that 38 per cent of prison suicides had a history of parental separation before the age of 16, not one prison suicide study has looked directly at the family backgrounds of prison suicides – a surprising omission given the significance attributed to family history in general suicide studies (Hawton and Catalan, 1987; Farmer, 1988; Morgan, 1979). Topp did not compare his figures for prison suicides with those for the general prison population, which leaves the finding rather bare. In the community, poor or turbulent family history is probably the single, most important predisposing factor to suicide in later life (Diekstra and Hawton, 1987).

Dooley reports only that 26 per cent of prison suicides were living alone or of no fixed abode before imprisonment; 62 per cent were living in some contact with others (including hostels or lodgings). For the rest, information was unknown. Backett similarly gives no details for family background, nor in this case of any indirect measure of family stability. Phillips combines marital status, home address and next of kin together 'as a crude indication of social stability' (Phillips, 1986:35) and finds that no differences appear between suicide, attempted suicide and the general prison population. This may be because the family backgrounds of most prisoners are unstable and unhappy. Measures of family discord, where they occur at all, are unsophisticated, tending to register the existence and timing of separation rather than the degree or repetition of conflict and breakdown. Recorded information will rarely be sufficiently detailed or consistent enough to allow such variables to be investigated.

The multiple constellation of factors relating to family history are a major concern of the literature on suicides out of prison (Goldney and Burvil, 1980; Diekstra and Hawton, 1987). It is likely that the disproportionately high level of family discord amongst prisoners is one of the prime causes of their collective high risk of suicide, a marked vulnerability demonstrated in many studies of prison suicides and prison suicide rates (Home Office, 1984; Winfree, 1985). Long-standing 'interpersonal chaos', particularly with a history of parasuicide, has been shown to identify one particular 'suicide syndrome' (Ovenstone and Kreitman, 1974).

Allebeck et al. (1988) found that substance abuse, antisocial behaviour and a restricted social network were all predictive of suicide in their cohort study of 50,465 young men (247 suicides). They found that: 'poor emotional control and early deviant behaviour predict suicide' (Allebeck et al., 1988:177).

Misconduct in school, alcoholism in the father and 'broken homes' were all significantly associated with suicide. Measures of low intellectual capacity and low social maturity were also found to be significantly higher in suicides than non-suicides. The significance of family history in prison suicides should be carefully studied.

Penal history

Previous convictions and experience of custody   Of those few studies that give details of criminal justice history, the findings tend to be somewhat contradictory. It may be that different 'types' of inmate suicide are appearing in the figures (see below).

Dooley found that 74 per cent of his prison suicide group had a history of previous convictions and over half (57 per cent) had been in custody previously (Dooley, 1990a). Backett found that 29 (88 per cent) of his prison suicides had a criminal history and 24 (73 per cent) had previous experience of imprisonment (Backett, 1987). Griffiths found that attempted suicides in prison had a greater number of previous convictions (Griffiths, 1990b).

Hatty and Walker found that prison suicides were less likely than other prison deaths or than the general prison population to have been imprisoned before: 52 per cent of prison suicides were known to have been previously imprisoned, and 60 per cent of the general prison population were likely to have been previously imprisoned. For 10/77 cases, no information was available (Hatty and Walker, 1986: 20–21).

The Massachusetts Special Commission found that 97 per cent of those suicides in lock-ups for which information was available (34/54) had previous arrest records. Many of the unknowns could have been first offenders, as with Hatty and Walker's study, as time delays in recording are likely (MSC, 1984). Bernheim concludes in his review of European, American and Canadian data that information relating to previous criminal justice history is superficial and contradictory (Bernheim, 1987:207). His argument cannot be refuted. Both those with previous convictions and previous experience of custody, and those without, appear to be at risk.

Circumstances of custody: penal status　One of the most consistent findings of prison suicide research has been that a disproportionate number of suicides occur amongst remand prisoners (Lloyd, 1990; Dooley, 1990a; Backett, 1987; Scott-Denoon, 1984). It is rarely mentioned in these studies that remand prisoners spend less time in custody than sentenced prisoners on the whole, and that their reception rate is significantly higher than for sentenced prisoners for this reason (O'Mahony, 1991). In addition, because local and remand prisons are generally larger (and more overcrowded) than other prisons, reception rates will be even higher. Far more prisoners are therefore exposed to risk during what is arguably the most stressful phase of custody.

Dooley found that 47.1 per cent of his prison suicide group were on remand at the time of death, significantly more than would be expected from the proportion of remand prisoners in the population. During the period of study (1972–1987) an average of 11.1 per cent of the prison population were on remand – 83 per cent were sentenced (47.5 per cent of his suicides were sentenced) and 4.3 per cent (5.4 per cent of his suicides) were convicted and awaiting sentence.

Backett found that 14 (42 per cent) of his prison suicides were sentenced and 19 (58 per cent) were on remand (approximately two-thirds of these were untried, the remainder were awaiting sentence). The average proportion of the prison population on remand during the period of the study was 14 per cent. In Norway, Hammerlin and Bodal found that 75 per cent of their 49 suicides occurring between 1956 and 1987 were on remand. They argue that the isolation of the remand population produces considerable mental, physical and social strain (Hammerlin and Bodal, 1988:4).

In Canada, Scott-Denoon found that 70 per cent of BC Correctional suicides occurred in the remand group, even though remand prisoners account for only 40 per cent of the total inmate population. (Remand prisoners will, however, account for a higher proportion of receptions into custody, as we saw in Chapter 1.) He concludes that remand prisoners are at greater risk of suicide, that suicide prevention programmes should be aimed at the remand population in particular, and that research should explore 'the dynamics at work in the remand inmate groups' (Scott-Denoon, 1984:xx).

From the available literature it is difficult to determine whether the increased rate of suicides during the remand period is due to the greater numbers of inmates exposed to risk during a time of maximum stress alone, or whether other factors may contribute to the excess. Scott-Denoon showed that when the admission rate is used, sentenced inmates in British Columbia had a suicide rate of 15.7 per 100,000 admissions and remand admissions had a suicide rate of 66.6 per 100,000

(Scott-Denoon, 1984: 94). He concludes that inmates on remand have a suicide rate four times that of sentenced admissions. This finding, based on small figures, and on a single location, would require further investigation before conclusions can be drawn.

Other possible explanations which have been offered for the apparently disproportionately high suicide rate on remand include the stressful nature of early confinement (Zamble and Porporino, 1988; Kennedy, 1984; Lloyd, 1990; Erikson, 1975), the tension and uncertainty of the pre-trial phase (Topp, 1979; Dooley, 1990a), the proximity of the offence, overcrowding, staff shortages, the instability of a continually changing inmate population (Gaes, 1985) and the high proportion of mentally disordered inmates on remand (Home Office, 1986a).

Offence The major concern of investigations into the offence for which prison suicides are charged or convicted is the over-representation (or otherwise) of offences of violence amongst the suicides. Gover first suggested that prisoners who were capable of doing violence to others, were also capable of doing violence to themselves (Gover, 1880:62). Studies of prison suicides suggest that inmates charged with or convicted of violent offences are slightly over-represented amongst those who take their own lives, but certain inconsistencies are apparent. It is apparent, for example, that young prisoner suicides are less likely to be imprisoned for a violent offence (see Chapter 3).

As seen in Table 2.2, prison suicides in Dooley's study had a significantly higher proportion of charges or convictions for violent or sexual offences. Hatty and Walker also found that homicide, assault and sexual offences were over-represented amongst prison suicides (Hatty and Walker, 1986:21). Scott-Denoon found

Table 2.2   Suicide by most serious charge or conviction

	All suicides (n=295) %	Sentenced suicides (n=140) %	Sentenced prison population %
Violence against the person:			
Murder	19.0	15.6	3.6
Other	17.3	23.5	15.2
Sexual offences:			
Rape	5.4	3.5	1.7
Other	4.8	1.4	2.9
Acquisitive offences:	33.6	39.0	61.3
Other offences:			
Arson	4.1	5.7	1.1
Criminal damage	4.1	2.8	1.5
Other	11.7	8.9	12.7

Note: $\chi^2 = 12.21$ d.f.$=3$ p<0.01, sentenced suicides v. sentenced prison population.
Source: Dooley, 1990a

that over half (51 per cent) of the 35 suicides in Canadian prisons between 1970 and 1980 were charged with or convicted of violent offences. Offenders imprisoned for violence account for less than one-third of the BC Corrections population (Scott-Denoon, 1984). The Correctional Service of Canada also found a significantly higher rate of suicide amongst offenders charged with violent crimes (76 per cent of all suicides' major crime type was violence against the person) (CSC, 1981:55).

Finally, in the US, Hayes' study found that just over one-quarter of jail suicides were charged with violent or personal offences. A much larger group (30 per cent) were charged with alcohol- or drug-related offences (Hayes, 1983:23).

It is possible that a single well-defined group of prison suicides – (domestic) murderers facing life sentences – contribute most of the difference in offence type between suicide and non-suicide groups. Eight of Scott-Denoon's 35 suicides, for example, faced murder or manslaughter charges (Scott-Denoon, 1984:48). If this group were removed from all studies (as an identifiable group in their own right) investigations into the characteristics of the remainder (the majority) of prison suicides may prove more meaningful.

Hatty and Walker found that prison suicides could be divided into types, each with slightly different criminal justice histories. Their data fell into three 'high-risk' groups, or clusters:

1 the previously suicidal, violent offender, remanded in custody prior to a court hearing;
2 the prisoner unfit to plead or facing the indefinite prospect of a Governor's Pleasure sentence, transferred to unfamiliar surroundings on a disciplinary measure;
3 the young offender, with a history of convictions for property offences (usually takes several convictions before a prison sentence is handed down for a property offence), with no job and no family for support.

Sentence length   When Dooley examined his sentenced group of suicides (140) he found that a significantly higher proportion were serving four years or more than the general prison population; over 25 per cent were serving life sentences (life-sentence prisoners make up 4.4 per cent of the prison population). The point made above, that murderers facing life sentences comprise a large and possibly distinctive sub-group of prisoner suicides (thus biasing the profiles of the rest) is borne out by Dooley's study.

Backett found that of those suicides amongst convicted prisoners, the majority were serving short sentences (for non-violent crimes such as theft). The longest sentence being served was four years. This is rather different from Dooley's findings, above.

As Lloyd pointed out in his literature review, few studies distinguish between inmates facing indeterminate and determinate sentences. Only Hatty and Walker provide this information, and they find that inmates with indeterminate sentences, including governors' pleasure, in particular, are over-represented amongst the suicides (Hatty and Walker, 1986:24).

Psychiatric background

Gunn *et al*. found in 1978 that the male sentenced prison population contained an excess of men with a previous psychiatric history, previous self-injury, alcohol or drug abuse and social isolation compared to the general population. These factors are all associated with an increased risk of suicide (Home Office, 1986a; Barraclough and Hughes, 1987).

Mental disorder/psychiatric contact

About a third of prison suicides are found to have received in-patient psychiatric treatment before their imprisonment (Lloyd, 1990; Phillips, 1986; Backett, 1987). Dooley found that 97 (33 per cent) of his prison suicides had a history of psychiatric contact and 80 (27 per cent) had previous psychiatric in-patient admissions:

> In the 97 cases where a previous psychiatric history was established the primary diagnoses were as follows: psychotic illness (including drug-induced psychosis), 21 cases (22%); depressive illness or reaction, 22 cases (23%); personality disorder, 25 cases (26%), alcohol or drug addiction, 13 cases (13%); other diagnoses or no diagnosis recorded, 16 cases.
>
> (Dooley, 1990a:42)

Gunn *et al*. (1978) reported that 22 per cent of the sentenced population (in 1973) had a history of psychiatric treatment. Coid illustrates through his literature review of psychiatric illness in the prison population that prisons have a higher level of psychiatric morbidity than the general population (Coid, 1984:79).

Dooley's finding that a third of his suicides had a history of psychiatric contact in his study is taken to indicate that an above-average proportion of prison suicides have a history of mental illness. A flaw in this argument, not raised by Dooley himself, is that the remand population (from which 47 per cent of prison suicides are drawn) have a higher level of psychiatric contact than the sentenced population (Taylor and Gunn, 1984; Gunn, 1991, pers. comm.).[5] In addition, even if prison suicides have a slightly higher level of previous psychiatric treatment than the general prison population alone, this is still considerably *lower* than that found in the histories of suicides in the general population. One important finding from Gunn's study is that (sentenced) inmates as a whole experienced a high degree of disturbance and psychological discomfort. The level of this distress was apparently maximal during the initial phase of imprisonment (Gunn *et al*., 1978; see also Backett, 1987; Zamble and Porporino, 1988 and Kennedy, 1984).

Backett found that 20 (61 per cent) of his prison suicides had a history of psychiatric contact; 11 (33 per cent) were identified as having received in-patient psychiatric treatment (in psychiatric hospitals in Scotland) prior to their imprisonment. Depressive disorders had been diagnosed in two instances. Other diagnoses (which were multiple in six cases) included schizophrenia (2), personality disorder (4), alcohol and drug dependence (5) and conduct disorder (1). Backett argues that, in contrast to the general population, the level of depressive illness amongst prison suicides is surprisingly low: 'in only one case from the prison records and two from the in-patient group could this diagnosis be found' (Backett, 1987:220). He suggests that: 'factors other than depressive illness may be important in those suicides which take place in prison' (Ibid.:220).

Studies of suicides in the community invariably find a very high level of psychiatric contact and in-patient treatment amongst their samples (Barraclough and Hughes, 1987; Barraclough et al., 1974; Sainsbury, 1988; Seager and Flood, 1965; Robins et al., 1959). Over 90 per cent of all suicides in the community show some history of psychiatric illness (Barraclough and Hughes, 1987; Sainsbury, 1988). Most studies also find high levels of depressive illness: it is the most common diagnosis at the time of death and is found in the histories of more than half of all suicides (Barraclough and Hughes, 1987; Barraclough et al., 1974). Most suicides in the community 'have a recognisable illness' and 'it is a treatable one' (Sainsbury, 1988:3). This is not true of prison suicides.

Alcohol and drug abuse

Dooley found that 29 per cent of his prison suicides had a history of alcohol abuse and 23 per cent had a history of drug abuse. The frequency of drug abuse in the histories of prison suicides has increased (see Topp, 1979; Griffiths, 1990b). Almost half (45 per cent) of the suicides in Backett's study were found to have alcohol- or drug-related problems. Death early in the period of custody was more likely amongst those with alcohol- or drug-related problems. Of these deaths, 60 per cent occurred within the first week (Backett, 1987:220; see also Hayes, 1983). Evidence in the medical files suggested that a third of them (five) were experiencing withdrawal symptoms at the time of (or immediately before) their suicide.

A study by Zamble and Porporino suggests that the abuse of alcohol and drugs by offenders prior to imprisonment is extremely high. Over half of their sample of inmates from Canadian prisons were thought to require treatment for alcohol abuse (Zamble and Porporino, 1988:62). Similar findings have emerged from UK studies (McMurran, 1986; McMurran and Hollin, 1989).

Alcoholism is known to contribute to suicide in the community, either directly or indirectly, impairing health and social functioning (Barraclough and Hughes, 1987; Chiles et al., 1986; Robins et al., 1959). Alcoholism is associated with depressive illness (Sainsbury, 1988) and can destroy careers and marriages (Barraclough and Hughes, 1987; Roy and Linnoila, 1986).

Previous self-injury and suicide attempts

Almost half of all prison suicides are found to have a history of attempts at suicide or self-injury (Dooley, 1990a; Backett, 1987; Correctional Service of Canada, 1981). Of Dooley's prison suicides, 43 per cent had injured themselves in the past; 22 per cent had injured themselves during the current period of custody. Only 10 per cent had used the same method as in the past; a third had taken some form of overdose and a third had cut their wrists or arms. Dooley suggests that the failure to achieve the desired result may have led to the use of a more lethal method, but adds that the range of available methods in prison is limited (Dooley, 1990a: 41–42).

Of Backett's prison suicides, 45 per cent had injured themselves in the past, in half the cases twice or more; 21 per cent had injured themselves during the current period of custody.

Scott-Denoon found that 16 of the 35 suicides in his study had recorded suicide attempts, gestures or threats prior to the fatal attempt. He argues that a current or previous self-inflicted injury is an indication of acute distress and is likely to be followed by a further, more serious injury or attempt (see Section II, this Chapter).

In the community, almost half of all suicides are found to have a history of previous suicide attempts (Barraclough and Hughes, 1987).

From individual to situational factors: the problem of prediction

Before considering the various situational and environmental factors found to be relevant to prison suicide, it is important to look briefly at the introduction of environmental variables into prison and prison-related research. The role of individual variables has dominated studies of suicides in prison, despite the development of interactive theories elsewhere in criminological research (e.g. Zamble and Porporino, 1988).

The first prison problem to alert researchers to the importance of the environment was absconding (Clarke and Martin, 1971; Banks et al., 1975; Laycock, 1977): 'As the research proceeded it became clear that, contrary to expectation, a view of absconding which emphasised the nature of the school environment was better supported by the findings than one which stressed individual differences' (Lodge, in foreword to Clarke and Martin, 1971:1). Studies of absconding began 'almost exclusively with the individual characteristics of absconders, the main focus being on personality variables' (Clarke and Martin, 1971:15). Environmental variables were only slowly introduced as factors such as time of the year, time after admission, location and the attitude of the staff began to appear as relevant to some of the statistics. It had been assumed that variance in absconding behaviour was due to individual differences. Clarke and Martin concluded from their review of research that 'personality differences contributed little to the aetiology of absconding' (Clarke and Martin, 1971:17). The role of environmental variables had been underestimated, despite the wide range in the absconding rates of different schools which could not be attributed to differences in admissions. An important finding was that absconding tended to occur soon after admission and after holiday periods, times thought to reflect anxiety and insecurity amongst boys recently removed from their familiar home environments. Time variations (seasonal and day-time) seemed to reflect an opportunity factor (for example, hours of darkness, staff on duty); there was also evidence that lack of parental visiting might lead to absconding.

Sinclair (1971) found that whether or not boys absconded or re-offended whilst resident in hostels (but not subsequently) was related to wardens' attitudes and training methods, rather than to factors in the boys' previous history (e.g. re-absconding was related to staff attitudes towards the absconders). He suggested that improvements to admission policies would reduce anxiety. Other recommendations included (unobtrusive) physical measures to reduce opportunities; the employment of more staff to increase communication between staff and boys; and the facilitation of regular visiting by parents to improve relationships with the home. Clarke and Martin concluded: 'the findings of this research indicate that more progress in the study of absconding is likely to be made through a deeper investigation of school regime and environment and particularly of staff attitudes and training methods' (Clarke and Martin, 1971:20).

In their study of absconding from open prisons, Banks *et al.* argued that 'high-risk' groups could be identified (younger inmates with longer criminal records, with 'medium'-length sentences, and convicted for burglary or theft; Banks *et al.*, 1975), but that these results did not indicate that inmates with such characteristics were *likely* to abscond. Most inmates, even in these categories, did not: hence the difficulties of prediction. The most that could be done, they argued, was that classes of inmate could be identified whose members may merit close individual scrutiny. An experiment temporarily excluding 'high-risk groups' from open conditions in the Northern Region failed: the result of this experiment was an increase in absconders from other categories. The authors argued that individual incidents may be foreseeable, based on an appreciation of domestic, personal and situational pressures.

In 1977, Laycock completed a further Home Ofice Research and Planning Unit (HORPU) study of absconding, this time from Borstals. She argued that an interaction model between individual and institutional factors may result in different factors predicting absconding within different institutions. She notes the gradual shift in emphasis from individual to environmental factors in the light of disappointing findings from early studies. Laycock confirmed that personality differences did not on the whole differentiate between absconders and non-absconders, but that the only individual characteristic that did was a record of previous similar behaviour. She did find several environmental variables to be significantly related to absconding from Borstals. First, the time in sentence was found to be early, suggesting that pressures felt in custodial situations were most strongly felt at the beginning. She found that absconders were unlikely to have discussed their problems with the staff.

Laycock argued that changes in the environment may determine the threshold at which young inmates abscond, so that as security is lower, and absconding increases, a different group of inmates would abscond. She argued that predicting *who* might abscond is more difficult than predicting when absconds are likely to occur. What might be possible, Laycock concluded, is to assume that certain sub-groups have a better predictability score than others so that, for example, a 'hard-core' of unpredictable absconders cannot be identified, but at an intermediate level some types of inmate will have a consistently higher level of absconding than others. These groups, and their predictability, may co-vary with security conditions, staff attitudes, admission policies and so on. Laycock concludes that research should be focused on different sections of the penal system, to see whether within absconders as a class, differentials at an institutional level affect our ability to predict, manage and prevent such behaviour in custody.

Situational factors in prison suicide research

The relevance of the above account to the case of prison suicide should be clear: environmental variables which have been found to be associated with absconding may be of equal importance in the study of suicides in prison. The role of individual differences has been so prominent in much of the research to date that environmental factors – or individuals' perceptions of environmental factors – have been neglected. The following account will bring together that research which has included situational variables, showing that many of the findings of absconding research could have been applied to prison suicide research long ago.

Method and timing of suicide

All studies find that about 90 per cent of prison suicides are accomplished by hanging and that they are most likely to occur at night.

Method

In Dooley's study, 90 per cent of the suicides were accomplished by hanging; other methods included cutting the neck (1.4 per cent), other cutting (1.4 per cent), smoke inhalation or burns (0.7 per cent), drug overdose or poisoning (3.8 per cent) or other methods (2.4 per cent) (Dooley, 1990a:41). In the USA, Hayes found that 96 per cent of 419 jail suicides died by hanging, using either their bedding or clothing as the means. Others used cutting, overdose or shooting (Hayes, 1983:471). Confirmation of the prevalence of hanging as a method can be found in Hatty and Walker, 1986; Scott-Denoon, 1984; Correctional Service of Canada, 1981; and Bernheim, 1987.

Time of day

Almost half of the suicides in Dooley's study occurred between midnight and 8 a.m. A quarter occurred between 8 a.m. and 5 p.m., a further quarter died between 5 p.m. and midnight (Dooley, 1990a:41). Hayes also found that most suicides occurred between midnight and 8 a.m. when staff supervision is at its lowest. The single highest rate (65 suicides/419) occurred between midnight and 3 a.m. Other peak periods were 3 a.m–6 a.m., 6 a.m.–9 a.m., and 9 p.m.–12 a.m. Scott-Denoon found a similar pattern, but warns that: 'There appears to be no "safe" time of day from a suicide prevention standpoint, and thus constant vigilance is the best rule to follow' (Scott-Denoon, 1984:xxii).

Day of week

Several studies find that the day on which the most frequent occurrence of suicides occur is a Saturday (Hayes, 1983; MSC, 1984). Others find that Sundays show a higher frequency (Scott-Denoon, 1984). Dooley found that the frequency of suicides on any particular day of the week did not differ significantly (Dooley, 1990a:41).

Time in sentence

The finding that suicides are most likely to occur early in the sentence has been consistent throughout prison suicide research. In Dooley's study, 51 (17 per cent) of the suicides occurred within one week of reception into prison; 84 (28 per cent) occurred within one month; 151 (51 per cent) within 3 months; and 227 (77 per cent) occurred within one year of reception into custody. The remaining 23 per cent (68 suicides) occurred after one year in custody (Dooley, 1990a:41).

Likewise Backett reports that the early stage of custody is a particular time of risk: four of the 33 suicides occurred within the first 24 hours of imprisonment; 13 occurred within the first week; and 20 within the first month. Two of the deaths occurred within a few days of the inmate's intended release (Backett, 1987:219).

Hayes found that over half of all jail suicides in the US during 1979 occurred within the first 24 hours of incarceration. An 'astounding' 26 per cent occurred within the first three hours (Hayes, 1983:470). More of those inmates charged with alcohol- or drug-related offences (a total of 97/419) died within the first three hours (56 per cent), and 84 per cent died within 24 hours of incarceration (Hayes, 1983:471).

Hatty and Walker confirm this trend (Hatty and Walker, 1986:26). Scott-Denoon finds a similar pattern, most suicides occurring early in custody (particularly amongst the remand group) and thereafter, declining in frequency as the time spent in custody increases. However, he warns once more:

there appears to be no time during a term of imprisonment that is safe from a suicide prevention standpoint ... there are many suicides that occur when the victim could be considered to be over the hurdle of adjustment and these are quite unforeseen by staff.

(Scott-Denoon, 1984:xxi).

Kennedy proposes that Clemmer's 'prisonization' thesis (Clemmer, 1940) can be applied to suicides occurring early in custody (Kennedy, 1984). The anxiety and depression associated with the transition from street to jail is particularly likely to precipitate suicide. Once the prisoner adjusts to his prison life, this 'transition trauma' may dissipate (see also Erikson, 1975). Although levels of anxiety increase again towards the end of a term of imprisonment, this time the levels of depression will be lower. Factors such as prior imprisonment may mitigate the effects of this trauma (Kennedy, 1984).

Zamble and Porporino show how the early stages of a sentence can leave inmates in a 'psychological and emotional limbo' (Zamble and Porporino, 1988:129).

Time of year

Dooley found an excess of suicides between July and September (p<0.04). He does not offer an explanation for this pattern, but agreed in a personal communication that this significant excess could be due to the summer holiday period, when specialist services are depleted, education departments are closed and staff short-ages are at their most severe (Dooley, 1990c). Other authors find peaks in the spring and autumn (Scott-Denoon, 1984; Hayes, 1983).

Penological factors

Location

A disproportionate number of suicides occur in special locations, such as prison hospitals, the punishment block and other areas of seclusion. In 1990, 25 per cent of prison suicides in England and Wales occurred in prison hospitals and 9 per cent in segregation units (Wool, 1991). Backett reports that 11 of his suicides were 'under observation'[6] at the time of their death. Four of the 11 had been identified as being at particular risk of suicide (Backett, 1987:219). In the 1983 Chief Inspectors' Report, about half the suicides were located in a hospital or medical wing (Home Office, 1986a:96). More importantly, almost all the 169 suicides considered in the Chief Inspectors' Report were located in a single room or cell (whether in the hospital or on ordinary location). It is possible that the dispropor-tionate number of suicides taking place in hospital or medical wings is simply due to preventive action, inmates identified as 'high-risk' being kept under medical observation.

Hayes found that 68 per cent of 419 jail suicides occurred in isolation. He concludes that isolation appears to be counter-productive in the prevention of suicides. A Canadian study found that the suicide rate in segregation and special handling units was far higher than that for ordinary locations, even though most (59 per cent) suicides occur in general locations (Correctional Service of Canada, 1981:12). Likewise, Scott-Denoon found that 30 per cent of BC correctional suicides occurred in segregation, observation and protective custody cells, which account for only 5.5 per cent of cell capacity. He concludes that these areas are places of high risk, and that staffing and training levels in these locations should reflect this fact (Scott-Denoon, 1984:114). The greatest number of suicides still occur in the general population cells (Scott-Denoon, 1984:117).

Some studies find a correlation between the level of security of an institution and the frequency of suicides, most occurring in maximum security establishments (Scott-Denoon, 1984; Correctional Service of Canada, 1981; Hatty and Walker, 1986). This could be an artefact of allocation procedures, which direct potential suicide risks away from lower security or open establishments, but this possibility is not raised in any of the studies showing such an association.

The effects of overcrowding

> Overcrowding has been proposed as the underlying cause of rapes, riots, hostage-taking and assaults.
>
> (Gaes, 1985:97)

Overcrowding is often assumed by commentators on the prison situation to be linked in some way to suicides (Home Office, 1984; Home Office, 1988b; Prison Reform Trust, 1983). Its effects on reception figures, average daily population, staff–inmate ratios, the availability of specialist resources and/or work and other activities or amenities (such as showers, food) and on relationships between inmates, are negative. Rates of illness complaints, levels of physiological stress and death rates have been found to be disproportionately high in overcrowded prisons (McCain et al., 1980). A single possible benefit in terms of suicide prevention may be the necessity of shared accommodation, as most suicides occur in single cells. McCain, Cox and Paulus drew a link between overcrowding and high stress levels, psychological impairment and high mortality rates. They found that large and overcrowded prisons have the highest suicide and attempted suicide rates, and numbers of psychiatric commitments (McCain et al., 1980). They use ADP as the basis of their calculations, however, which presents a serious flaw in their analysis (see below).

Overcrowding is easier to identify than depression or loneliness, and easier to rectify (Gaes, 1985:97), but the association with prisoner suicide may be a superficial association, masking more complex problems thereby left unexplored. Gaes argues that 'crowding may act as an intensifier of stressful conditions that have been precipitated by other causes'. There is some evidence that social density (number of occupants in housing quarters) has more impact than spatial density (space per person) (Gaes, 1985:109; McCain et al., 1980). From the literature, it appears that overcrowding alone is rarely a direct precursor to suicide. It is other problems, concealed by overcrowding but exacerbated by it – such as unwanted interactions, noise, feelings of helplessness, lack of clothing, food, medical and other specialist care, changing hierarchies, administrative and other problems that might contribute to the suicide rate. There is some evidence that overcrowding may lead to increased misconduct and assault rates (particularly amongst the young;

Gaes, 1985; McCain *et al.*, 1980), and that males react negatively to overcrowding whereas females may respond positively (Gaes, 1985:103).

One of the most important results of research in this area is the discovery that the effects of overcrowding are moderated by coping ability and social support (Gaes, 1985: 104–5), so that *for certain individuals*, overcrowding and all that it entails may be an essential link in the chain producing 'the onset of a suicidal crisis', but by itself, it is an inadequate explanation for high suicide rates.

It should also be borne in mind that those prisons with the most marked overcrowding are those prisons with the highest reception and discharge figures. This will increase the proportion of inmates in the population who are new receptions, and reduce the average levels of time served. Thus more inmates are arriving at the gates at a high-risk period, to be replaced by more 'at-risk' inmates at a high rate.

Prison-induced stress

Sperbeck and Parlour found that suicidal referrals in correctional facilities in Alaska differed from non-suicidal prisoners in that suicidal referrals 'seemed to have a much higher incidence of secondary stressors above and beyond the basic shame and discomfort of incarceration shared by almost all inmates' (Sperbeck and Parlour, 1986:96). Such secondary stressors included marital and financial crises. Such crises may render the prison experience unbearably stressful. Backett argued in his Scottish study that prison-induced stress may be a critical factor in prison suicides. He had suggested that 'other factors than depressive illness may be important in those suicides which take place in prison' (Backett, 1987). He suggests that it is possible to view prison suicides as the result of varying degrees of stress rather than formal illness. In accordance with Gunn's and colleagues' (1978) evidence that a high degree of disturbance and psychological discomfort is experienced by the prison population as a whole, Backett argues that the level of this stress changes according to the varying aspects of incarceration. Gunn found that the level of distress experienced by prisoners appeared to be maximal during the initial phase of imprisonment, diminishing as inmates adjusted to prison life (see also Erikson, 1975). Most suicides occur during this initial phase, at a time when (identifiable) stress factors are most numerous, and inmates face the greatest amount of uncertainty. This results in a *'continuum of distress'*, rather than a specific illness or depressive condition with recognisable symptoms. In this case, Backett suggests, suicide may take place if and when a critical threshold is exceeded. This threshold may vary, and depends on a balance between the factors themselves and the individual's resources to cope with them.

Two concepts require definition in order to proceed further with the notion of prison-induced stress: the concept of stress itself and the concept of coping. Monat and Lazarus refer to stress as 'the field of negatively toned emotions such as fear, anger, depression, despair, hopelessness and guilt' (Monat and Lazarus, 1985:3). The stress arena 'refers to any event in which environmental demands, internal demands, or both *tax* or *exceed* the adaptive resources of an individual' (Monat and Lazarus, 1985:3). Humans may respond positively to stress, or they may respond negatively. This response depends on both the nature and extent of the stress and their own coping resources: 'coping refers to efforts to master conditions of harm, threat or challenge when a routine or automatic response is not readily available ... Coping refers to adaptation under relatively difficult conditions' (Monat and Lazarus, 1985:5).

Examples of stress factors from Backett's study include withdrawal from drugs, or adjustment to prison life. Maris described the significance of 'role transitions' or 'rites of passage' in suicide, showing how changes in social roles have consequences requiring new skills and abilities for successful transition (Maris, 1981:45). If these skills cannot be mastered, the individual may succumb to the 'crisis' thereby encountered. Entry into prison is clearly one 'rite of passage' inmates have to cope with. One experience of poor adjustment is likely to make the next adjustment harder: 'It is the *repeated* disruptions and stresses of life transitions or of failed transitions that can wear down one's will to live' (Maris, 1981:47).

Prison stresses may be experienced by the whole population, with suicides and attempted suicides being located variously at the far end of a continuum of perceived stress and coping ability. Such a continuum might be referred to as 'prison-induced distress'. Thus the focus of questions relating to suicide in prison is shifted from the personal characteristics alone of inmates who commit suicide in custody, which has contributed in limited ways to our understanding, to a consideration of those factors which may exacerbate individual vulnerability to suicidal behaviour during a custodial sentence and the nature of that vulnerability. Other 'stress factors' identified in previous studies (e.g. Sykes, 1958; Goffman, 1968; Sapsford, 1983), are the loss of freedom, autonomy and personal safety: the removal from a familiar environment; restriction of movement; compliance with (at times incomprehensible) rules and regulations; subjection to an impersonal decision-making process (e.g. parole); loss of control over outside events; and violence and victimisation (see also Johnson, 1976 and Bowker, 1980). Most studies suggest that the maximum impact of prison-induced stress is felt at the beginning of the custodial experience, but thereafter different events may continue to be accompanied by severe discomfort. Johnson and Toch argued that this stress could have a destructive effect on the institution and its staff, both in the long-term (accumulating a society of severely damaged people; contributing to recidivism) and the short-term (most immediately, contributing to suicide or self-injury):

> If a prisoner is placed in an unbearably stressful situation with no means at his disposal to cope with this overwhelming experience, he may direct his feelings of hopelessness towards himself. This 'self-destructive breakdown' (Toch, 1975) has been identified as unique to the prison setting, and it is seen as an index of the personal difficulties that face prisoners.
>
> (Johnson and Toch, 1982:82)

Backett suggests that one useful way of investigating the relevant factors in prison suicide is to compare them with suicide in the general population 'to see whether similar factors operate in the two settings'. In the general population, the decision to commit suicide 'is influenced both by their psychological state and the situation in which they find themselves' (Backett, 1988:74). Just as situational variables are likely to play a part in prison suicides, so they must do in the community at large, an observation often forgotten by commentators and researchers on suicides in the community. The majority of those who commit suicide in the community are found to be suffering from a clearly identifiable mental illness (usually a depressive illness, often with alcohol dependence (Backett, 1988)), but the majority of people who are mentally ill do not commit suicide. The presence of depressive illness renders the individual psychologically vulnerable, but still it requires some additional factor to precipitate the suicidal act.

The differences between prison suicides and others (Backett, 1987; 1988) suggest that 'different vulnerability factors may operate in a prison setting'. Furthermore, Backett argues:

> if depressive illness is infrequently found in prison suicides then there will be little point in developing a prevention strategy aimed at diagnosing and treating this illness. It may be more appropriate to examine possible precipitants to suicide and in this context most attention has been paid to the stress associated with imprisonment.
>
> (Backett, 1988:76)

Differences in 'coping ability' or adjustment to imprisonment have engaged the attention of psychologists and penologists recently (Porporino, 1983; Porporino and Zamble, 1984; Zamble and Porporino, 1988; Sapsford, 1983). Backett suggests, in accordance with considerable evidence, that prisons contain, 'an excessive number of people with poor or limited coping skills, and it is within this group that are found those particularly vulnerable to the effects of stress' (Backett, 1988: 77). This literature has not been systematically applied to the problem of suicides in prison (with the exception of earlier suggestions made by Johnson, 1976), but an investigation of the application of this literature to our understanding of suicides in prison will be undertaken in Chapter 4.

Motivation

Few studies investigate possible motivations for suicide in custody. Classifications of suicidal types have been drawn up (Hatty and Walker, 1986; Phillips, 1986) but these classifications are profiles and do not include considerations of possible motivating factors. This approach to suicide in prison describes their characteristics but does not provide possible causes of the behaviour. At best, a few studies report the possible motives attributed to the suicides, usually by staff such as governors and medical officers, and in Gover's case, also by chaplains. The lack of fit between others' attributed motives, and those given by people making suicide attempts has been the subject of considerable research in its own right (Bancroft and Hawton, 1983; Hawton, 1986; Morgan, 1979; Hawton and Catalan, 1987). The mis-match between attributed motivation and actual or subjective motivation found in these studies should alert us to the limitations of studies of motivation based on recorded information alone.

In Gover's early study, requests were made of the governors and chaplains for the 'supposed motive' for each of the 81 suicides occurring between 1872 and 1979. In only half the cases could answers be given. Gover discovered the range of motives attributed to these 40 suicides could be divided into several categories: fear (14), depression (6), shame (9), passion (3), unsoundness of mind (2), drink (4) and remorse (2). 'Fear' included fear of penal servitude (10), fear of imprisonment, fear of losing a pension and of rearrest. Depression was sometimes attributed to family discord or to a severe sentence. 'Passion' included jealousy and revenge. Almost a quarter of the suicides were attributed to shame. Gover distinguishes between shame and remorse, adding that the small number of suicides attributed to remorse: 'may be regarded as confirmatory of the truth of the common saying that men do not suffer so much from consciousness of guilt as from the consequences of discovery' (Gover, 1880:61–62).

Smalley only infers that emotional shock plays a significant part in the causation of suicides in prison from the fact that almost 40 per cent of the 86 cases he analysed were first offenders, and a disproportionate number occur early after reception (Smalley, 1911:41). Topp argued that the anticipation of a long sentence may increase the propensity to suicide and that a number of suicides may have been making attempts to elicit sympathetic attention.

Few of the contemporary studies claim to be looking for the causes or motivation for prison suicide. They look for a risk-profile, so that the suicide-prone can be identified and prevented, by physical restraint: that is, by means of isolation, removal of all dangerous objects and intermittent observation (SHHD, 1985). Research has been directed at the prevention of suicide by individual and situational measures, not at understanding or treating the causes.[7] Just as the search for the causes of crime has been abandoned by many criminologists in favour of situational crime prevention (Clarke and Mayhew, 1980; Clarke and Cornish, 1983), the search for the causes of suicide in prison has never been at the forefront of research.

Of the contemporary studies, Dooley has made one of the few attempts to assess possible motivating factors. In order to do this, Dooley used accounts of the events leading up to the deaths provided by coroners' inquest reports, prison files, suicide notes (where available) and comments made by staff or other inmates. The various motives found were divided into four categories: factors relating to the prison situation, outside pressures, guilt for the offence and mental illness (Dooley, 1990a:40). Factors relating to the prison situation included:

– *imprisonment being intolerable* (unable to face the possibility/length of sentence; unable to cope with the regime; fear of intimidation, actual or perceived victimisation by other inmates);

- *lack of communication* (no visits/letters; failure of a visitor to arrive, etc.);
- *the inability to cope with confinement* due to low frustration tolerance.

Outside pressures included:

- *threat to a close relationship* (divorce, separation, 'Dear John' letters, ostracism after family finds out about offence, etc.); and
- *receipt of bad news* (domestic problems, failure of appeal, etc.)

Dooley found that motives could be attributed to 91 per cent of cases: 40 per cent were apparently motivated by prison pressures, 15 per cent by outside pressures, 12 per cent by guilt for the offence, 22 per cent by mental disorder. Over three-quarters of the 'guilt for offence' group (= 28 suicides) killed themselves on remand, at night. Most were charged with or convicted of a homicide offence. In almost a third of this group there was a sexual component to the offence. The 'mental disorder' group were more likely to have received previous psychiatric treatment and to have injured themselves before, using potentially lethal methods. They were also more likely to be single, living alone or of no fixed abode prior to arrest. Finally, Dooley found that the 'outside pressure' group:

> tended to be more typical of the prison population than the others, that is, they were more likely to have been charged or convicted of an acquisitive offence, to have previous convictions, and to have been married or living with others before imprisonment.
>
> (Dooley, 1990a:42)

Dooley concludes that: 'the single commonest motive for prison suicide is the inmate finding the prison situation intolerable' (Dooley, 1990a:44). But he adds that individual psychological factors, such as feelings of guilt, and mental disorder, come a close second.

The only other study to include a discussion of motivation is Scott-Denoon's BC Corrections study in which the author infers motivation from prison files, coroners' inquests, psychiatric reports, comments made by staff, other inmates, and in this case, families. He reminds us of the important point that: 'Almost by definition we accept that the culminating or precipitating event is most likely not the single motivator but perhaps the last or final motivator in a complex pattern of pressures or perceived pressures' (Scott-Denoon, 1984:68). The author then presents primary and secondary motivators in his analysis, but in only nine of the 35 cases in the study is he confident of the identification of primary motivators. He argues that the loss of a significant person is an important factor, together with fear, and alcohol- or drug-related problems (Scott-Denoon, 1984:69–70).

Outside, hopelessness, depressive illness, alcoholism, loneliness, ill health, bereavement and poverty have been found to be associated with suicide (Barraclough and Hughes, 1987; Roy and Linnoila, 1986; Diekstra, 1987). Few 'explanations' of suicide are offered in these studies; these associations are assumed to speak for themselves.

Summary

Suicide rates are higher in prison than in the (equivalent) community, although methods of calculating these rates have been inadequate to date. Using an 'exposure to risk' equation, it is clear from at least two studies that prison suicides occur more frequently than suicides in the equivalent general community. Rates have been increasing in the UK and elsewhere at a rate faster than any increase either in the average daily population or in reception rates (Dooley, 1990a). Importantly, there is little evidence to link prison suicides with depressive illness (Backett, 1987). Studies aimed at the identification of high-risk groups are flawed and contradictory. They are often based on inadequate or small samples, and the range of variables they consider is narrow and inconsistent. However, several compatible features of prison suicide emerge.

It appears that prison suicides are associated with youth, the early twenties being a particularly high-risk age group. They are usually male – although female suicides do occur – and white. They are usually single, or lacking stable and supportive relationships. The nature of their relationships is of more significance than its status. The family background of prison suicides, so important to studies of suicides in the community, are not considered in any recent studies. Many prison suicides have had previous experience of custody and have a high number of previous convictions. Remand prisoners are particularly at risk, although about half of all suicides occur amongst sentenced inmates in the UK. Authors have not tended to consider the disproportionate numbers of remand prisoners passing through remand centres at a time of maximum risk.

There is some evidence that suicide occurs with more frequency amongst inmates charged with or convicted of violent offences, particularly murder or manslaughter, although most prison suicides, in most countries, are imprisoned for acquisitive offences. It is possible, however, that different types of prison suicides occur, those charged with offences of murder forming a distinct group which bias the profile of the remainder. Three different types of suicide identified in the literature appear to be:

1   the psychiatrically ill;
2   the serious offender (e.g. murderer) facing a life sentence;
3   the unpredictable young offender sentenced or facing charges for acquisitive offences and showing similar characteristics to the general prison population, according to variables so far explored.

The different profiles for each of these groups (which are 'ideal types' and which may not be mutually exclusive) may account for the fact that few reliable patterns relating to background factors such as criminal justice history, offence and sentence length occur amongst prison suicides as a whole. A recent Home Office report (1984) suggested that investigating selected groups of prison suicides separately may offer a helpful resolution to this problem.

Prison suicides may be slightly more likely than the general prison population to have received in-patient psychiatric treatment. They are far less likely than the general population of suicides to have a history of depressive illness and/or psychiatric treatment, however. Virtually all suicides in the community are found to have a history of depression and psychiatric treatment. This is true of only a third of all prison suicides. Other factors than those normally associated with suicides in the community may therefore play a part.

The level of alcohol and drug abuse amongst prison suicides is high. These deaths tend to occur very early in the sentence. The role of alcohol and drug abuse amongst suicides in the community is also high. It is not known whether prison suicides show a higher level of such a history than the general prisoner population. About half of all prison suicides have injured themselves before, about a quarter during the current period of custody. Most suicides die by hanging, very few die by any other method. At least half of all prison suicides occur at night, usually in the early hours of the morning. There may be an excess of suicides at the weekend. All studies agree that suicides are disproportionately likely early in the sentence, or soon after reception. There is no time during a term of imprisonment which is safe, however. Suicides occur at a disproportionate rate in special locations – such as in segregation units or on hospital wings. Isolation does not alleviate risk, and may be counter-productive. There is some association between the level of security in establishments and the frequency of suicides. This may be an artefact of allocation procedures, which divert potential suicide risks away from open establishments.

Overcrowding alone does not appear to contribute to the suicide rate, although its consequences, such as the high proportion of receptions, competition for scarce and specialist resources, staff shortages and so on, may intensify stressful conditions originally precipitated by other causes. The apparent motivation for prison suicide appears to be fear or loss: fear of other inmates, of the consequences of one's crime, of imprisonment, and loss of a significant relationship, such as lack of communication or divorce. Shame, guilt and mental disorder play a relatively minor role (numerically), particularly amongst the young. The most common emotion in suicides outside is hopelessness–helplessness or *ennui* (Diekstra, 1987:30–31).

As shown in this chapter so far, the young prisoner suicide may differ in important respects from other (groups of) prison suicides. This possibility will be considered in more detail in Chapter 3. The following sections will discuss suicide attempts and self-injury in prison, suggesting that the common underlying characteristics of these activities may be as significant as their differences.

SECTION II: ATTEMPTED SUICIDE AND SELF-INJURY

In view of ... the fact that over 50 per cent of those prisoners committing suicide between 1958 and 1971 had a history of previous attempts (Topp, 1979), we are surprised that there have been so few studies of deliberate self-injury occurring

in prison ... Government reports (Home Office, 1984; 1986) have repeatedly commented on the need for research into attempted suicide occurring in prisons.
(Wool and Dooley, 1987:297)

In the community, attempted suicide and self-injury are usually considered in isolation from suicide, as separate phenomena having a limited association with completed suicide (Hawton, 1986). Little is known about the nature and extent of self-injury or its relation to suicide. In prison, where greater surveillance is possible, and the available means of self-harm are restricted, it may be argued that the nature and motivation of such behaviour is unique in this environment. Far from being predominantly female behaviour involving a limited danger to life, as self-injury is assumed to be outside, serious self-injury amongst young males in custody is frequent, and may endanger life without prompt intervention. Over a dozen studies investigate suicide attempts or self-injury in prison (Wool and Dooley, 1987; Griffiths, 1990b; Cullen, 1981; Cookson, 1977; Coid et al., 1990a, b, Wilkins and Coid, 1990; Albanese, 1983; Bernheim, 1987; Orlowski, 1986, Toch, 1975, 1982; Johnson, 1976; Johnson, 1978; Johnson and Toch, 1982; Correctional Service of Canada, 1981). Some of these are reviewed by Lloyd (1990); other earlier and theoretical studies have been reviewed by the Correctional Service of Canada (1981). Many are exclusively record-based (the exceptions are Coid et al., 1990a, b; Wilkins and Coid, 1990; Toch, 1975; Johnson and Toch, 1982; and the studies by Johnson). Some deal exclusively with women prisoners (Coid et al., 1990a, 1990b; Wilkins and Coid, 1990; Cullen, 1981 and Cookson, 1977). These studies tend to differ in approach and content from those dealing with mixed or all-male samples, and will be discussed in more detail in Chapter 7. Likewise, there are a growing number of studies dealing exclusively with young offenders (Thornton, 1990; Power and Spencer, 1987; Johnson, 1978). These studies are discussed separately in Chapter 3.

None of these studies provide an adequate operational definition of 'attempted suicide', and few distinguish between attempts at suicide and other less clearly motivated self-inflicted injuries. Many take officially recorded attempts at suicide as the basis of their sample (Wool and Dooley, 1987; Correctional Service of Cananda, 1981). Most of the studies are describing a wide range of behaviour. The important question of the relationships between self-injury, attempted suicide and completed suicide is never adequately addressed.

Prison suicide attempt and self-injury rates

Few studies attempt the difficult task of estimating rates of self-injury or suicide attempts in prison. Recording is poor and haphazard (Toch, 1975; Home Office, 1990a; 1990d; see also Chapter 4). Definitions of the various behaviours are unreliable and unclear (Stengel, 1970; Kreitman, 1977; SHHD, 1985). Annual figures are provided in prison department reports, but these figures are so seriously flawed as to be almost meaningless (Home Office, 1990d; Toch, 1975). Estimations in official reports are occasionally made on the basis of an assumed ratio of attempts to completed suicides outside, but again, this method has no validity, as most attempts and self-inflicted injuries in the community remain undiscovered and go unrecorded, and there is no evidence that the ratio would be similar in the prison situation.

Few studies provide estimates of the rate of suicide attempts in custody (or provide enough data to allow estimations to be made). The rates are high, however (Correctional Service of Canada, 1981; Toch, 1975), and they are particularly high amongst young inmates (Thornton, 1990; Power and Spencer, 1987). In a study of coping behaviour amongst a sample of 133 male Canadian inmates, Zamble and Porporino found that 13 per cent of their subjects has attempted suicide; 29 per cent had seriously thought about suicide (Zamble and Porporino, 1988:40). Some estimates of suicide attempts and self-injury amongst young offenders are given in Chapter 3. Rates of attempted suicide and self-injury in the history of prisoner populations have been investigated, and the few studies that provide this data confer, reaching a figure of between 16 and 17 per cent of all inmates in their sample or establishment having a record of attempted suicide or self-injury (Albanese, 1983; Griffiths, 1990a). Details of the severity of the injury are never given, and it is impossible to know whether the injuries occurred in custody or outside.

Descriptive aspects

By far the most common method of self-inflicted injury in prison is wrist-cutting (Jones, 1986; Wool and Dooley, 1987; Power and Spencer, 1987). This method is noted to be less lethal than the method used in most completed suicides: hanging (Correctional Service of Canada, 1981). Other methods include arm-cutting, cutting other parts of the body (legs, abdomen, throat, etc.), attempting hanging, overdosing, hitting, swallowing foreign objects (batteries, bed-springs, razor blades, glass), re-opening stitches, inserting items in the body, burning and refusing food[8] (Jones, 1986; Wool and Dooley, 1987; Cookson, 1977). The seriousness of the injury incurred can range from the superficial (requiring no treatment) to potentially lethal damage resulting in loss of consciousness and permanent damage, such as brain damage (Albanese, 1983). Outside, by far the most common method of self-inflicted injury is by overdose (Hawton, 1986; 1978; Hawton and Catalan, 1987). Only 5 per cent of patients admitted to hospital for self-inflicted harm use any other method (such as cutting, gunshots, jumping from a height and jumping in front of a moving vehicle, Hawton, 1986:151).

Almost all studies find that the average age of self-injurers is younger than both the average age of completed suicides and that of the general prison population. Self-injurers are also more likely to be single than either completed suicides or the general prison population (Phillips, 1986; Correctional Service of Canada, 1981). Self-injury is associated with closed or maximum security establishments (Correctional Service of Canada, 1981), and with special locations, such as segregation units and psychiatric units. It is also associated with inactivity (CSC, 1981) and a disproportionately high number of disciplinary reports, often for assaults and other serious disciplinary offences (Jones, 1986; Toch *et al.*, 1989). A high number of previous convictions is associated with suicide attempts and self-injury in prison (Griffiths, 1990b). Alcohol and drug abuse is also found to be associated with these behaviours (Correctional Service of Canada, 1981). The incidents occur earlier in the day than completed suicides, when staff availability is higher. Some studies find that a low level of education is associated with self-harm in prison, although the level of intelligence does not differ from the rest of the prison population (Correctional Service of Canada, 1981). Rates of self-injury are found to be high early in custody (Albanese, 1983).

Motivation

In Wool and Dooley's study, explanations most frequently offered for the suicide attempts were, that a close relationship was threatened, that a visit had not materialised or that prison was intolerable. Guilt and boredom were also cited more than once. The authors conclude that young men are particularly emotionally vulnerable when imprisoned, especially on remand. They suggest that a threat to any personal relationship occurring at this time 'may tip them into a state of mind which causes them to make a suicide attempt' (Wool and Dooley, 1987: 300). Isolation or difficulties in communication may contribute. In addition, stress induced by various aspects of prison life – for example, staff shortages (especially in remand centres), may add to the emotional pressures felt by those inmates least able to cope with the demands of custody.

The act of self-injury has been described as arising from feelings of 'melancholy tinged with self-contempt' (Cooper, 1971). Toch describes 'self-destructive break-downs' as expressions of frustration, self-doubt, personal agony and the search for relief (Toch, 1975). He divides self-destructive acts according to their origins, some arising from difficulties in coping, others from difficulties with self-perception, and with self-control. Isolation, boredom and 'a sense of resourcelessness' all contribute to the sense of hopelessness and pain associated with self-harm (Toch, 1975:38–9): 'It is a back-to-the-wall, dead-end desperation, an intolerable emptiness, helplessness, tension. It is a *physical* reaction, and a demand for release or escape at all costs' (Toch, 1975:40).

SECTION III: SUICIDE, SUICIDE ATTEMPTS AND SELF-INJURY – CONTINUITY OR DISCONTINUITY?

> Recent reviews have suggested that it is possible to extrapolate from findings of attempted suicide to completed suicide ... and Ottoson (1979) has concluded 'that they are expressions of a common suicidal process'.
>
> (Goldney and Burvil, 1980:2)

Studies and authors differ in their approach to the question of the relationship between suicide, attempted suicide and self-injury in custody. The most pervasive view, found in the literature and in common (and professional) attitudes towards the issue, is that there is very little overlap between them (Wool and Dooley, 1987; Power and Spencer, 1987). Psychiatric literature expresses the same opinion (Stengel, 1964; Kreitman, 1977; Morgan, 1979), although there is some recent evidence that those whose deliberate self-harm most resembles completed suicide are those most likely to go on to commit suicide (Lloyd, 1990; Pallis *et al.*, 1984; Hawton and Catalan, 1987). The importance of this argument is the acknowledgement that there may be different types and degrees of self-harm – a possibility rarely accounted for in research design – and that there does appear to be a clear overlap between self-injury and (future) suicide. The possibility of a *continuum of self-destructive behaviour* has rarely been raised in the context of prison suicide research. An important oversight in the struggle to treat the behaviours as separate has been the evidence that there are common causes to the two behaviours. As we shall see in Part II of this book, the causes expressed by prisoners describing their activities as suicidal are the same as those causes relating to less lethal types of self-harm. In understanding the behaviour, therefore, and in order to alleviate the distress associated with it, the whole continuum should be addressed.

The only English study that seriously attempts to distinguish between the general prison population, suicide 'attempters' and successful suicides was carried out by M. Phillips of the Prison Psychological Service. This study was carried out at HMP Brixton, and published as a Directorate of Psychological Services (DPS) report in 1986. It was based on the 32 successful suicides and 129 attempts occurring in Brixton between 1973 and 1983. Although the study is of limited general application (it is based exclusively on one unrepresentative institution), it is detailed and useful.

In this study, the prison suicide group was defined by the verdict of the Coroners' Court, and included all those for whom hospital case papers were available (n=32/34). The 'attempters' were defined by incidents of non-fatal self-injury leading to the completion of an F220, used to record and notify such an injury. The normal sample consisted of a 1 in 200 sample of the nominal index cards for the population of Brixton (n=411) from 1975 to 1984.

Phillips (1986) found that the two suicidal groups differed from the 'normal' prison sample in terms of age, length of stay and type of offence. However, she concluded, although these differences were statistically significant, they were not sufficient to allow the groups to be successfully discriminated at a level that would be of any practical value in terms of identifying those at risk of suicide. In accordance with other studies, most of the successful suicides were by hanging, and most occurred in the hospital wing.

She found that the average age of the normal sample was 31.1 years; the suicides were significantly *older* (36.8 years) and the attempters somewhat *younger* (29.3 years). The suicide groups tended to be incarcerated for longer and for more serious offences than the normal prison population, but almost 30 per cent of the attempts and 22 per cent of the actual suicides occurred within the first seven days. *Half* the suicidal incidents occurred within the first month. A significant proportion of the suicide group were widowers.[9] Phillips divided the types of offence with which the three groups were charged into three categories; 'those against the person', 'those for gain', and 'miscellaneous'. She found that suicides were significantly more likely to be charged with a 'person' or 'miscellaneous' offence than the other two groups. Attempters were more likely to be charged with a 'person' offence and less likely to be charged with a 'gain' offence than were those in the normal sample.

A discriminant function analysis was performed on the three sample groups in order to force them to be as statistically distinct as possible. Phillips found that the attempted-suicide group had the least accurate predicted membership, and over-lapped a great deal with the normal sample. Almost half the cases were misclassified. A quarter (23 per cent) of the normal sample were wrongly classified as suicides, suggesting that considerable difficulties are encountered in attempts to make such predictions, even after detailed research has been carried out.

All the individuals who used cutting as a method were in the attempted-suicide group; they were significantly younger than the suicide group, and were more likely to have been charged with an offence for gain. They were less likely than would have been expected to be on medical location or special watch. This suggests that attempters (especially self-cutters) could be an unusual and complex group, comprising cases that are especially difficult to predict. They differ from the 'prison suicide' in significant ways.

Phillips argues that 'since hanging is clearly the most effective way of committing successful suicide', these cases could be seen as a more serious attempt. Wool and Dooley (1987) drew the same conclusion from their study. They analysed 111 consecutive Prison Department Attempted Suicide Reports (those leading to the completion of a Form F220), occurring in a one-year period (October 1983–September 1984) in the prisons of the Midlands and South West Regions of England. During this one-year period, 111 episodes were reported. Most (58 per cent) involved remand prisoners; 65 per cent of the incidents involved young offenders aged between 16 and 21. Over 80 per cent of incidents involved prisoners below the age of 26 years. Most attempts were by cutting the arms (72 per cent), although 18 per cent attempted hanging. This sub-group were regarded as a separate category, in view of the fact that suicide in prison is overwhelmingly accomplished by hanging. The 20 episodes of hanging were committed by 19 prisoners, a large majority of whom were on remand (65 per cent). This would indicate, the authors argue, that these attempts were more likely to be serious.[10] Just less than half of the hangings (45 per cent) occurred in young offender establishments. Wool and Dooley suggest that mentally disordered groups may be more likely to make determined attempts, given that mental handicap and psychosis was mentioned in seven of the 20 explanations for these attempts.

Phillips eventually found that although attempted suicides who used hanging did not differ significantly from self-cutters, they were overall more similar to successful suicides than were the attempters as a whole. Phillips attempts to classify the suicides and suicide attempts into 'types', concluding that there are some differences between suicides and attempted suicides, but that these differences are unreliable. Her typology was as follows:

Suicides:

a) *non-criminal 'normal'* who suddenly commits a serious interpersonal offence; he is older and commits suicide later in his sentence; few precons, offence against person, home address and no psychiatric history.
b) *unstable substance abusers* – previous hospital admissions, miscellaneous offence (e.g. arson or criminal damage); early in sentence.
c) *criminalised disturbed group* – 'gain' offences, preconvictions, previous attempts and frequent present psychiatric diagnosis.

Attempted suicides:

a) *violent offenders* – offence against person; few hospital admissions, not on medical location.
b) *young criminals* – early attempt; gain offence, average preconvictions, few previous attempts or present psychiatric diagnosis.
c) *disturbed group* – miscellaneous offence, high psychiatric incidence; special location.

(Phillips, 1986)

The findings from this study, although based on rather small numbers, are compatible with those from other studies, confirming that attempts tend to occur early in the sentence, are often characterised by the presence of some psychiatric history and/or previous attempt, and may be classified according to method of attempt. However, Philips concludes, such results are not strong or consistent enough to allow prediction of suicidal incidents or individuals. Significant differences found between the two suicidal groups and the normal population of Brixton prison could still misclassify a large number of 'normals' as 'at risk', and fail to identify many inmates at risk of suicide. She concludes, with others, that individual prevention strategies are probably the least effective approach to suicide management, and that general preventive measures – from reducing opportunities to improving conditions and regimes, offer far more scope for success.

Differences and similarities between suicides, suicide attempts and self-injurers: the appeal function and the appeal effect

In prison (and outside) self-injury not severe enough to endanger life is frequently assumed to be a manipulative, attention-seeking gesture (Toch, 1975; Consumers of Mental Health Services, 1988). Suicide attempts that brush with death are often assumed to be mistakes. Completed suicides may be interpreted as attention-seeking gestures that 'went wrong', or accidents (SHHD, 1985). Many of the self-inflicted deaths in Dooley's study and in prison department statistics received 'open' or 'misadventure' verdicts for this reason.

Cookson described an incident involving a female prisoner who was told that her husband had been involved in a car crash. She could find out no details of the incident. It was only after she had cut herself that someone found out what had happened and told her, 'which illustrates the instrumental aspect of self-injury' (Cookson, 1977:345). This combination of action and outcome is often used to illustrate the manipulative or attention-seeking element of self-injury:

> The explanation most frequently given by staff is that the self-injurer is 'attention-seeking'. It is an unfortunate fact about most institutions, suffering as they do from chronic staff shortage, that whereas 'good' conformist behaviour goes un-noticed and unrewarded, 'bad' behaviour will evoke an immediate response from staff who, unable to watch everyone at once, must adopt the strategy of scanning the scene for anyone who stands out from the crowd.
>
> (Cookson, 1977:333)

In fact, this instrumental interpretation of motive has many flaws. Zamble and Porporino show that most inmates (and most offenders) constitute a group unlikely to employ behavioural or coping strategies that involve planning or considerations of future outcome. Their frequently maladaptive behaviour is *reactive* rather than *purposive* (Zamble and Porporino, 1988:51–69; see also Chapter 4). Inmates are more likely to describe their self-injury as a compulsive act (Toch, 1975) carried out in desperation, often after staff (and others') unresponsiveness to other modes of appeal:

> Stengel and Cook find the suicide attempt frequently was the only effective alarm signal to mobilize long overdue medical and social help ... Removal of the person from a conflict situation, prevention of divorce or other undesired action by a loved one, and other social situations can stimulate employment of suicidal attempts as appeals.[11]
>
> (Johnson, 1973:240)

It is when the appeal function of self-injury fails to achieve any effect that despair is likely and a more dangerous and desperate state of mind may ensue (Johnson, 1973:240; Chiles *et al.*, 1986). Those incidents with such a 'function', however unstrategically considered, attract the least sympathy from staff: the appeal effect of such behaviour is proportionately reduced.

The Samaritans report that 90 per cent of (particularly young) suicide attempters or persons threatening suicide express the view that they are glad they did not die, once the attempt is intercepted, or the crisis over. A feeling of conflict about the intended outcome, or of temporary despair is clearly present in almost all suicides (see also Morgan, 1979). Diekstra concludes: 'The common cognitive state in suicide is ambivalence' (Diekstra, 1987:31).

A study of patients admitted to London hospitals for attempted suicide found that attempts were made in such a way that intervention was always possible

(Stengel and Cook, 1958). The authors concluded that the urge to live is always present alongside the urge to die. Self-destruction is not the only motivation in a suicide attempt (Johnson, 1973:239); this does not mean it is not present. Albanese contends that the finding (both in and out of prison) that about half of all suicides have a history of self-injury is sufficient to indicate that non-fatal self-injury is not necessarily 'manipulative': 'For this reason it is useless to ask 'Is this person a manipulator?' It is more useful to group all self-injurers together and ask questions which can generate useful information such as, "Why is the person injuring himself?"' (Albanese, 1983: 65). Similarly, Wicks argues: 'Unless correctional administrators become willing to discard the suicidal manipulator model and show interest instead in the reason underlying *all* self-injurious behaviour, little will be learned about the mutilators and such destruction will continue' (Wicks, 1974: 250).

Suicide and self-injury have traditionally been investigated as separate behaviours, with separate (but overlapping) populations (Stengel, 1964; Stengel and Cook, 1958; Johnson, 1973). Given the increased likelihood of suicide once an injury has been inflicted (Paerregaard, 1975; Hawton, 1986), it would be more useful to see suicide – both in action and intent – as a continuum along which one step may prove to be the first stage of a pathway to despair (O'Mahony, 1990; Maris, 1981). Responding positively at the first step, and providing alternatives, may divert from the destructive route along which the prisoner is setting.

Chapter 3

Young prisoner suicides and suicide attempts

A special case?

Young offenders might be a special case; their stay in prison might be their first lengthy period away from home and their first experience of custody. Moreover, bullying and scapegoating are probably more rife amongst youths than amongst older people.

(The Chief Inspector of Prisons' Thematic Review of Suicide in Prison (Home Office, 1984:14))

SECTION I: SUICIDE AMONGST YOUNG OFFENDERS IN CUSTODY – A SPECIAL CASE?[1]

One of our number has expressed particular concern about the arrangements for the prevention of suicide among young prisoners, and it may be that separate arrangements are appropriate, given the different nature of regimes in young offender establishments.

(Prison Reform Trust, 1983:3)

Studies differ as to whether the under-21 age group are at particular risk of suicide. Circular Instructions tend 'not to distinguish between arrangements for adult and young prisoners' (Prison Reform Trust, 1983:3). Lloyd argued that young offenders in custody appear to be less at risk of completed suicide than other groups (Lloyd, 1990). Recent research and events, however, have highlighted the special risks posed by young offenders, who are increasingly likely to use hanging as a method of self-destructive behaviour, both in prison (Wool and Dooley, 1987) and outside (McClure, 1984b). The evidence suggests that the early adult years are a particularly at-risk time (Hatty and Walker, 1986; Hayes, 1983). Hatty and Walker (1986) found that prison suicides in Australia were heavily concentrated in the early adult years (20–24). The suicide rate for young offenders in custody is higher than the equivalent rate outside (Flaherty, 1983; Hayes, 1983; Dooley, 1990a).

As seen in the previous chapter, it is the remand population who are (numerically, at the very least) most at risk of suicide. Young offenders make up a third of the remand population on any one day (see Table 3.1); 22 per cent of the sentenced prison population are under 21. The proportion of under-21 annual receptions is disproportionately high, as the sentences served by young offenders tend to be shorter than those served by adults. They provide a large 'pool' of potential suicide risks.

The most recent study of suicides in prison in England and Wales included 295/300 consecutive prison deaths receiving suicide verdicts (Dooley, 1990a). The details of those suicides involving young offenders were extracted from the data in this study and kindly supplied by the author of this study, at the request of the researcher. They are presented below.

Table 3.1   Sentenced and unsentenced young offenders as a proportion of the total prison population 1988

	Male no.	Female no.	Total no.	Young offenders no.	%
Remand	9,982	430	10,489	3,439	(33)
Sentenced	37,006	1,276	38,282	8,346	(22)
Totals	46,988	1,706	48,771	11,785	(24)

Source: Prison Statistics England and Wales, 1988

Young offender suicide in England and Wales 1972–1987

Thirty-one (10.5 per cent) of the 295 prison deaths receiving suicide verdicts occurring between 1972 and 1987 and studied by Dooley (1990a) were of prisoners aged under 21. All of the 31 deaths by suicide died by hanging. Some of the deaths were clustered in particular establishments. Young prisoners are more likely to be located in particular establishments, or wings within particular locals and remand centres, however.

It has been possible, using Dooley's figures, and Prison Statistics for England and Wales, to show how young-offender suicide rates compare with all suicides in prison between 1972 and 1987.[2] Using the same calculations as those shown by Dooley (1990a) for all prison suicides, it is clear that the rate of young offender suicides has increased since 1972, and that this increase is slightly larger than that shown for all prison suicides.[3] In addition, by showing more detail about the nature of the young offender prison population at these times, it can be seen that much of the increase could be attributed to the increasing proportion of remand prisoners in the young offender prison population: the sentenced young offender population has increased only slightly since 1972; the remand population has increased by over a half (see Table 3.2). The percentage increases for all suicides in prison between 1972 and 1987 are given in the last column.

From the details given in this table, it is clear that much of the increase in the young-offender prison population has been amongst remand prisoners. The average daily population of sentenced young prisoners has actually fallen since 1976–1979. Since 1972–75 the number of remand receptions has increased by almost one-third;

Table 3.2   Young offender prison statistics and suicides 1972–1987

	1972–75	1976–79	1980–83	1984–87	Increase (%)1972–75 to 1984–87	Increase (%) for all adults and YOIs
Total receptions (annual averages)						
remand	22,728	25,496	27,595	29,690	(31)	
sentenced	20,123	25,191	27,837	26,101	(30)	
Total	42,851	50,687	55,432	55,791	(30)	(23)
Average daily population						
remand	1,935	2,032	2,241	3,029	(56)	
sentenced	8,971	10,161	10,397	9,786	(9)	
Total	10,906	12,193	12,638	12,815	(18)	(22)
Suicides	5	6	8	12	(140)	(121)
Suicides per 100,000 receptions	2.9	2.9	3.6	5.4	(86)	(80)
Suicides per 100,000 ADP	11.5	12.3	13.4	23.4	(103)	(81)

Source: Prison Statistics England and Wales, 1972–1988

the average daily population of young remand prisoners has increased by over a half. Young offenders are being remanded in custody in greater numbers in 1984–87 than in 1972–75, but they are also spending longer there (and in more crowded conditions, often in local prisons intended for adults).

Young offender suicides: description

Half of the 31 suicides were on remand at the time of death (the figure for all suicides was 47 per cent); five (16 per cent) were convicted and awaiting sentence, and 10 (32 per cent) were sentenced. The corresponding figures for all suicides were 5 per cent and 48 per cent, respectively. In other words, 11.4 per cent of all those suicides by sentenced inmates receiving verdicts of suicide were accomplished by young offenders; 11.5 per cent of remand suicides were accomplished by young offenders; *31.3 per cent of suicides amongst convicted prisoners awaiting sentence* occurred amongst young suicides. All of the ethnic minority deaths received suicide verdicts.

Almost half of the suicides were accomplished by young offenders charged or convicted with burglary and theft (45 per cent compared with 34 per cent of all suicides). Few of the young offender suicides were charged with or convicted of offences of violence, compared with the sentenced prison population, or with all prison suicides. Half (of those sentenced inmates receiving suicide verdicts) were serving sentences of between 18 months and three years. Only four inmates (13 per cent) had a recorded history of psychiatric treatment. This is substantially less than that found in the records of all prison suicides. Over half had a history of self-injury (55 per cent); 19 per cent had injured themselves during the current sentence. Over a third (39 per cent) of the suicides occurred in a single cell, but nine of these deaths occurred in multiple cells (29 per cent).

Timing

No particular pattern was apparent regarding the day of death (four deaths occurred on a Monday, nine on a Tuesday, six on a Wednesday, seven on a Thursday, five on a Friday, five on a Saturday and nine on a Sunday). Most of the deaths occurred between midnight and 8 a.m. Most (65 per cent) of the deaths occurred within three months of reception into custody, but many (10) occurred after that. More young offenders committed suicide earlier in the sentence than adults (with the exception of the first few days). Few young offenders committed suicide after one year of their sentence.

Young offenders differed slightly in terms of apparent motivation for the suicide from all prison suicides. Almost half of the young offender suicides (45 per cent) were attributed to prison pressure, slightly more than all prison suicides. Guilt for the offence was less likely to be a major motivation, and mental illness was slightly less likely to be the main motivating factor.

Distinguishing characteristics of young offender suicides

To summarise, young offender suicides differ from the total group of prison suicides in the following respects:

Young prisoner suicides have increased slightly more than all prison suicides. They are more likely to cluster in particular establishments; they are more likely to occur amongst convicted unsentenced inmates; they are more likely to be charged with or convicted of acquisitive offences. They are likely to be serving slightly shorter sentences and to end their lives within one month or at most one year of reception into custody. Young offender suicides are much less likely to be found to have received psychiatric treatment (13 per cent as opposed to almost a third of all prison suicides). Gunn found that violent, sexual and drug-related offences were more often associated with psychiatric disturbance than were property offences (Gunn et al., 1978:318). The offences of these young suicides and the infrequent presence of a psychiatric history, together suggest that psychiatric illness plays a minor role in their deaths (SHHD, 1985; Dooley, 1990a; Fawcett and Mars, 1973; Diekstra, 1987). Slightly more of the young offenders have a past history of self-injury, but they are no more likely than all suicides to have injured themselves during the current sentence. They are slightly more likely to die between midnight and 8 a.m. (55 per cent as opposed to 47 per cent of all suicides). Almost half of the suicides are attributed to prison pressures (40 per cent of all suicides were so ascribed).

Several other studies support the argument that the under-21 age group differ in significant respects from adults, and may have a different susceptibility to suicide in prison. Their offences are found to be less serious: usually property offences (Hayes, 1983), their attempts more frequent (Phillips, 1986), and they are more likely to occur in clusters (Grindrod and Black, 1989; SHHD, 1985; Home Office, 1988c). As we saw in Chapter 2, Australian research shows that when prison suicides are divided into types, one 'atypical' but high-risk group emerges which departs from the profiles otherwise associated with prison suicides. This atypical group (found by Hatty and Walker, 1986 and Australian Office of Corrections, 1985) is the young offender with a history of convictions for property offences. He is male, single, with no job or family support; he has a history of self-injury.

There is some evidence that young suicides are more likely to occur in isolation or segregation areas (Hayes, 1983). Young prisoner suicides may differ from adult suicides in other respects, such as impulsivity (Fawcett and Mars, 1973), and the influence of 'contagion' (Diekstra, 1987). They are likely to have less ties (children, spouse, etc.) than the adult population. Importantly, the suicides of young offenders may be more 'situation-specific' (Dooley, 1990a; Diekstra, 1987).

SECTION II: SUICIDE ATTEMPTS AND SELF-INJURY AMONGST YOUNG PRISONERS

What does emerge from several studies is the tendency for the young to be greatly over-represented in terms of suicide attempts and self-injury in custody. In the UK, 65 per cent of 111 attempted suicides reported to the Midlands and South West Regions between 1983 and 1984 were by young offenders (Wool and Dooley, 1987). In most prison-suicide and attempted-suicide studies, suicide attempt groups are found to be younger than prison suicide groups, and are more likely to use cutting as a method (Phillips, 1986; Correctional Service Canada, 1981). Young offenders in Wool and Dooley's study were more likely than adults to use hanging as a method of deliberate self-harm. In a UK study by Thornton (1990) one in 20 inmates in 21 closed male YOIs from three prison regions were found to have injured themselves during the current sentence. Similarly, Power and Spencer (1987) investigated the large number of young inmates declaring themselves to be suicidal or injuring themselves deliberately in one institution in Scotland in order to explore possible motivating factors.

Rates

Rates of suicide attempts and self-injury are notoriously difficult to assess with any reliability, as shown in the previous chapter (Lloyd, 1990; Wool and Dooley, 1987; Toch, 1975). A recent study of sentenced young offenders in closed male YOIs provides the most comprehensive estimates of the percentages of sentenced young offenders who have made attempts or injure themselves in custody (Thornton, 1990), but these figures cannot be translated into rates per 100,000 ADP or annual receptions as the author does not give enough information about the dates of the study or the regions (three out of four) included in the study (see Table 3.3).

Table 3.3   Percentages of attempted suicide and self-injury amongst male sentenced young offenders

		Attempted suicide %	Self-injury %
Current sentence:			
	remand	2.7	4.7
	local prison	0.9	1.1
	YOI	1.6	3.1
	Totals	5.2	8.9
Previous institutions		1.8	4.3
Outside		8.3	13.0

Source: adapted from Thornton (1990:8)

Thornton's study consisted of 440 young offenders in 21 closed YOIs from three prison regions. He used the data from personality questionnaires and structured interview schedules administered by the Young Offender Psychology Unit. He found that one in eight of the young offenders had a history of self-injury. One in 12 reported having injured themselves during their current sentence (including remand). About half of these inmates reported that they intended to kill themselves. His study does not distinguish between types, degrees or frequency of self-injury.

Although the outside figures are quite high for both attempted suicide and self-injury, Thornton points out that the 'exposure-to-risk' factor will have some impact on the figures: the young men will have spent considerably longer outside than in prison. The average time spent in the current YOIs was approximately 110 days. Not all inmates will have spent time on remand. However, it is apparent that 'a disproportionate number of suicide attempts occur on remand and in local prisons immediately after sentencing':

> Thus the uncertainty associated with the sentencing process and the adjustment period immediately after it would seem to be high risk periods. Nevertheless it would seem that about sixteen YOI inmates in a thousand go on to attempt suicide even after this high risk period is over.
>
> (Thornton, 1990:9)

Young offender suicide attempts and self-injury: description

Wool and Dooley analysed 111 consecutive Prison Department Attempted Suicide Reports (those leading to the completion of a Form F220) occurring in a 1-year period (Oct 1983–Sept 1984) in the prisons of the Midlands and South West Regions of England. These forms are known to be a serious underestimation of the actual number of suicide attempts occurring in prison department establishments (see Chapter 4). Most of the incidents (58 per cent) involved remand prisoners. Twenty per cent were located in young offender establishments; however, 65 per cent of the incidents involved young offenders aged between 16 and 21. Most (over 53 per cent) of these young offenders were in local prisons and remand centres at the time of their injuries. Over 80 per cent of the incidents involved prisoners below the age of 26 years. Both Thornton (1990) and Wool and Dooley (1987) report a higher rate of self-injury and suicide attempts during the remand period. Wool and Dooley (1987) argue that the high proportion of suicide attempts occurring during the remand period may be due to staffing levels in local and remand prisons:

> At this time of maximum vulnerability and isolation for an inmate there is little continuity of staffing on the wings, with the result that prisoners are not able to get to know staff and confide in them. Similarly, staff cannot so easily detect an inmate's reaction to bad news or, indeed, whether he is distressed for any reason.
> (Wool and Dooley, 1987:300)

The availability of and relative ease of access to specialists (such as probation officers, psychologists and visiting psychiatrists) in training establishments is limited; 'listening ears' may be even harder to come by in local and remand centres.

Wool and Dooley conclude from their study that a high risk of attempted suicide is associated with youth, being on remand or recently sentenced, and having a history of mental or physical illness. They do not discuss the young-offender suicide attempts separately (although they do look briefly at the method used in those incidents which occurred in YOIs separately, but this only includes a small proportion of the attempts made by young offenders). It is possible to calculate that 53 per cent of the young offenders were on remand at the time of their injury.

Most attempts were by cutting the arms (72 per cent), although 18 per cent attempted hanging. This sub-group were regarded as a separate category, in view of the fact that suicide in prison is overwhelmingly accomplished by hanging. The 20 episodes were committed by 19 prisoners, a large majority of whom were on remand (65 per cent). These attempts are assumed to be more likely to be serious. Just less than half of the hangings (45 per cent) occurred in young offender establishments. Wool and Dooley suggest that mentally disordered groups may be more likely to make determined attempts, given that mental handicap and psychosis was mentioned in seven of the 20 explanations for these attempts. Explanations most frequently offered for the group as a whole were, that a close relationship was threatened, that a visit had not materialised, or that prison was intolerable. Guilt and boredom were also cited more than once.

The authors conclude that young men are particularly emotionally vulnerable when imprisoned, especially on remand. They suggest that a threat to any personal relationship occurring at this time 'may tip them into a state of mind which causes them to make a suicide attempt' (Wool and Dooley, 1987:300). Isolation or difficulties in communication may contribute. In addition, stress induced by various aspects of prison life: for example, staff shortages (especially in remand centres), may add to the emotional pressures felt by those inmates least able to cope with the demands of custody. They end by suggesting that 'any change in regime that decreases stress and fosters links with family, friends, etc. may go some way to decreasing the rate of completed suicides in prison' (Wool and Dooley, 1987:301). It would appear from this research that the nature and causes of self-injury and attempted suicide in prison are in many ways similar to what we know of completed suicides.

Some would disagree: Power and Spencer (1987) argue in their study of 76 consecutive young inmates aged between 16 and 21 placed on strict suicide observation (SSO), that suicidal and medical intent in parasuicide (a verbal threat of suicide, or a self-inflicted injury) are particularly low. They see self-injury as a separate problem from attempted suicide. Most inmates exhibit minor wrist lacerations, although some set fire to their cells, swallow objects or use 'the unpredictable and dangerous method of feigned hanging' (Power and Spencer, 1987:227). Descriptive and demographic data were collected from the 76 inmates on SSO using a semi-structured interview. A suicidal intent scale and a medical lethality scale were employed by the institution's clinical psychologist to assess the level of risk shown by each inmate. The time of the study was unlikely to be representative, as the establishment was facing an unprecedented epidemic of potentially suicidal behaviour on the part of inmates, resulting in swift allocation to strict suicide observation (SHHD, 1985).

The authors found that almost half of their sample had made verbal threats only, without actually injuring themselves: 31 per cent lacerated their wrists or forearms, 8 per cent set fire to their cells, or to furniture in the cells, 7 per cent swallowed objects such as glass, batteries, needles or paper-clips and 5 per cent 'feigned hanging'. In only 4 per cent of cases was medical lethality found to be high (that is, 'requiring specialised medical care or urgent intervention without which there would have been a significant threat to life' (Power and Spencer, 1987:229)). Two of the four hanging attempts and one of the wrist lacerations came into this category. In 4 per cent medical lethality was found to be moderate (requiring treatment, but no threat to life). One wrist laceration, and two cell fires came into this group. In 92 per cent of the sample, no specialised medical treatment was required. Two hanging attempts, five swallowed objects, four cell arsons, 22 wrist lacerations and all 37 of the verbal threats came into this category.

According to the scale employed by the authors, 94 per cent of the 70 inmates exhibiting minimal medical lethality scored nil on the self-report suicidal intent scale. The authors omit to discuss the possibility that admitting suicidal intent may result in prolonged placement on strict suicide observation (SSO), a fate most inmates wish to avoid. The inmates also had low scores on the 'objective' intent-circumstances scale (Beck *et al.*, 1974). All of the self-report intent scores were much lower than the intent-circumstances scores. In the high-lethality group, the intent-circumstances score was seven, and the self-report score was four (out of

11). Cell arson may be associated with a higher-than-average intent. The authors argue that threats of suicide are taken seriously in custody. The few inmates exhibiting high suicidal intent are more likely to be regarded as psychiatrically disturbed. Feigned hanging is a most dangerous method of exhibiting parasuicidal behaviour, and these incidents could result in 'quasi-suicides' or unintentional deaths. This argument is repeated often in the literature. It is difficult to find evidence to either support or refute it.

Thornton (1990) argued that the 'quality of an inmate's personality is the best predictor of self-injury during a sentence'. Inmates with a neurotic personality are more likely to injure themselves in custody. He proposes that: 'a history of attempting suicide can be treated as a diagnostic indicator of a vulnerable personality, one particularly likely to develop depression within the custodial setting' (Thornton, 1990:4). Previous self-injury, then, is a good predictor of future self-injury. It also predicts future depression during a sentence, however, so that 'false positives' (inmates falsely identified as potential suicide risks) may actually require the special treatment intended for inmates thought to be at most risk of suicide. The link between depression and self-injury is often ignored (Anthony, 1973). Thornton provides evidence here that self-injury is often an expression of vulnerability and misery.

Young offender suicide attempts and self-injury: motivation

Wool and Dooley (1987) argue that suicide attempts are motivated by 'some form of emotional stress relating to poor communication with family and friends' (p. 297). Of all attempts, 43 per cent were apparently motivated by domestic worries – including close relationships being threatened, visits or letters not arriving, or other bad news. A quarter of the attempts were due to prison pressures, such as boredom, or finding the prison situation intolerable. Five per cent were due to an apparent psychotic illness; 16 per cent were attributed to some other emotional disturbance, such as fear, guilt or temper. In 9 per cent of cases the reason was unknown, or not given on the Form 220 (F220). Isolation and difficulties in communication may contribute to the distress felt by those undergoing domestic worries.

Power and Spencer found that half of their sample attributed their parasuicidal behaviour to 'anticipated friction with fellow inmates' (Power and Spencer, 1987:231). SSO provided an escape from such threats. Eighteen per cent said they had experienced some form of emotional upset (for example, a consecutive sentence, the death of a relative, etc.) before the incident. Other motives included manipulation:

> 28% of parasuicidal inmates reported a degree of manipulation associated with their behaviour; for example, deciding to opt out of the regime by being placed on SSO; expecting to avoid loss of remission following placement on mis-

conduct report; or expecting transfer to more convivial surroundings such as the prison hospital.

(Power and Spencer, 1987:231)

The authors conclude that the motivations for prison parasuicidal activity include 'avoidance of subjective situational threats' and are similar to Johnson's 'floundering dependants' ('a weak personality especially vulnerable to the pressures of confinement and aggressive inmates') and 'fear of inmates' ('those inmates accused of being informers or otherwise defined as enemies of other inmates') groupings (Johnson, 1973:264).

Johnson found that his sample of 143 young 'crisis-prone' (self-destructive) inmates differed significantly from their 168 adult counterparts in three ways: they were disproportionately prone to crises reflecting an inability to maintain self-control and composure in solitary confinement (isolation panic); they were more prone to crises indicating 'last-ditch efforts to reinstate flagging social supports' (self-certification, or 'neurotic dependency' in the author's words, Johnson, 1978) and finally, they were disproportionately prone to 'crises which marked a declaration of psychological bankruptcy in the face of social pressures and threats' (fate avoidance) (Johnson, 1978:463). Johnson's study was based on semi-structured interviews exploring the 'events feelings and concerns leading to the self-destructive act or acts' (Johnson, 1978: 462–3). He found that: 'youths displayed distinctive patterns of psychological breakdown related to concrete coping tests posed in the prison environment and self-esteem problems posed when imprisonment strained interpersonal links or undermined feelings of social competence' (Johnson, 1978:463). He argues that segregation proves more unmanageable for young inmates than for adults because of their especially strong needs for social contact and support: 'The conditions of solitary confinement can directly undermine preferred coping strategies. Some adolescents rely heavily on activity as a mode of adaptation. Their goal is to immerse themselves in prison life and to ignore disquieting outside concerns' (Ibid.:466).

Many adolescent prisoners feel an intense need for support from significant others (Johnson, 1978:469) and yet their links are often unreliable and transitory:

A key problem for many adolescents, however, is that their relationships lack depth and maturity. Ties to family are often substantially weakened (even dissolved) by histories of one-way involvement, in which the person has manipulated, abused or taken loved ones for granted. When support (predictably) fails to materialise in prison, these men feel helpless.

(Ibid.:470)

Their self-destructive behaviour may be a last resort in a degenerating relationship: a bid to achieve some response from distant but significant others. To this extent, it is seen as manipulative and egocentric – the young inmates feel resentful and rejected:

But such self-destructive conduct is not undertaken dispassionately. The need for support is painfully real. The person knows he has alienated loved ones; self-injury represents an extreme move designed to communicate genuine distress and establish one's legitimacy as a candidate for help.

(Ibid.:471)

Young inmates quickly feel abandoned and helpless – an abandonment they may have helped to bring about. Their self-destructive conduct may have strong and ancient roots:

repeated efforts to gain care and attention may alienate precisely those persons from whom the individual wishes to secure love. When such behaviour results in repeated incarceration, it may strain family bonds to the breaking point. The person who desperately seeks love may thus find himself abandoned when he most needs family support.

(Ibid.: 472)

This need for attention is immediate and urgent; relationships with staff may mirror those outside, inmates forcing a response from the impersonal prison environment by 'breaking down' (Toch, 1975; Johnson, 1978). Sometimes these bids result in (short-term) gain; more often, they do not accomplish much; they may have negative results. At the very least they reinforce the inmates' feelings of worthlessness: 'To get results, he must resort to extreme measures' (Johnson, 1978:474). If support is not forthcoming, either from the immediate surroundings or from outside: 'His crisis may thus escalate from one of panic, where intervention is possible, to one of hopelessness' (Ibid.:480). Johnson concludes that prison creates special problems for young offenders, a particularly vulnerable group (see also Johnson, 1976): 'Many youths need social support, shared activity, acceptance ... Prison ... is an arid human environment, presenting obstacles to adaptation and threats to self-esteem. It symbolizes community rejection, closes off opportunity and stunts interpersonal growth' (Ibid.:481).

The particular problem of bullying presents serious problems for many young offenders in custody, contributing greatly to the pressures they experience throughout a period of imprisonment:

For a comparatively large group of youths, however, the norms of prison contribute to an environment rife with pressure. Many such persons must strive to avoid victimization, hide personal suffering and otherwise maintain a low profile. Among the more sheltered and naive offenders, prison pressures may prove unmanageable and spawn psychological breakdown.

(Johnson, 1978:462)

Rates of bullying and victimisation in young offender establishments and in prisons which accommodate young offenders are high and may be increasing (Johnson, 1978; McGurk and McDougal, 1986; Shine et al., 1990; see also Bowker, 1980). Bullying and 'baroning'[4] are particularly likely during reception and during the first few days after arrival on a new wing (Shine et al., 1990). Young inmates may be particularly susceptible to threats or attacks from others, having few of the resources and skills necessary to avert such behaviour (Johnson, 1976; Bowker, 1980).

Epidemics

'Waves' of suicides in and out of prison, are largely associated with youth (Grindrod and Black, 1989; SHHD, 1985, but see also Home Office, 1987; Home Office, 1988c). Explanations for this phenomenon include the 'contagion' theory: that one suicide provides the trigger for another, and the imitation theory: that real or fictional suicide models have an effect (the Werther Effect[5]) on others – particularly the young (Schmidte and Hafner, 1988).

Reports into multiple prison suicides in the UK emphasise that the deaths were unconnected and that each had an individual explanation (McHugh, 1989, pers. comm.). A suicide 'cluster' refers to an excessive number of suicides occurring in a close temporal and geographic proximity (Gould, 1988:1). Cookson and Williams argued in a recent report that the suicide clusters in Leeds prison could have been random, according to a statistical model designed to test the randomness of rare events (Cookson and Williams, 1990). The sample and the time frame they employ is far too small for legitimate use in this way.

In the community, there has been a more determined research effort into the role of contagion and/or imitation in suicide. Schmidte and Hafner found that imitation effects were clearly observable for long periods, particularly in the 15–19-year-old male group, following a twice-broadcast six-episode weekly serial showing the railway suicide of a male student. Young male suicides increased by up to 175 per cent during the 70-day period to follow the first episode. The effects were still apparent in older groups, but decreased, so that no effects were observable for males over 40 and females over 30 years (Schmidte and Hafner, 1988:665).

Similarities between the specific characteristics of the 'model' and the observer play an important role in learning by modelling. Self-esteem may moderate vulnerability to modelling. State anxiety, low assertiveness and poor coping ability have also been shown to be associated with suggestibility (Gudjonsson, 1988:159). Schmidte and Hafner define learning by modelling as: 'the acquisition of new patterns of behaviour through the observation of the behaviour of one or more models (Bandura, 1976)' (Schmidte and Hafner, 1988:666).

Newspaper and television reports of suicides (particularly of celebrities) have been shown to have some impact on the number of suicides occurring shortly afterwards (Gould et al., 1987; Gould, 1988; Schmidte and Hafner, 1988), particularly amongst adolescents (Gould and Shaffer, 1986). Fictional suicides and suicide attempts have similarly been shown to have some impact:

> More recently, Ellis and Walsh (1986) investigated the effects of an episode of the English soap opera 'Eastenders' in which one female character took an overdose of drugs. In the week after the broadcast 22 patients with an overdose

were admitted to the emergency department in which the authors worked. The weekly average for the ten preceding weeks had been 6.9, while that for the ten preceding years had been 6.7.

(Schmidte and Hafner, 1988:667)

Not all studies show a positive association between models of suicide – real, reported or fictional – and increased suicidal behaviour in the following period (Modestin and Wurmle, 1989). Those that do show that the effects are particularly strong where similarities (in age, sex and social status) exist between the model and the imitator (Schmidte and Hafner, 1988:673) and that it is the overall frequency of suicide that changes and not just the method chosen (Schmidte and Hafner, 1988:675).

Modestin and Wurmle argue that 'the imitative influence of suicidal behaviour plays a role primarily in adolescents' (Modestin and Wurmle, 1989:512). Their results suggest that, '"epidemics" do not necessarily occur because of the effects of modelling, but ... the occurrence of multiple suicides may have a different common cause' (Modestin and Wurmle, 1989:513). In institutions in particular, multiple suicides may be more likely for reasons directly related to the institution: 'micro-social influences such as organisational instability, lowered staff morale, weakening of the relational system of the staff, and shortcomings in leadership have all been identified as being of importance at the time of such epidemics' (Modestin and Wurmle, 1989:513).

The absence of key (or constant) staff may be associated with a disproportionate number of suicides in a short period (Langlay and Bayatti, 1984), as may clusters of changes and social tensions. In prison, the presence of 'suicide fever', organisational changes, low morale, a harsh subculture and common domestic problems have been found to be associated with clusters of young prisoner suicides (SHHD, 1985; Home Office, 1990c; McHugh, 1989, pers. comm.).

Summary

A recent increase in the number of young offender suicides, particularly whilst on remand, can be explained in part by an increase in the numbers of young offenders 'exposed to risk' during a period of remand. The frequency of young offender suicides has increased slightly more sharply than all prison suicides, according to all different base measures (absolute numbers, receptions and ADP). Half of the young prisoner suicides occurring between 1972 and 1987 were charged with or convicted of burglary or theft and half of those sentenced were serving sentences of between 18 months and four years. Over half of the young offender suicides occurred on remand. Some had a history of previous self-injury, 19 per cent during the present period of custody. Over a third of the suicides occurred in a single cell, and over half were carried out between midnight and 8 a.m. Almost two-thirds of the deaths occurred within three months of reception into custody, and almost half were attributable to prison pressures. It appears that psychiatric history plays a less prominent role in young prisoner suicides than amongst adults. Young prisoner suicides may for this and other reasons (e.g. impulsivity) be more situation-specific than suicides amongst the general prison population.

Chapter 4

A change of direction

How the punishment hurts, how it feels, the suffering and the sorrow, these are elements most often completely lacking in the texts.

(Christie, 1981:15)

INTRODUCTION

The previous chapters looked at rates and explanations of suicide, suicide attempts and self-injury in prison, and in particular, amongst young prisoners. Most of the information on which such rates and explanations are based is derived from record-based research. Official figures, prison department files and other sources of recorded information provide the source for most of our current understanding of the field. Only Johnson (1978), Johnson and Toch (1982) and Thornton (1990) talk to the inmates themselves, or use any other source of information besides records.

Few studies reflect critically upon this information as a data source, assuming that it provides at least an adequate basis from which to draw conclusions about the nature and extent of either suicide or self-injury in custody. Little is known about recording practice or record content, apart from a few precautionary statements about their possible limitations (Burtch and Ericson, 1979; Dooley, 1990b; Johnson and Toch, 1982). There are many factors which play an important part in the recording of information on suicide and self-injury, such as inquests, time, training, priorities and staffing levels. No satisfactory explanation for suicides in prison has been found, nor has there been any more useful way of detecting those inmates who may be at risk of suicide than the limited and often contradictory 'suicide profile'. This profile assumes a uniformity of characteristics amongst prisoner suicides which is not borne out by a closer look at the available information. Individual perceptions of potentially stressful situations have not been considered.

The aim of this chapter is to illustrate the serious problems inherent in previous research, by discussing questions of the reliability of suicide verdicts, both in and out of prison, and other recorded information, statistical and otherwise. It goes on to suggest that efforts to predict the suicidal individual have been of limited use in practice, and in the understanding of the notion of vulnerability to suicide. Research on coping behaviour in prison provides a more promising approach to the study of the nature and causes of suicides in prison.

Limitations of previous research

There are five major limitations in research to date on suicide, attempted suicide and self-injury in prison. These are:

1 the inadequacy of figures on suicides;
2 the inadequacy of incident figures on suicide attempts and self-injury;
3 the lack of any control group;
4 the inadequacy and inappropriateness of recorded information;
5 the focus on a prediction of the suicidal inmate.

Suicide figures and records, based as they are on the outcome of coroners' inquests, provide an inadequate data source for any analysis of rates or explanations of suicides in prison. Only one study (Topp, 1979) takes this into account when drawing up a 'prison suicide profile'. As we shall see below, this has unfortunate consequences for the results of record-based research. A recent study by Dooley (1990b) illustrates this point. Secondly, the recorded data on suicide attempts and self-injury are notoriously weak, and cannot be assumed to bear any valid resemblance to the 'true incidence' of such behaviour. Thirdly, many of the studies do not include control data from the general population or from the prison population from which suicides and suicide attempters are drawn. Thus, it is impossible to know whether characteristics found to be associated with prison suicides and suicide attempters are simply reflections of the characteristics of the general prison population. Fourthly, the contents of prison department files are often incomplete or contradictory; they exist for reasons entirely unrelated to research, and they have been shown to constitute an unreliable source of information. Lastly, the aims and theoretical approaches of studies of suicide and suicide attempts in prison have been weak, concentrating on the prediction of the 'at-risk' inmate rather than on any understanding of the origins of his or her behaviour. Prison suicide research has remained insulated from sociological critique, from psychological studies of cognitive appraisal or coping behaviour and from careful theoretical reflection.

These limitations will be illustrated below, together demonstrating the current gaps in our understanding. Although many of these gaps will remain with us for some time, it is hoped that the research outlined hereafter, and its methodological approach, may at least suggest ways of moving forwards from here, and that its own findings suggest where some of the answers may lie.

SECTION I: SUICIDE FIGURES – THE FLAWS

There is an important distinction between the knowledge that someone ... probably ... committed suicide, and the *legal requirement* that one be *sure* that he both intended the outcome, and had the capacity to take the action. In a court of law, one must be satisfied of the *intent* and of the *capacity*. A suicide is – historically – the murder of oneself, and the law requires it to mean just that.

(Coroner, 1989, pers. comm.)

One of the assumptions of prison suicide research implicit in virtually all of the studies so far discussed is that 'prison suicides' are in fact a meaningful and valid group comparable to suicides amongst the general community. These two groups – suicides in prison, and suicides in the community – are compared for similarities and differences, and those differences that have been discovered then become the subject of further research and speculation. So, for example, recent studies (Backett, 1987; Dooley, 1990a) have taken as their starting point the consistent finding that not only are the rates in prison higher than rates in the community, but the profile of the prison suicide is significantly different. The prison population may be said to be 'suicide-prone': that is, predominantly male, socially rootless, uneducated, unemployed, poor and from unstable social and psychiatric backgrounds. Traditionally, this proneness to suicide amongst the prison population has been assumed to explain its prevalence (Topp, 1979; Home Office, 1984). This assumption, however, is an example of an 'ecological fallacy', whereby researchers have assumed that those prison suicides which occur are drawn (exclusively) from this 'pool' of suicide-prone inmates. Amongst prison suicides, there are a surprising number of apparently 'low-risk' cases: the young, those serving short sentences, those with no psychiatric history, those with jobs, homes and families. Prison suicides lack to some extent the psychiatric history normally associated with suicides out of prison. This finding suggests that *other* factors than, say, psychiatric illness, or long-term depression (normally associated with suicide), may play a part in those suicides which occur in custody (Backett, 1988).

So, if the profile, and therefore probably the causes of inmate suicide are different from the typical suicide, here lies the primary research question: to what extent could 'institutional factors' (the regime, prison stresses, fear, isolation, the prospect of a long sentence, loss of contact with the family (Backett, 1987; Dooley, 1990a) be said to play a part? This is typically where the record search begins: life histories are compared, coroner's records are sought, medical records are searched, historical data are collected, coded and analysed. As prison suicide research has progressed, more situational variables have been added to the list of predictive factors, and research has cautiously begun to suggest that the suicidal inmate may after all be difficult to predict, but the suicidal situation may be less so.

The implications of this development have only moderately, if at all, been translated into prison suicide prevention procedures, which remain firmly committed to predicting suicide-prone inmates on reception or, more recently, during a sentence, something which they inevitably fail to achieve. The most recent instructions (CI 20/89) have, to their credit, moved in their approach from the identification of the 'suicide-prone' inmate, to the recognition of the 'onset of a suicidal crisis'. This change reflects the growing acknowledgement that suicide-prone individuals do not exist in a social/environmental vacuum, but may become 'suicidal' as a result of particular circumstances and events, sometimes building up over a substantial period of time. At the last count (before the implementation of the most recent Circular Instructions) it was found that only 16 per cent of all prison suicides are identified as being 'at risk' before they succeed in killing themselves (Dooley, 1990a). It is not known how many potential suicides are identified and prevented. This proportion of successfully identified 'risks' has remained constant since the early 1970s (Topp, 1979), before most of the contemporary research on suicides in prison was carried out, suggesting that increasing research on the characteristics of individual suicides has not contributed greatly to its prediction, or prevention. As we have seen already in Chapter 2, the successful identification of an inmate at risk of suicide by no means ensures his or her successful prevention.

The increasing awareness of the importance of the environment both in this context and in others may improve the identification of the 'onset of risk' if reliable patterns continue to emerge. Many of the 'risk' situations in suicide research are the same risk situations as those discovered in other areas of prison research: post-reception, pre-release, after bad news/bereavement, pre-parole decisions, etc. as we saw in Chapter 2. If any identifiable situation is conducive to suicide, it is also conducive to absconding, and other prison problems and disturbances. These collective 'symptoms' of prison/prisoner malaise are often referred to as indications of the prison climate: 'As long as prison overcrowding, suicide, murders and riots persist, the search for improvements must continue' (Wormith 1984:392).

It cannot be argued that there is no psychiatric element in or predisposition to suicide in those who succeed, both in and out of prison; but what should be acknowledged is that just as outside, it is more usually a combination of (psychiatric) vulnerability, situational stress and individual perceptions which trigger the final suicide act than either component alone.

This increasingly situational approach to prison suicide research has been a valuable and meaningful line of inquiry, which has been critical. It has provided significant insights into the stresses of prison life (e.g. pre-release; the immediate impact of custody) and it has brought the issue of prison suicides into an arena with a growing tradition in sociological penology. There is an important problem, however, which arises when trying to make sense of the basic figures on suicides in prison.

It appears that certain basic questions about the validity of suicide *verdicts* in prison, have never been adequately addressed. If there are serious problems with suicide verdicts, particularly if they affect their comparability in and out of prison, this will also have serious repercussions on the validity of the sort of record-based research already referred to. This oversight may be surprising in the light of well-known sociological critiques (Atkinson, 1982; Douglas, 1967; Taylor, 1982) suggesting that suicide figures are sociologically 'constructed' and organised by certain background expectancies which operate to repair the generally ambiguous and disorganised fabric of everyday life. Suicides which 'look like' suicides, become suicides. It would appear that prison suicide research has remained insulated from such sociological critiques. Instead, largely clinical or official research has continued unperturbed by questions of definition, validity and reliability. Researchers have only rarely included other categories of non-natural deaths besides those actually receiving a verdict of suicide in a coroner's court, in their investigations (Topp, 1979; Dooley, 1990b).

It is not only the category of suicide which should raise doubts in the researcher's mind, but also the contents of any explanation of the death which then follows. As Atkinson (1982) and Taylor (1982) are at pains to illustrate, suicides are constructed on the basis of a largely circular process of interpretative reasoning based on the coroner's and others' assumptions about what a suicide 'looks like'. Once a preliminary verdict of suicide is reached – often on the basis of expected facts such as mode and situation of death (e.g. hanging, following the death of a spouse), confirmatory evidence is 'found' in the person's history: depression, suicidal intent, isolation, and so on. Taylor refers to this as 'digging' – to reveal what we think of as a suicidal problem. These problems then become the major source of information at inquests – and the major source of information in research. This evidence, and its construction, has more to do with our legal (and psychological) requirement of proof of *intent*, needed before a suicide verdict can be brought, than with the real-world suicidal action that is by now several steps away from the final reports. An example: a hanging follows several unsuccessful – or superficial – attempts at suicide. The jury return a verdict of 'death by misadventure' following a strong directive by the coroner. The evidence was selected, the summing up was strongly weighted in favour of the latter interpretation; the inmate had 'done this kind of thing before', an attention-seeking gesture gone wrong. Does this verdict constitute a 'social fact'? This social fact, if such, disguises possible disagreement between pathologists, dispute as to the verdict, selective evidence given by 'coroner's witnesses' and wide discretion in the final 'telling of the tale'. The judicial attitude towards suicide is summed up as follows: 'Suicide is not to be presumed. It must be affirmatively proved to justify the finding. Suicide requires an intention' (Chambers and Harvey, 1989).

Coroners' inquests and deaths in custody: a process

A verdict of suicide can only be brought by a coroner. All deaths thought to be unnatural are referred to a coroner, who may then authorise an inquest. All deaths in custody require an inquest; they must also be held with a jury. This takes place in the coroners' court, but few similarities exist between criminal or civil, and coroners' courts. The criminal and civil courts are essentially adversarial, and their purpose is to establish proof of liability – or, in a criminal court, guilt. The main purpose of the coroners' court, on the other hand, is to inquire into a death, establishing the physical cause, and 'to present a verdict, from an established range of verdicts, which is consistent with the facts'. In the words of a coroner:

The purpose of the inquest is to establish, *who* the deceased was, *where* they died, *when* they died, *why* they died – or perhaps more correctly, *how they came by their death*. What is very important is not to attach blame to anybody. It is just to establish the facts, and that is a very important distinction.

(Coroner, 1989, pers. comm.)

There is no prosecution and no accused. In contrast to the adversarial procedure of criminal courts, the coroners' procedure is inquisitorial. If questions concerning personal liability emerge during the inquest, then it may be adjourned, 'either for the person involved to be present and/or represented, or for the DPP to investigate and/or institute proceedings in the criminal courts' (Scraton and Chadwick, 1987:16). As Scraton and Chadwick point out:

Until recently the coroners' court could indicate liability and coroners were able to commit people for trial. These powers no longer obtain but a coroner still possesses immense discretion to make recommendations. For example, deaths which occur in the course of leisure pursuits ... will often carry a coroner's recommendation concerning clothing, equipment or instruction. Similarly, deaths at work are regularly subject to recommendations concerning safety precautions.

(Scraton and Chadwick, 1987:16)

Coroners may be trained in medicine or law (or both). There is a possible dichotomy between the use of medical evidence and legal argument, which raises doubts about the consistency with which the two disparate professions undertake their task. They are appointed by local authorities, after practising for at least five years in their specialist field, and normally serving as a deputy coroner for some time. They work within a specific geographical location, holding a position of authority, carrying broad powers and extensive discretion:

The apparent professional expertise which they possess, together with their extensive powers in their courts and the sole responsibility for summing up a case and directing the jury accordingly, provide coroners with immense authority in the handling of controversial cases.

(Scraton and Chadwick, 1986:17)

They work closely with the police in the course of their investigations, relying on the coroners' officer to gather and present much of the evidence at an inquest. The other main agent upon which the coroner depends is the pathologist – who is formally independent, but instructed by the coroner. The pathologist provides a medical opinion, suggesting ways in which the person might have died given 'what is known'. The interplay between 'opinion' and 'professional expertise' in all three agents has been well documented (Scraton and Chadwick, 1987:17). There is often dispute at all stages of the investigation. There is also a significant argument that all three agents: coroners, pathologists and coroners' officers, have an inevitably 'special relationship' undermining any claims of autonomy and independence from 'established interests'. Either way, verdicts are not 'facts', but a product of a long and complex process beset with negotiations and interpretations.

On a structural level, then, there are two levels on which inquests can be seen as problematic. First, it may be that they are inappropriate as a means of inquiry in particular controversial circumstances: 'This ... raises the question of the deficiencies of coroners' investigations and courts in a *structural* sense as they relate to a range of controversial deaths involving the police and prisons' (Scraton and Chadwick, 1986:21). Secondly, there are organisational elements in the process leading up to a verdict which make suicide as a category fairly equivocal: certainly incomplete, if not meaningless. Rather like 'crime' as a category, it may be that the 'homogeneity' of 'suicides' as a group is artificially restricted to its legal definition as such: deaths for which a suicide verdict is successfully applied at inquests become suicides.

What is crucial is whether these issues of description and explanation – the process – differ in the prison context from those which occur in the general community. For example, Atkinson (1982), Douglas (1967) and Taylor (1982) all refer to hanging as the one virtually conclusive 'suicidal' mode of death in the community: 'Hanging, particularly once homicide has been excluded, is probably the most unequivocal suicidal cue' (Taylor, 1982: 77–8). Most (90 per cent) suicides in custody are accomplished by hanging (Dooley, 1990a) – that 'most unequivocal cue'. However, two features of prison hanging must be considered. First, many unnatural deaths in custody with verdicts other than suicide (open verdict, death by misadventure, etc.) have involved self-strangulation. Secondly, many serious attempts at hanging are never defined or understood as suicide attempts: other explanations are found (attention-seeking, misadventure even sexual asphyxia). Hanging in prison, then, is not a 'most unequivocal suicidal cue'. Is this because the behaviour differs, or because the interpretation of the behaviour differs, in this new context? It is a pity (for prison sociology) that Atkinson, Taylor and Douglas never became interested in prison suicides.

Proof of intent is required before a verdict of suicide may be brought. Is this proof less likely to be found in prison? In other words, are more open verdicts, or other unnatural death verdicts brought in the prison situation? A recent study by Dr Enda Dooley (1990a; 1990b) into consecutive prison suicides over the last 15 years suggests that many probable suicides are officially classified as 'open verdicts' or other non-natural deaths. (This is also true of suicides outside prison, albeit for different reasons: Chambers and Harvey, 1989; Barraclough and Hughes, 1987; Chambers, 1989.)

Between 1972 and 1987 there were 442 unnatural deaths in prison: 300 of these were given verdicts of suicide; 142 were given other verdicts. In a recent article (Dooley, 1990b), Dooley was asked to judge which of the unnatural group were in fact 'probable suicides'. He found that 52 (out of the 142) – that is, one-third – were a result of consciously self-inflicted injuries. In other words, they were likely suicides, according to the evidence. This group did differ in significant respects from the suicide-verdict group. There were a higher proportion of females, suggesting that women may be less likely to be given a suicide verdict; fewer of the deaths were accomplished by hanging (although the figure was still 71 per cent, against 90 per cent of those deaths receiving suicide verdicts), there was a more frequent history of self-injury during the sentence (45 per cent, against 22 per cent of the suicide group), and these deaths were more likely to have occurred during the day. These findings suggest that it may only be those suicides which 'look like' suicides which have any certainty of being recorded as such. Even then, many consciously self-inflicted deaths will receive other verdicts – 'lack of care' (although this is quite rare), 'misadventure', 'accidental' or 'open'. Who gets left out of such statistics? It appears that there may be systematic patterns biasing the figures, and therefore the profiles of prison suicides. Important information concerning both young offender suicides in particular, but also concerning all prison suicides, is masked by restricting research-based profiles to deaths receiving suicide verdicts.

A coroner was asked whether he thought recorded suicides were an underestimate of the true rate, this was his reply:

> I would have thought that the evidence for suicide in prison was pretty clear, in that they're hangings. I mean, not many people tear up sheets and hang them on the bed or the back of their window or door or something, and then die by mistake. So I would have thought that it's pretty accurate. I mean, *outside*, you would probably say that it is a slight underestimate because, you know ... many open verdicts *are* suicides. Well, I mean, coroners *know* that. As I explained to you before, they've got to be *satisfied* about the *evidence*, you know ... It isn't just a case of some psychiatrist thinking to himself, well, the coroner is full of nonsense, the silly fool ... the coroner probably knew it was a suicide, *too*, but the evidence wasn't there to satisfy the court of law.
>
> (Coroner, 1989, pers. comm.)

This is a common assumption, also found in most of the prison suicide literature: that suicides in prison are, if anything, likely to be a more accurate picture of the real rate than suicides in the general community, because of the conditions of surveillance and containment. However, Dooley's findings, and the above commentary, cast serious doubts on this assumption.

There have been suggestions in the sociological literature (Fenwick, 1984) that certain pressures may be exerted upon coroners to bring, for example, an open verdict in the case of a possible prison suicide. There are other suggestions that families may exert pressure away from a suicide verdict, out of guilt, shame or denial, or that the police may prefer a suicide verdict, as an open verdict remains an 'unsolved case' on their books. Alternatively, there have also been suggestions that the Home Office dislike the suicide verdict, and encourage the use of alternatives (Broderick Report, 1971; Knapman and Powers, 1985; Coroners Rules, 1984). Is there any truth in this claim? One coroner's response: 'Absolutely ... *no* evidence of that at all! No evidence of that at all! That would be totally outside of the law!' (Coroner, 1989, pers. comm.). Open verdicts are 'brought when the evidence is insufficient to reach a conclusion, and that, quite simply, is that!'

There appear to be no particular instructions or guidelines issued to coroners, but what they do receive (from the Lord Chancellor's Department) is a list of suggested verdicts: 'It is only a list of suggested verdicts, and the coroner can in actual fact return any verdict he wishes ...'. Coroners differ in their preferences, some steering juries away from open verdicts, others steering them away from 'suicide' – unless the jury is sure, beyond reasonable doubt, that the death was in fact a suicide. Verdicts of 'misadventure' and 'accidental death' or 'open' are common. The only alternative verdict which is uncommon is 'lack of care' – a verdict implying that the death would not have occurred if the inmate had received the (usually medical) attention he should have received. Only three verdicts of 'lack of care' were brought in cases of prison deaths between 1972 and 1987 (Dooley, 1990b).[1]

Suicide rates: suspending judgement

Just how objective and accurate – or reliable – is a suicide verdict? Is it more reliable in prison, or less? How many self-inflicted deaths in prison are given other verdicts, such as 'misadventure', 'open' or 'accidental'? Some authors suggest that many unnatural deaths receiving other verdicts than suicide, are in fact suicides (Holding and Barraclough, 1975; Pescosolido and Mendelsohn, 1986). This corresponds to the proportion of unnatural deaths found to be 'probable suicides' by Dooley (one-third; Dooley, 1990b). Without suggesting that coroners' deliberations are intentionally collusive, there are legitimate questions to be asked about the validity of prison suicide rates in the light of what is known about the legal reasoning and requirements inherent in their production. If the assumption that prison suicides are a more reliable category than suicides amongst the general community is flawed, this is a relevant consideration in terms of the validity of both previous and current research, whatever the explanation. The same problem is true of community suicide research, which also relies upon suicides identified by legal requirements. Barraclough found that unnatural-deaths differed in significant respects from deaths receiving suicide verdicts. He concluded from this that unnatural deaths were therefore not likely to be suicides. He does not discuss the possibility that his profile of a 'suicide' may be flawed as a result of those suicides not receiving suicide verdicts appearing amongst his unnatural-deaths group (Barraclough and Hughes, 1987). In this context, it is important to note that the Prison Department began to publish statistics on self-inflicted deaths as well as those attracting suicide verdicts at inquests, in 1990.

SECTION II: RECORD-KEEPING IN PRISONS

A second problem concerns the record-based approach to suicide attempts and self-injury in prison. Just as with suicide, but for slightly different reasons, both the statistics and the contents of the records from which data is taken, on which most current research is based (Wool and Dooley, 1987; Phillips, 1986) are seriously flawed. The only studies to acknowledge this limitation are Jones (1986), and Toch (1975). As with most statistical information on which criminological research is based, the requirements for recording such information are clearly unrelated to the requirements of research: they are collected for another purpose entirely (Kitsuse and Cicourel, 1963).

The statistics

'Paper-work' is one of the most frequently heard complaints from staff about routine tasks in prison service life. Every aspect of prison life from the inmate's first reception into custody – his property card, his record, his category and so on, to the aggregate details of time spent out of cells, or in education and at work, to the weekly reception and discharge figures, is monitored. Most of this monitoring is necessary and desirable as without systematic recording, property would go astray, staff would not know who they had in the establishment and checks could not be made on the operation of regimes. However, the purpose of the monitoring, and its meaning, is sometimes questioned by those charged with the task of completing the relevant forms. The sheer scale of the documentation required is vast, and occasionally elicited sarcasm from staff: 'If there's one thing I can tell you about a dead inmate, it's that we can't bury him until he's worth his weight in paper!' (Governor Grade). Suicide attempts and self-injury statistics are amongst the most problematic of these information sources.

Recording of self-injury

Instructions to Prison Department establishments require staff to complete a form (F213) every time an injury occurs in prison. This might be an accident, a fight, an unknown cause or self-inflicted. The form is simple and short, requiring only the time and nature of the injury.[2] In addition to the (F213), a hospital incident book is kept at all Prison Department establishments, where a constant diary of all happenings on the hospital are recorded, mainly to inform other staff and to ensure that information is passed between shifts. This book is often the best place to find a record of self-injury incidents: staff are better at informing themselves than informing 'outsiders'.

Recording of suicide attempts

Where an attempt at suicide occurs, a form F220 should be completed. This is a much more complex form than the F213, requiring staff from various departments (hospital, discipline staff, chaplain, governor) to write up to a paragraph, giving reasons for the incident, and any background information felt to be relevant. Establishments differ in their propensity to raise an F220 (Home Office, 1990d), most only doing so where the incident is considered to be rather serious. The decision to raise an F220 is usually made by the medical officer, sometimes in consultation with the hospital or other staff. The total number of F220 forms raised each year at each establishment is submitted to Headquarters. These become one of the available Prison Department annual 'attempted suicide' statistics. The form requires information on the inmate's offence, sentence, age, previous convictions, earliest date of release, date and method of attempt; it then elicits opinion about the incident from the medical officer, chaplain, welfare officer, governor, and a report of any inquiry. It requires a great deal of searching out for information, and chasing up of the relevant staff. There is a lot of work involved in its completion, and it might take several days to 'do the rounds'.

In practice, the F220 was rarely completed, or seen in records, partly because many self-inflicted injuries were not clearly 'suicide attempts'. However, in many cases the incidents were difficult to assess and some would certainly have resulted in death, were it not for the chance intervention of a member of staff. Two factors affected the decision whether or not to raise a form. The first was the tendency to assume that no attempt that was unsuccessful, however serious the injury, was a 'genuine attempt'. The operational definition of an attempt at suicide was in this case 'one that succeeds'. A second reason was that staff did not want to raise the form: it was long and involved, time-consuming and contributed to figures which reflected badly on individual establishments. The (four-page) form involved many different staff having to inteview the inmate, or remember detail they found difficult to retrieve. Sometimes, their knowledge of the inmate was simply not sufficient to contribute – very little contact had taken place.

During the research, on more than one occasion, the F220 was referred to as the 'nearly a dead inmate' form. In some establishments, emergency transfer to outside hospital would be required before the form was raised. In others, however, a regular proportion of those self-injury incidents referred to the prison hospital would lead to the completion of an F220.

A second form on which serious attempts at suicide may be recorded is the Incident Report Form (CI 18/1988: The Reporting and Management of Incidents and Follow-up Action).[3] It is completed by governors of establishments. It is divided into 'minor' and 'major' incidents, and is coded for computerisation. 'Death of an inmate' or 'Suicide of an inmate' are both major incidents (the others are concerted indiscipline, escapes, hostage-taking, roof-top demonstrations, assaults, food-refusal and so on). An attempt at suicide is recorded as a minor incident, unless it is thought that it will attract unfavourable publicity. It may then, like other minor incidents, be treated as a major incident. This form is submitted to region, where figures are compiled on the various incidents occurring in establishments from year to year.

F220s and Incident Forms, raised by different staff groups (and grades), may not coincide. Governors decide to raise Incident Forms; medical officers raise F220s. Regional and national figures on prison suicide attempts, if they are available, do not necessarily add up. This is confirmed by studies in other countries, where similar discrepancies between medical and security reporting systems and personnel exist (Albanese, 1983). The F220, upon which annual figures and the only UK research on suicide attempts in custody is based, are infrequently and haphazardly completed (Home Office, 1990d).

The content of records

A second problem inherent in record-based research is the unreliability of the information available in records. Information may be incomplete (Dooley, 1990a), incorrect (Dooley, 1990b, 1990c) or selective (see also Zamble and Porporino, 1988; Griffiths and Rundle, 1976). Files may contain contradictory information, and it is apparent that an inmate's understanding of events and decisions (which go unrecorded) may be different from those recorded in his or her file. Information contained in files was often negative, and rather different from the 'whole' story, when related by the inmate. Files read before the interview always presented a grimmer picture of the inmate than the interview and other contacts with inmates subsequently presented.

Record-based studies miss a great deal of valuable information relating to suicidal activities in prison. Certain situational or 'institutional' factors may appear in documentary material available to the researcher, such as overcrowding, hours out of cell, location, staff–inmate ratios and so on. But this conception of 'the prison' as a series of identifiable and recordable 'institutional factors' is seriously limited, as other recent areas of prison research illustrate (McDermott and King, 1988). Organisational and relational aspects of 'the prison' are as real and important in terms of life inside as are visible and quantifiable factors such as hours spent out of cells, timing in sentence, and so on. The prison itself 'does' very little in terms of its impact on prisoners: 'the prison itself does not do anything ... it just sits there. What really matters are the "subtle specifics of each prisoner's participation in prison life"' (Wormith, 1984:427).

So 'what goes on' in prison may be unavailable in *any* form of documentation – however carefully collected, and despite the increasing volume and availability of this sort of material. Similar criticisms of retrospective, record-based suicide and suicide-attempt research can be found in studies in the community (Hawton and Catalan, 1987).

SECTION III: SUMMARY AND THEORETICAL CONSIDERATIONS

It is clear that there are serious difficulties inherent in relying upon statistical information alone when trying to assess the incidence of various types of behaviour in prison. Part of the problem lies in the uncertainty over what actually constitutes a suicide attempt. This issue has never been satisfactorily resolved, and definitions will continue to differ. In addition, however, there may be factors discouraging staff from raising all the relevant forms every time an incident occurs – the wish to keep incidents out of the 'attempted suicide' category wherever possible, the time involved, the general dislike of complex forms and the (possibly limited) amount of information available on the inmate concerned:

> Doctors and prison officers are, of course, not unbiased in these cases. It would not be surprising if, unconsciously, they preferred to blame misadventure for a death which could possibly have been prevented by them, had they taken a different view of the situation.
>
> (Stengel, 1971:14)

Even suicides, so often taken to be 'unequivocal', cannot be assumed to be so. Record-based information may be incomplete, biased and unreliable. The search for the suicidal profile has dominated research to date, and has restricted the theoretical approach to the subject. A preoccupation with the 'individual' is conceptually limited, and has been questioned in many other areas of the prison world:

> This 'individualisation of blame', together with allegations or assumptions of 'pathology' in the aetiology/motivation of disruptive behaviour undoubtedly appeals to popular stereotypes, and mirrors a similar long and now somewhat discredited theme in the history of criminological theory, from Lombroso in the 19th Century to 'dangerous offender'/'sexual psychopath' legislation in the second half of the 20th Century.
>
> (Bottomley, 1990:12)

Any exclusive or superficial concern with the environment, however, is equally flawed. Outside of prison suicide research, in other areas of prison life, a more meaningful and promising avenue can be found. Research which incorporates the subjective perceptions of the subjects, and which assumes a critical interplay between individual and environment, offers a fresh start for prison suicide research. A study of prison coping behaviour by Zamble and Porporino provides an appropriate framework for answering some of the primary research questions raised so far.

Coping with custody: asking the inmates

Zamble and Porporino argue that the interaction between situational or environmental factors and the individual's coping ability will be a crucial determinant of prison behaviour. Coping ability is related to many aspects of behaviour and lifestyle, including the use of time and relationships with others (Zamble and Porporino, 1988:25). Sperbeck and Parlour argue that 'subnormal coping skills' are often associated with (or are the result of) other disorders, such as borderline personality disorder (Sperbeck and Parlour, 1986). Toch showed that many self-destructive and disruptive inmates have 'sharply limited coping skills' and that self-laceration may be seen as a 'declaration of bankruptcy' (Toch *et al.*, 1989:174–5, *passim*; see also Johnson, 1976). Zamble and Porporino's investigation into coping behaviours in prison included an analysis of the lifestyle and behaviour of inmates when they were in the community. The authors found that inmates had spent considerable amounts of time outside in 'idle passive-spectator activities'

(Zamble and Porporino, 1988:43). Many appeared to live in a perpetual present, in the company of friends (see also Diekstra, 1987). Their lifestyle was loose and unstructured: 'Most subjects described *passing* their time rather than *using* it, in the company of others' (Zamble and Porporino, 1988:44). Their living arrangements and relationships were impermanent, casual and unsatisfactory. The use of alcohol and drugs was high: 'the average pattern was one of casual, unplanned days, with greater dependence on friends than family or work, little focus and no goals' (Zamble and Porporino, 1988:47).

Most of the subjects did not report that they experienced these background features of their lives as a problem, but they did show 'substantial deficiencies in the way they coped with problem situations':

> When faced with a problem, they usually attempted to deal with it directly and immediately, but their attempts were mostly unplanned, scattered, and impulsive ... Some responses were used repeatedly, even though they were totally ineffective in remediating the problem, or were even harmful.
>
> (Zamble and Porporino, 1988:54)

In short, the authors conclude, 'coping was a disaster area for most subjects'; they found 'the same gamut of ineffective, inappropriate or exacerbating responses in every sort of situation' (p.55). There are many modes of coping behaviour, some of which are more effective than others: active, cognitive, behavioural and avoidance (Gudjonsson, 1988:160). Coping ability lies at the root of many other behaviours and traits, including susceptibility to influence from outside sources (Gudjonsson, 1988). Mood can affect the ability to call upon or implement one's coping strategies (Williams and Scott, 1988; Moore *et al.*, 1988). Even temporary depression can have a debilitating effect on the ability to generate facilitative thoughts and strategies. *Reactive* problem-solving, with little planning or anticipation of future results characterised the coping strategy employed by most of the subjects in Zamble and Porporino's study: avoidance, escape, alcohol and drug use or other palliatives comprised the range of alternative coping strategies most often used. This description of their behaviour shows an instrumentalist view of self-injury to be inconsistent with the whole range of many offenders' behaviour. Reactive, non-purposive behaviour describes their actions more appropriately. These strategies are referred to by the authors as 'low-level' modes of coping. With these methods, problems endured, or were exacerbated. Most imprisoned offenders, they conclude, are maladaptive. Sperbeck and Parlour argued that suicidal behaviour is often an *extension* of the impulsive and unrestrained emotionalism associated with seriously impaired coping skills (Sperbeck and Parlour, 1986). In prison, problems are more difficult to resolve, as the range of options (including escape, palliatives and avoidance) is limited.

Poor coping is associated with instability in relationships and residence, with low proportions of time spent in work and 'directed activities', and with 'lack of planning and infrequent thoughts of the future' (Zamble and Porporino, 1988:70). Zamble and Porporino argue that offenders may differ little from others on most measures of background characteristics, but that they do show poor coping ability. These coping characteristics are mediated by such factors as social class and previous experience of custody. It is hypothesised in the present research that young inmates may be differentiated according to the *extent* of this poor coping ability, and that those inmates least able to cope with the special environment of prison will be those most at risk of suicidal thoughts and actions during a sentence.

Coping with custody: Zamble and Porporino's results and their applicability to the investigation of vulnerability to suicide in prison

The isolation and boredom of many of the inmates in Zamble and Porporino's study made it 'easy to understand why they were so willing to talk with us' (Zamble and Porporino, 1988:82). Restrictions on time, facilities and physical movement created strain amongst their subjects. Many reported sleeping problems, anxieties, feelings of hopelessness, depression and of constantly missing people. A third of their subjects scored six or higher on the Hopelessness Scale. The Hopelessness Scale (Beck *et al.*, 1974) is a 20-item questionnnaire found to be strongly associated with suicidal ideation. The subject assigns 'true' or 'false' to a series of statements expressing hope or hopelessness. A mean score of 9–12 is found to significantly differentiate depressed and suicidal patients from controls (see Zamble and Porporino, 1988; Williams and Scott, 1988): 'Scores as high as we found are undeniable indications of depression, and even possible suicidal tendencies' (Zamble and Porporino, 1988:85).

This emotional disruption is *reactive*, that is, it may be temporary and externally caused, rather than endogenous and likely to be described as 'clinical'. Most inmates felt miserable during the early stage of custody. The authors argue that this misery could provide a 'window of opportunity' through which the 'winds of change' may blow (Zamble and Porporino, 1988:89). Without hope, or constructive choices, their misery may turn to despair. Instead of opportunity, inmates face chronic problems of separation from loved ones, inactivity and anxiety: 'After the drama of arrest and trial, life settles into a mundane level where the uniformity is punctuated by petty confrontations, minor deprivations and bureaucratic restrictions' (Zamble and Porporino, 1988:91).

Williams shows how depressed and suicidal patients see their life situation and their past, through a 'window of despair', with over-generalised negative memories superseding positive or specific memories – a cognitive bias lowering the threshold of vulnerability to feelings of hopelessness (Williams and Scott, 1988). Alone, isolated or unable to sleep, this preoccupation with negative life events may encode perceptions of the present and the future. The 'fact of imprisonment dominates prisoners' lives', and yet their ability to cope with these facts has never been adequately investigated in relation to prison suicide.

Zamble and Porporino argue that inmates cope with prison problems in the same way that they cope outside – by escape, avoidance or maladaptive behaviour (Zamble and Porporino, 1988). Some cope relatively well, by desensitising themselves to pain (forgetting the outside) or by just 'doing their time', and awaiting release. For some, it is possible to settle into the way of a sentence, drifting along, making a few friends or maintaining regular contacts with family and friends outside. Most problems remain, however, and 'alarming' levels of depression and anxiety found at the early stages of the sentence, remain elevated (with some decrease) throughout. Some of the initial effects of imprisonment dissipate over time: 'The shock, disruption, and novelty of a new term in prison after a while turns into the familiarity and boredom of consistent routine' (Zamble and Porporino, 1988:111).

Most of the emotional disturbance found later in the sentence will have been imported from their pre-prison lives, according to Zamble and Porporino, if levels of pre-prison alcoholism and poor coping skills in all areas of their lives are taken into account. Measures of loneliness and boredom remained high throughout the sentence, even though measures of most other dysphoric emotional states (depression, anxiety and guilt) seemed to reduce slightly. Their mean levels were still elevated 'even though they had dropped to within the normal (subclinical) range' (Zamble and Porporino, 1988:119). The authors do not elaborate on the feelings of boredom and loneliness, nor do they indicate how these feelings might be distinct from depression. Inmates continued to cope by 'narrowing their attention to the present moment' (p.122). Relationships with other inmates may be kept deliberately superficial, so that sudden transfers, releases or movements do not result in more separation and feelings of loneliness. The survivors show signs of, 'the coldness and self-containment of men who have been cut off from intimate contacts with other people' (Zamble and Porporino, 1988:123).

Having a number of friends in prison was associated with lower measures of dysphoric emotion (depression amd anxiety). None of the other expected variables such as sentence length or current offence showed any relationship to measures of depression, anxiety or anger. In other words, background factors were unhelpful 'predictors' of emotional states, whereas *cognitive appraisals* (such as reported problems and feelings of boredom) were strongly associated with emotional states. The authors conclude that: 'coping theory allows a considerable advance in predictive and explanatory power beyond that possible with previous models' (Zamble and Porporino, 1988:142).

They show that inmates' expectations and appraisals are better indicators of their condition than 'inadequate behavioural assumptions' may be. They suggest that refinements to coping theory provide the most likely path to a better understanding of many types of prison behaviour. 'The most common consistency in suicide is with life-coping patterns' (Diekstra, 1987:33). Sapsford argued in 1983, after Cohen and Taylor (1972) that tests of ability and measures of psychological deterioration would not reflect the pains or harms of imprisonment: 'We need to look more closely at attitudes and beliefs; what prisoners do, and what they think' (Sapsford, 1983:5).

In the remainder of this book, it is hypothesised that young prisoners who injure themselves and/or attempt suicide during a sentence will show poorer coping skills than those inmates who do not engage in self-destructive behaviour. The research reported in the following chapters will investigate whether aspects of imprisonment, poorly understood in previous prison suicide research, may contribute to 'the onset of a suicidal crisis', particularly amongst these poor copers, or vulnerable inmates. Differential coping ability may help to distinguish potential suicide risks from the general prison population, many of whom show characteristics which, outside of prison, might suggest a vulnerability to suicide. There will be other types of prisoners who are at risk of suicide, for a variety of (sometimes related) reasons. What follows constitutes a first attempt to construct a model around which we can begin to understand this process. It is only by engaging in meaningful interactions with the prisoners themselves, in the context of a long and semi-structured interview, that this information can be sought (Toch, 1975). Understanding the real and diverse pains of imprisonment, and the inability of many inmates to cope with them, may lead us to reconsider assumptions based on previous studies of the effects of imprisonment that prison does little or no lasting harm (Walker, 1983; Bukstel and Kilmann, 1980). This latter argument may be based on a flawed conception of harm (see Cohen and Taylor, 1972; Christie, 1981; Mathieson, 1965 and Wormith, 1984).

Part II

Talking to staff and prisoners

Chapter 5

Investigating suicides in prison

it is as inhabitants of this human world that we ... must finally recognize that there is a certain kind of scientific 'objectivity' that can lead us to know everything, but to understand nothing.

(Fromm, *Beyond the Chains of Illusion*, 1962:viii)

SECTION I: THE PROBLEM

This chapter sets out the strategy employed throughout the research conducted in the search to understand suicide attempts amongst young prisoners, discussing methodological and theoretical issues arising from it. The reader is reminded of the theoretical and practical research aims, and of the serious gaps left by previous studies. Some preliminary issues of definition, description and explanation are raised, and the particular nature of the research problem considered. The rest of the chapter outlines the methods chosen, justifications for this approach, and relates precisely how the research was carried out. Finally, the experience of carrying out this investigation is discussed, reflecting on the research process in the prison setting, and raising themes such as reflexivity, gender effects and ethics.

Aims

The aim of the fieldwork was twofold:

1 To explore the nature and incidence of suicide, suicide attempts and self-injury amongst young offenders in custody, and to seek an interpretative understanding of them;
2 To understand the problems faced by staff in the management and prevention of suicides in custody.

There are two elements to the problem to be understood, then. First, its nature; and second, the particular problem of its setting. At the outset, the phenomenon must first be defined, described and interpreted. What is self-injury, and when does it 'become' a suicide attempt? Is it part of a continuum towards suicide, or is it distinct from it, with different motivations and interpretations?

An initial aim was to explore the nature and extent of the problem – an essentially *descriptive* task. Is there a particular pattern to the incidents which occur in custody? How frequent is it; who does it, when and how? Are there differences between groups – male and female, repeat 'cutters' and single incidents?

A second aim was to understand or *explain* these incidents. What factors contribute to the likelihood of self-injury and suicide attempts in custody? To what extent are incidents 'imported' via the characteristics of the inmates, or 'produced' by the institutional pressures and problems generated by the actual experience of imprisonment? Crucially, what accounts do inmates themselves give of their behaviour? Can a better understanding of the problem be achieved by asking those involved what motivates or triggers these incidents? Is it to some extent determined by the (sub-) culture of young offender institutions? How do other inmates explain suicide attempts in custody?

What sort of problem does self-injury pose for the prison staff? How do they explain and manage it? Staff are responsible for identifying 'genuine' attempts, and distinguishing these from incidents which may have other motivations. How far do they see the problem in the same way as those engaged in such behaviour? How do they cope with 'cries for help' and attempts at taking one's life whilst in their care? Are there aspects of 'the suicide problem' in prison which are overlooked, or misunderstood, by instructions designed to deal with it?

Nature of the phenomenon

Suicides in custody are relatively rare, and can only be studied in retrospect, after explanations have inevitably been constructed (Douglas, 1967; Atkinson, 1982; Taylor, 1982). This process, and the retrospective nature of the inquiry, as well as the absence of the subject, and the issue of which 'suicides' receive suicide verdicts, renders such research highly problematic (see the discussion in previous chapter).

Suicide *attempts*, particularly in the controlled environment of a prison, offer an alternative source of understanding, as the subjects themselves can be asked about the incident, as well as related topics and events leading up to it. There are still problems to be addressed. One is the argument that genuine suicide attempts always succeed, and to that extent there is no such thing as a 'suicide attempt'. This argument has little evidence to support it (Stengel, 1964; also Kreitman, 1977 but see Bernheim, 1987), and is particularly unlikely in the prison setting, where attempts are sometimes prevented by the intervention of an officer (or an inmate), and a rapid transfer to hospital. Many attempts are 'genuine' to the extent that, without the (sometimes highly unexpected) intervention of officers, death would be certain. Others reflect the ambivalence often reported in suicide attempters, being neither clear attempts to end one's life, nor unequivocally 'safe' gestures. The nature of the phenomenon under study evades the neatness of categorisation, and it is therefore impossible to define a 'suicide attempt' in advance of the data collection.

Self-injury, on the other hand, occurs frequently in young offender institutions

(SHHD, 1985; Grindrod and Black, 1989; Home Office, 1988c); the 'continuum' of self-destructive acts can range from superficial scratches and cuts not requiring stitches to serious hanging attempts resulting in loss of consciousness. The lack of any valid or reliable previous operational criteria suggested that entering the research setting with definitions already formulated would be unwise (Schneid- man, 1985; Chambers and Harvey, 1989; Kreitman, 1969; Stengel, 1970). The definition adopted for the purposes of this research was pragmatic: any self-in- flicted injury serious enough to result in treatment in the prison hospital was included in the study. Decisions about suicidal intent were made later. The operational definition of a requirement of hospital treatment was chosen because of the difficulty of locating minor incidents, most of which went unrecorded, and the focus of the research, which was primarily aimed at understanding self-injury in relation to suicide attempts. This attempt to concentrate efforts at the 'serious' end of the spectrum still resulted in a wide range of incidents, and did include three which were later excluded in the light of the interview.

Understanding the problem I: previous research

There are two major problems in much of the previous research on suicides and attempted suicides in prison:

1 The reliance upon official and documentary sources of data alone;
2 The frequent lack of any control group.

To take the first problem, few studies have ventured to ask either inmates them- selves, or those closest to them – the prison staff – 'what happened and why'. The methodological and theoretical orientations of such research has remained at the level of individual differences, searching in vain for a 'profile' of the suicidal inmate, usually in the histories of those who have killed themselves in custody. Factors relating to the institution, or to the subjective experience of the inmates, have been overlooked, or studies have failed to ask, 'what lies between the stimulus and the response?' (Burgess, 1982).

Secondly, previous studies have generally failed to show whether any of the factors found to be associated with prison suicide are factors characteristic of suicide attempters and completers only or of the particular prison population from which they are drawn (Lloyd, 1990). The same comparison is required of qualita- tive data. In finding that the experience of imprisonment is painful in particular ways for some prison suicide attempters, it is necessary to show that this is in fact a distinguishing characteristic of suicide attempters before any conclusions can be drawn, as it may be the case that the experience of imprisonment is equally painful (or otherwise) for many other inmates.

Research and writing in other areas of prison life (particularly coping studies) offer a promising entree into the arena of suicide attempts in custody (Sykes, 1958; Zamble and Porporino, 1988; Toch et al., 1989), as we have seen in previous chapters. Together these studies suggest that it is the inner life of the individual we need to understand. How do those making attempts in custody understand and explain their own actions? Can we learn anything more, or anything new from those we seek to comprehend? It is a major oversight of previous research that the thoughts and reflections of the subject group themselves have been neglected. Arguably the most valuable source of information is the inmates concerned. Some would argue that the change of approach from record-based, empirical data to a more systematic focus on the subjective, qualitative aspects of experience represents one of the challenges of feminist methodology to 'malestream' criminology (Gelsthorpe and Morris, 1988). An ethic of *listening*, and trusting the subject's account, perhaps distrusting traditional conceptualisations, could be seen as following from a feminist epistemology (Harding, 1987:2). Whilst the influence of feminist writers in criminology (and elsewhere) has undoubtedly played a part in the development of my own methodological preferences, it is largely from other sources than feminist writing itself (such as left-realist and radical criminology, mainstream qualitative texts and prison sociology as far back as Cressey, 1961 and Sutherland, 1937) that these influences have come.

A further source of valuable information, apart from for the purpose of comparative data, is other inmates: those who experience the same environment; those who, whilst not injuring themselves during the custodial sentence, are closest to the culture and context in which others do. How far is there an institutional or cultural 'explanation' for self-injury, suicide attempts or suicide in custody? Do other inmates contemplate these acts themselves – have they ever come close? What stopped them? Why do they think other inmates do these things? Are there, in fact, systematic differences between the subject group and other inmates, not just in terms of personal or background characteristics, but in terms of *how they perceive the prison experience*, the subjective world of their environment?

It is the prison officers – those in daily contact with inmates – who face the task of identifying potentially suicidal inmates throughout the sentence; the officers who deal with the aftermath of a death, who respond to suicide attempts of all degrees and varieties, and who cope with repeated self-injuries, at any time of the day or night. On the coal face, as it were, they are expected to act with skill and confidence in an arena where they are seen, and see themselves, as unskilled and untrained. The doctor casts the final judgment: is the inmate at risk of a (further) suicide attempt or not? Perhaps the staff could have a more valuable role to play in the detection and prevention of suicides in custody than the selection of candidates for psychiatric assessment. Perhaps there are other (better) questions they could ask than, 'are you feeling suicidal?'[1] Prison staff are the other neglected group in the arena of prison suicides – despite the obvious wealth of experience and reflection available, their views have never been sought in any systematic way.

There is a further dimension that requires exploration if the problem is to be understood in the custodial setting: officers (and others) sometimes express ambivalent feelings towards those who attempt suicide or injure themselves in custody. Can this be understood? Are there aspects of the problem *as it is experienced by prison staff* which underlie these conflicting emotions – or fear? How do they see themselves in a climate of increasing numbers of successful suicides, widely publicised, and condemned. Could their role in any prevention policy be different?

There are three major sources of information available, which have previously been neglected: self-injuring or 'at risk' inmates, other inmates, and prison staff. It seemed that talking and listening would be crucial. The next methodological question was then: how best to do this, and where? But first, what kind of explanation was being sought?

Understanding the problem II: prediction or explanation?

There are three possibilities in prison suicide research: prediction, explanation or the recognition of vulnerability. The notion of prediction has been criticised both in the literature and in practice for two reasons. First, it is an imprecise art: it over-identifies those who may not be suicidal ('false positives') and under-predicts those who do go on to commit suicide ('false negatives'). Prediction of the suicidal individual thus diverts attention away from the rest of the population, leaving only those identified as reaching a suicidal crisis to be prevented, by whatever means. The individual prediction approach has not succeeded in either understanding or preventing suicide. It also has inherent limitations in the study of human social action.

A second alternative aim of research is explanation. To what extent can any notion of causal explanation be legitimate? Human action is neither guided by laws, nor determined, except perhaps in Matza's 'soft determinism' sense (Matza, 1964). Positivist notions of causal explanations deprive human actions of the freedom and subjective meaning inherent in them, and have historically (at least in many areas of criminology) given way to more complex, interactive interpretations. Sparks has observed in this context that much of the intellectual history of the social sciences in the twentieth century, criminology prominent amongst them, is the history of the critique of positivism and especially of the application of a positivist notion of causation to the understanding of human activity. Areas of criminological research which are still very much under the influence of positivist explanations of behaviour include 'official' research, prison psychology and criminal career studies. These approaches may still have more influence over policy than the results of non-positivist research (Sparks, 1990, pers. comm.). A notion of explanation in which the subjective meaning of action, and a grasp of the complex of meanings in which a course of action emerges, is required. Weber's concept of 'verstehen', as 'explanatory understanding', and Walker's notion of 'possibility explanations' are useful here. These concepts help to separate the aim of prediction from the aim of explanation: 'Prediction requires a degree of certainty without necessarily any explanatory force, whereas explanation requires a degree of plausibility and adequacy at the level of meaning without necessarily any predictive power at all' (Bottomley, 1979:76). Social science inquiry has historically been preoccupied with a motivation to control and predict (and improve). Hempel argues that equally, research may be motivated by the desire to understand, by 'man's insatiable intellectual curiosity, his deep concern to *know* the world he lives in, and to *explain*, and thus to *understand*' (Hempel, 1966:95). To that extent, the research seeks to understand, where understanding assumes such concepts as empathy and appreciation, in contrast to the traditional correctionalism associated with 'causal' understanding (Matza, 1964). This is the notion of explanation towards which the research aims: 'These explanations should be judged primarily according to the extent to which they render intelligible the behaviour under examination, with an intelligibility that is compatible with the subjective meaning of the behaviour for the actors involved' (Bottomley, 1979:77). Bottomley argues that an analysis of reasons and motivations play a central part in the elucidation of subjective meaning. As an explanation, its adequacy does not depend on empirical generalisations: 'The explanation does not imply that if the same circumstances occurred on another occasion the man would act similarly' (Lessnoff, 1974:88, in Bottomley, 1979:77). What it does require, is that the possibility explanation derived satisfies the researcher's curiosity to understand (Walker, 1977:1). Walker argued that sophistication may interfere with common sense (Walker, 1977:2). It is an argument in this book that an exclusive preoccupation with measurable modes of explanation and understanding alone have deprived the research topic of an important type of understanding. Quantitative methods of data collection and analysis are an essential component of our understanding in this field. This approach should be supplemented, however, by a rigorous examination of the meaning and validity of such data. The gaps exposed can only be filled by the application of other (qualitative and ethnographic) methods of research. Sophistication and discipline in exploring the field are required, but the complexity lies (and should be permitted to lie) with the subjects, rather less than with the research methods. Explanatory understanding is therefore a central aim of the book; the prediction of suicidal inmates is not. A related secondary aim is to move towards a diagnosis of vulnerability, that is, to understand which inmates may be vulnerable to suicidal feelings during a sentence, without knowing whom amongst them may go on to make an attempt. The use of the word 'vulnerable prisoner' as used by the Home Office (1989b) is strictly meant to indicate vulnerability to attack or abuse by other prisoners (that is, inmates on Rule 43, see Chapter 6). Other sorts of vulnerability (such as that outlined in this book) are not included under this term, and are not normally embraced by the special provision available in vulnerable prisoner units. This is unfortunate, given the report's recommendation that: 'The prison staff have a vital role to play in helping potential vulnerable prisoners to cope successfully with life on normal location. It is important that key staff should be designated to keep a discreet eye on such prisoners' (Prison Department, 1989:28).

The 'personal officer' approach is explicitly suggested as a valuable and effective way of meeting the counselling needs of these prisoners, and their potential suicide risk is mentioned, amongst other problems they might have, such as social skills needs, high levels of anxiety and domestic problems. Prisoners on Rule 43 (6) are not amongst the highest-risk groups (contrary to common opinion) for suicide or suicide attempts, so this approach should go beyond prisoners segregated on Rule 43. The set of recommendations and guiding principles outlined in this report are exactly the kind necessary for all prisoners potentially at risk of suicide. Avoidance of recourse to Rule 43 (6) is a major feature of the report's recommendations – a recent instruction about the avoidance of isolation in stripped conditions has been issued (Home Office Directorate of Prison Medical Services, 1990).

There may be a group of inmates who are most at risk of suicidal thought and action, should certain thresholds be exceeded. These inmates are in a wholly separate sense, vulnerable. We may not be able to predict their behaviour, but it would be possible to reduce their collective risk of suicide.

SECTION II: THE PROCESS

The research on which this book is based included a fieldwork project carried out in young offender institutions in England and Wales, and involved spending considerable amounts of time talking and listening systematically to inmates and staff about incidents of suicide, suicide attempts and self-injury in which they were involved, or about which they had comments to make. The information collected included 180 tape-recorded interviews which were transcribed, coded and analysed; the collection of information already available in records and reports; lengthy informal discussions with inmates and staff and participation in all aspects of prison life.

The fieldwork comprised four periods of five weeks each in two male and two female centres. The four establishments were selected by the Prison Department, after some negotiation, on the grounds of suitability and convenience to all parties. One of the original four chosen (Aylesbury) was later exchanged for Portland, because of 'operational pressures'.

In view of all the circumstances and the potential importance of the 'institutional' variable, it appeared that a small number of individual institutions would provide a sufficiently large sample of recent or current suicide attempts and incidents of self-injury, particularly if 'closed' establishments were selected, and if they provided full-time medical provision for other young offender institutions in the region. This would result in inmates from neighbouring (and not so neighbouring) establishments being received on transfer in the event of an incident requiring treatment and full-time medical observation. One establishment from each of the four prison regions was selected.

In each establishment, some time was spent corresponding, visiting and familiarising myself with the institution's routine organisation. An induction period was arranged during the first week, to facilitate meetings with key staff, to make arrangements for office space and for keys to be issued.[2] This time was spent establishing trust, credibility and access (cf. Sparks, 1989:14–15) and gathering background data about the establishments. Notices went out to staff alerting them to the research, and inviting comments and questions. A liaison officer served as the main co-ordinator of arrangements, providing a welcome source of information and communication, and the essential 'tour' of the establishment. At Glen Parva the liaison Officer was a Governor grade; at Styal, Portland and Bullwood Hall they were officers (a senior officer (SO) and two principal officers (POs), respectively). This was in fact felt to be more appropriate, and diplomatic, as the fieldwork was nearer to the 'ground' from the very beginning. At no point was there any reluctance from any quarter within any of the four establishments to co-operate with the project. Contrary to expectations staff and inmates welcomed the opportunity to talk to 'someone who wanted to listen'.

Choosing methods

A central aim of the research was to adopt a set of strategies that would be most appropriate to the subject being studied. The particular nature of the prison setting as a research field is discussed later in the chapter. Methodological triangulation (Denzin, 1978), or using different (complementary) methods to study the same events, can improve both the validity of the data, and its interpretation, as the imperfections of each method are compensated for by the particular strengths of others. So the inadequacies of recorded information can be compared with the data derived from interviews, and vice versa. Possible interpretations can be discussed with staff and inmates, or elaborated according to experience. Insights gained from participant observation can be checked against the aggregate data; on the other hand, most of these aggregate data are only meaningful through experiences gained from 'immersion in the field' for long periods, both before and during the interview data-collection phase. Attitudes and opinions expressed during interviews can be checked against action, and each source of information can be accumulated as part of a growing understanding of the whole. Corroboration is never flawless, however: problems of validity and bias still remain. Indeed, '*differences* between sets or types of data may be just as important and illuminating' (Hammersley and Atkinson, 1983:199). Harding argues that:

> A research *method* is a technique for (or way of proceeding in) gathering evidence. One could reasonably argue that all evidence-gathering techniques fall into one of the following three categories: listening to (or interrogating) informants, observing behaviour, or examining historical traces and records. In this sense, there are only three methods of social inquiry.
>
> (Harding, 1987:2)

By this account, the methods chosen for this research comprised all three available methods: interviews, observation and record-based data. Four main complementary techniques through which data could be sought effectively were chosen:

1 semi-structured interviews with inmates and staff
2 data from inmate files
3 descriptive data from establishments
4 observation and participation

The various methods chosen were considered to be complementary and appropriate for the problem to be understood. In addition, they constituted practical, realistic and opportunistic choices, given the setting, and the available sources of information.

Inmate interviews

The survey method – that is, the interview or questionnaire – has traditionally been used as an efficient and systematic research tool in particularly large-scale research as a means of collecting large quantities of 'good' highly standardised and analysable data in a short time (Bulmer, 1977; Davis, 1971; Moser and Kalton, 1971; Mann, 1985). This largely quantifiable source of information is then used to make convincing generalisations about the subjects concerned. The survey (opinion polls, for example, or crime surveys, self-report studies and so on) is a standard research technique; its results are usually statistical, and as such, they are taken seriously. It may be used to collect data for description, explanation or prediction, enabling the accumulation of a body of data specifically designed to test underlying hypotheses.

However, the data collection instrument in survey research may range from a closed format, pre-coded, postal questionnaire to a discursive, open-ended interview schedule for qualitative analysis. Each type has its advantages and limitations. In this research, where possible, the natural advantages of the survey method has been assimilated into the questionnaire design: the information is systematic, largely quantifiable and it can be efficiently collected. However, the purpose of the interview was to explore the subject's own experience of self-injury and suicide attempts in custody; to get at the subject's inner life (Park, 1925) to penetrate the subjective world of definitions, experiences and reactions and relate this to action. A discursive interview was required: a fairly long, facilitative questionnaire, sensitive to the feelings and anxieties of the subject. A life-history is perhaps too grandiose a term to use in this context, but the methodological and theoretical approach to the research design is borrowed largely from ethnomethodology, permitting some balance between 'objectivism' and 'the internal, covert and reflective elements of social behaviour and experience' (Denzin, 1978). 'In the life-history is revealed, as in no other way, the inner-life of the person, his moral struggles, his successes and failures in securing control of his destiny in a world too often at variance with his hopes and ideals' (Burgess, 1982).

The interview was shaped after pilot work which included discussions with groups of inmates. It was grounded in the research field; it progressed from structured to semi-structured questions. By way of introduction, I explained my role and interests, pointing out that the interview was both voluntary and confidential, and that there was no need to answer questions that made the subject feel uncomfortable. Every effort was made to obtain the 'informed consent' of the participants, whilst it must be acknowledged that this is a problematic concept in the custodial context (Taylor, 1985, pers. comm.). Permission was requested to leave a tape-recorder on during the interview, as I explained that we would both talk faster than I could write, and that I wished to transcribe the interview later, so as to accurately represent the subject's own view. No subject refused. (One asked if he could have a copy of the tape, as he had never heard himself talk in such depth before! I enquired on his behalf, but this was not allowed.) I explained my position in the establishment, assuring subjects that the information given to me during the interview would not affect any decisions to be made about their sentence, but would remain with me.

The tape-recorder allowed a more interactive and natural interview style, although some notes were taken (cf. Lofland, 1971:89), and time was left at these points for subjects to offer elaborations spontaneously. Occasional silences whilst making notes was an effective 'prompt'. Moser and Kalton noted that tape-recording sets the interviewer 'free to concentrate on the interview' (Moser and Kalton, 1971:281). They also warned, however, of the risk of reducing response rates and accuracy of reporting, particularly on sensitive subjects, but these problems were not encountered, as far as it was possible to know. One subject even warned me half way through the interview that he thought the tape was about to end. I assured him that it continued to record on the reverse side, at which he returned, satisfied, to the topic of discussion. (Staff occasionally did this, too.)

The interview comprised several sections:

1 criminal justice history
2 personal and family background
3 the current sentence
4 details of injury, if any
5 reflections on the prison experience

It began with largely factual questions, checking details already covered by the file. Where a difference arose, clarification was sought in the interview, if required. Few differences did arise, and those that did were usually errors or omissions in the record (for example: marital status; the file may have recorded 'single', where the inmate was either recently married, or had got engaged. (See also Dooley, 1990b and Griffiths and Rundle, 1976 for the weaknesses of data from prison files.)

Later sections of the interview consisted of largely open-ended questions about the current sentence, any recent episode of self-injury, and questions about the prison experience. An autobiographical sketch was sought, leading the subjects from their recent past and circumstances, in through the prison gates, along the landing and into their cell. How did all this feel, how would they describe these experiences; what had been the background to a recent suicide attempt? Had it ever occurred to them before? When? What was going on in their lives to make them feel so bad? Is that what it was like this time, or was this different? Could they say, in their own words, what they were feeling at the time – and why? Could they describe to me what happened?

The questions were worded as simply as possible, using their language. Certainly in the prompts, increasingly, a common language emerged. *Their account* of their lives, their feelings and experiences, was sought. The questions provided a framework, and guided the subjects in time from 'out there' to 'in here' – to now, and to a series of reflections on the experience of custody, both for themselves and for others. The questionnaire was a resource for us both, to hinge these reflections on, to allow the stepping-stone path to be trodden, often with relief. Where a suicide attempt had occurred, the subjects articulated pain and despair – but, never left without a response (the most terrifying, yet common reaction to the expression of suicidal feelings) – further questions were used as a guide, steering them through the pain, recognising and describing it, then moving on. Giving it words – words that were meaningful for the subject – was a relief. Between us, we were understanding.

The length of the interviews ranged from half an hour to two hours, the average for the subject group taking about 50 minutes. The 'non-response' rate was nil – no inmates refused to participate in the research. Many commented that they were glad to, expressing some satisfaction in being presented with an opportunity to talk openly about themselves. The interviews became more discursive, as the research progressed, and I could probe further and learned to prompt in different ways, as ambiguities or subtleties of meaning emerged. Official records began to look more and more unsatisfactory as file information was compared to the interview material, not always because it was wrong (although this was not unusual), but because it was inadequate.

Other instruments used

The questionnaire was supplemented by an additional source of data: a 'Hopelessness Scale' (Beck et al., 1974), completed at the beginning of the interview. This was self-completed, where possible, sometimes with oversight, or minimal discussion. The scale consisted of 20 statements about the past and the future to which the respondent was asked to circle true or false. A hopelessness score of nine or above has been found to be strongly associated with suicide (Williams, 1986; Beck et al., 1989).

The samples: definition and selection

The subject group

At each establishment, the subject group consisted of:

1 all inmates who were referred to the prison hospital during the time of the fieldwork (or in the preceding month) for treatment for self-inflicted injury;
2 any others to whom my attention was drawn by word of mouth, where staff (or inmates) thought that a particular inmate was a 'good case' usually because of recent self-injury or occasionally, suicide threats.

The first group were traced via hospital records (the daily occurrence book, and institutional records of self-inflicted injury).

Criteria for selection

All injuries requiring hospital treatment were included in the research, in order to understand the problem in all its varieties, and to see whether 'serious' attempts could be identified, and differentiated from other incidents. For the purposes of the data collection, all (knowable) incidents requiring treatment were included. Where incidents competed for attention, preference was always given to the more serious attempts. This was rare, however, so the subject group were as far as possible, 'purposive' (McNeill, 1989) and exhaustive: that is, they were not a sample, but consisted of all available cases over a period of up to five weeks. Similar choices had to be made about how far to go back in tracing recent incidents which had occurred before the placement. If they were serious, and preferably recent, and if the inmate was still present, they would be interviewed.

The subject group therefore included a variety of self-injurers, ranging from almost fatal hangings rescued by a hair's breadth, who were interviewed within days (or hours) of the incident, to 'repeat cutters' who had not injured themselves for several months, but who had a serious institutional history, and continued to present some risk to the staff. The total sample included 50 inmates. Three further interviews were carried out at Styal with adult women, who were serious enough self-injurers to justify additional interviews, but these cases were excluded from the data analysis on the basis of age (they were over 21).

The comparison group

A census of all the inmates in each of the four fieldwork establishments was drawn up, based on the prison record (index) cards kept in each of the administration offices. This usually provided information on the inmate's name, number, location in the prison (although this frequently changed, and was not always correct), age, address, ethnic origin, offence, sentence length, sentencing court, earliest date of release (EDR), parole eligibility date (PED) and latest date of release (LDR). This list was drawn up during the first few days of each placement (now no longer necessary to carry out by hand, as inmate index cards are computerised!). The comparison group was selected from this list. An estimated maximum (e.g. of up to 20) based on the expected number of subject cases at that establishment was chosen, and this number was selected randomly from the total available population, at intervals along an alphabetical list. No further selection was felt to be appropriate, as the young offender population in closed YOIs had already been pre-selected on the most significant variable: age. To some degree, they are also pre-selected on other variables, for example, offence type, history and sentence length. As comparisons on all variables were of potential significance in the research, any further selection or 'matching' would have been premature. Sentenced inmates only were included in the 'pool' so that at Glen Parva, for example, the available pool of inmates was 400. Beginning at any point between one and 20, one inmate in 20 was selected to provide a group of 20 inmates from the general population. Two inmates were lost because of a sudden transfer, and one failure to return from home leave.

As the main focus of the study was on the nature and causes of suicide and attempted suicide (as understood from as many sources as possible), and the available time was limited, the comparison group were interviewed only in equal numbers to the subject group that materialised, despite their much larger numbers in the population. Statistical comparisons based on background characteristics would form a part of the analysis, but of central interest here were the differences between the subject and comparison groups concerning their subjective description of the prison experience.

Staff interviews

Some priority had to be given to the inmate interviews, in terms of time and numbers, as the data required was directly related to them. After experience in the first establishment, it was decided that a 10 per cent minimum sample in each institution would be interviewed, with representation from all grades. In order to obtain the maximum amount of information across a broad range of staff, more interviews were carried out wherever possible (particularly in the first establishment). Informal but lengthy discussions were also carried out with officers throughout, and with specialist staff (works instructors, auxiliaries, clerical staff and so on) (see the section on observation and participation, p.116).

Interviews would often be arranged after a discussion with a small number of staff, for example, in the centre office of a wing, so that by the time the formal interview had started, both the interviewer and interviewee had a clear idea of the range of likely questions and the issues requiring additional discussion. Again, the final questionnaires were amended in the light of piloting and initial discussions. Both staff and inmate interviews quickly became more focused as 'warming up' questions were found not to be needed. The first major finding of the project was that everyone had plenty to say.

Staff interviews ranged from half an hour to three hours: the higher the grade, the longer the interview, generally (with one or two notable exceptions). The average time was 40 minutes. It was not feasible to attempt a strictly random sample of staff, so availability and willingness determined the sample to some extent. Shift patterns and work commitments in prison render any notion of selecting prison officers for pre-arranged interviews wholly unrealistic. Instead, it was more diplomatic to spend whole days on particular wings, waiting for officers to find themselves in a position to talk freely for a considerable amount of time. Even then, interviews were often interrupted by phone calls and knocks at the door. Officers were far more likely to make the time during a day, if some acknowledgement was shown of the pressure they often work under. Every effort was made to draw on staff from all areas of each establishment, and from all grades. Only two officers showed any reluctance to be interviewed, suggesting others in their place.

In addition to the formal interviews, which were not always easy to arrange, carry out or complete, officers were asked informally for their views on the various aspects of the problem, sometimes in groups, whilst carrying out other routine duties, or during breaks. Themes emerged again and again, and copious notes were taken during and after these discussions. It was typical for officers to show some initial concern about the potential time involved in a formal interview, but then to proceed to devote long periods of time and effort explaining how they saw the problem, once they became engaged. The same approach to the officers as that adopted for the inmates was taken – unconditional positive regard, and some genuine sympathy for their own predicament. Showing some understanding of issues pertinent to them (Fresh Start (see Introduction, note 4)), overtime bans, fears of litigation and accountability, frustrations relating to their role, and so on) overcame any initial hesitation they might have had to speak freely. Many times, officers commented, 'it is nice to speak to someone who really wants to know'. Attitudes expressed during the interviews were compared with those expressed informally during discussions, so that some check could be made on the representativeness of the formal interviews.

The spread of experience amongst the various staff interviewed was broad, with senior staff tending to have been in the service somewhat longer, as expected. The basic-grade prison officers ranged from new entrants with less than one year's experience, to officers with over ten years in the service. It had not originally been intended to ask officers how long they had been in the service – only how long they had been at the present establishment. But as every officer mentioned 'years in the service' during the first round of interviews, it was incorporated into the interview schedule! It was evidently a matter of some importance to officers.

Each interviewee was asked what their present rank and job in the establishment was and what other establishments he or she had worked at. Staff were then asked to outline briefly their daily work routine, particularly in respect to the inmates, and in more detail, which stages during the sentence they would contribute to, such as reception procedures, report-writing, attending boards, taking applications and any welfare responsibilities. This information was for background information, enabling the researcher to understand exactly how each establishment was organised, and how responsibilities were divided. The first part of the interview, then, was a mixture of structured and open questions about the job of each particular officer or staff member. This served as an introduction to the remaining semi-structured questions, and provided clues as to which aspects of the suicide prevention procedures might be most relevant to each staff member. For example, a reception officer would then be asked in particular about the reception screening process: how many trainees were received, how often, at what stage during the day, when they would be seen by the medical officer, and so on.

Data from files

Despite the limitations of documentary sources as data (discussed earlier), there are still several uses to which this large source of information can be put. File information, if used in conjunction with other methods, can be used as a validity check on interview material (and vice versa); case-record data can serve as a probe, indicating important areas of questioning in the interview. Perhaps most of all, it can serve as an indication of 'organisational and institutional processes' (Kitsuse and Cicourel, 1963), containing valuable descriptive and 'decision-making' material about the inmate's behaviour in prison, reactions to it and attitudes towards it.

Inmates' files comprised the prison record, wing record and in 39 cases, the medical record was offered by the staff. These documents covered many areas of interest. A file-schedule was prepared, and used as the introductory section of the interview as a means of extracting the most relevant data. These areas consisted of:

- background information (e.g. social enquiry report and criminal history)
- current (and previous) sentence details
- disciplinary record
- progress through sentence
- staff reports (parole, house reports, reviews)
- contact with probation officer responsible for throughcare
- visits and letters
- notice of past or present suicide risk (F1996) or referral for assessment (F1997), and response

Information was not always complete, up-to-date, correct or available; sometimes contradictory information was present in the file, and the amount of information available in each inmate's record varied tremendously. Those with the longest custodial histories, and the worst disciplinary records inevitably had the largest files, some of which were literally bulging with assorted papers, and had to be held together with ribbon. Occasionally, press cuttings reporting the offence were included in the record, or copies of letters that had been censored (for example, one indicating suicidal feelings to a girlfriend). Suicide notes were found in three files.

The 'successive layers of error' intervening 'between the actual event and the recorded event' (Merton et al., 1956; Bulmer, 1980) normally associated with official criminal statistics, is as true of prison records as it is of criminal records, suicide verdicts and other official or documentary sources of evidence. They are originally collected for other purposes entirely (Moser and Kalton, 1971: 241), hardly intended for the use of researchers and interviewers: 'An offender's record, then, may never reflect the ambiguous decisions, administrative discretions, or accommodations of law enforcement personnel; a statistical account may thus seriously distort an offender's past activities' (Kitsuse and Cicourel, 1963:138).

Case-record material, however, serves as 'a valuable supplement to data obtained by direct study' (Moser and Kalton, 1971:242), and it was used as such.

Observation and participation

During the fieldwork phase a log and diary was kept, recording all observations, conversations and activities. A census or 'day profile' of the population was drawn up, and various sources of information about the establishment were tapped: Board of Visitors' (BOV) reports, internal reviews, correspondence, bulletins, psychology department statistics, regime-monitoring figures and so on.

At all four establishments, group discussions were held with small numbers of young offenders, either as part of an education (life and social skills) class or as an additional evening discussion group, to which all those able and wanting to attend were invited. At Styal and Bullwood Hall particularly, there were so few young offenders that the available supply was quickly exhausted. This problem was exacerbated at Styal, where there was no available interview space in each house (the dining room was used when empty), so that individual interviews were particularly difficult to conduct. Group discussions, on the other hand, were easy to arrange, and were well attended. Several of these were therefore carried out in the evenings, sometimes at the request of the inmates themselves. They were negotiated so as not to conflict with any of the 'soaps' – in fact, the researcher was usually invited to stay and watch them after the discussions!

During the piloting of the questionnaires, discussion groups were held at which the questions and language used would be discussed. I would explain the aims and methods of the research, asking for opinion and comment about the questionnnaire, and a prison problems scale which had informed the inmate interview schedule (Zamble and Porporino, 1988), discussing the questions, and the range of possible answers. At the first establishment, Glen Parva, this was done most systematically, with suggestions and corrections being incorporated into the final versions of the questionnaires. Where new information arose at the other three, a note was taken, or the new discovery would be used as a prompt in further interviews. Often the participants would fill in the prison problems scale, for example, then we would discuss the results, and the 'other problems' category. All group sessions were recorded, and comprehensive notes were made after each session with the aid of the tape. Other more informal involvements in institutional life included participation in education classes, association, mealtimes, choir practice, playing table-tennis, group discussions, playing games and watching television; observation of meetings (for example, Boards of Visitors, Senior Management, Labour Board), reception procedures, adjudications, officer training sessions, pre-release courses and most other aspects of everyday prison life. Copious notes were taken during most of the day. Occasional weekends and evenings were spent in each establishment, and long lunches or even lodgings with staff keen to expound about the topic provided a thorough immersion in the field for the purposes of background information.

Data analysis

At the end of the fieldwork phase, which lasted 15 months in all, final transcripts were completed, a coding schedule was devised, based on the range of answers given, and as much of the data as possible was coded and analysed using SPSSX (Nie *et al.*, 1989). Qualitative material was retained in detailed case histories, notebooks and in quotation booklets, and guided the data-handling and analysis throughout. The data was looked at in aggregate, before being refined and re-coded in the light of the patterns that emerged.[3] The four quotations booklets eventually filled during the transcribing process contained examples and illustrations of the range and type of answers given to each question, and provided an essential guide to the writing-up process.

SECTION III: THE RESEARCH EXPERIENCE[4]

In his address to the Prison Chaplaincy Conference (September, 1989), Canon Eric James used a theme he applies to all human predicaments: 'We would all benefit from subjecting ourselves to what we subject them to ... We could do with more *sitting where they sit*' (James, 1989). This comment conjured up a particular interview with a young woman who had injured herself repeatedly in prison. We had sat in her cell, she had been stripped of her clothes, her furniture had been removed, and she was dressed only in an indestructible nylon tunic. We sat on her bare bed, the indestructible blanket on the floor. The room was cold, her skin was purple and red, broken by cuts all over her arms, legs and face. She was wearing bright blue eye shadow – this she had been allowed, and she had wanted to look more presentable before the interview. Even though I was clothed, and warm, I sat where she sat – and she apologised for the discomfort this might cause me.

During this research project, inmates were interviewed in strip-cells (or 'protected rooms'), in their own cells, in the laundry, in the TV room, in the hospital, down the block, in probation officers' interview rooms, in officers' offices, in the dining room, in the library – and even in the outside hospital. The interviews comprise the core of the research. Informally, the research involved going to art exhibitions, to chapel and carol services, sitting in on groups about incest, sex offending and pre-release, reading out the inmates' stars on association, holding our own discussion groups, playing games and learning how to make soft toys. With the staff, I attended training sessions, POA meetings, attended management meetings, became a 'sounding board', attended one or two prison officers' Xmas parties and drank a great deal of tea.

One of the realities of the research process which becomes disguised by the process of organised writing up at the end is the emergent nature of the project, as it changes and grows, or develops throughout. Many of the themes to emerge in the writing of this book were not apparent at the outset, appearing at various stages and becoming incorporated into the fieldwork, or into the range of questions asked. An example of this learning process and change in emphasis which – in retrospect

– occurred in many places, was amongst the staff. Prison staff forced a change of perspective on me, as I entered into their world, an outsider. One of the many lessons of the research for me was that staff were willing enough to discuss the topic on the agenda, but they often came to ask whether *staff* suicides, staff depressive illness, staff stress and problems formed any part of the research. It was sobering to admit that this was not part of the initial research question I had set out with. Obviously staff issues and problems were being looked at as part of the context in which suicide prevention procedures were being carried out, but it had not occurred to me as the researcher to frame these questions in terms of staff suicides – nor, in fact, to collect statistics and other relevant data about them. Inspired by increasing examples of parallel troubles, I did begin to 'listen' to this theme more as the research progressed, as anecdotal evidence about numbers of staff suicides accumulated – only to find that the information was not available in any retrievable form (Howard League, 1990). 'Exactly!', replied my eager informers and interrogators, 'no-one worries about the staff'. A feeling identified by Carroll in 1974 – 'we're the ones that have to come in and put up with all this shit. No-one gives a damn about us' (Carroll, 1974:55) – continues to emerge amongst prison staff today. This point was often raised during suicide prevention training sessions, and during the discussions and debates which followed.

In the end, the reader should perhaps be aware that the staff chapter of this book (Chapter 8) took on a rather different shape to that anticipated by the preparation and reading carried out early in the research. Very few of the themes that ultimately emerged could have been anticipated from the literature, or from previous experience. As a result of this, my own methodological commitment to the value of exploratory techniques of research grew.

The research role

For staff and inmates alike, the role of researcher is that of observer, and listener. The most difficult aspects of the researcher's role are the 'don'ts': don't get involved, don't take sides, express opinion, breach confidences or react to very much at all; don't be mistaken for a probation officer, social worker, psychologist, volunteer or governor grade – or 'someone from the parole board' ... or identify with any of the last; don't be dependent on the staff, but never overlook them; don't get in the way, but don't neglect to explain yourself, sometimes apologetically, to each individual when they ask: 'Who did you say you were, exactly?'

Carefully prepared advance notices to staff helped – but evidently do not replace the personal explanation, and justification for one's continual presence, and the slightly uncomfortable combination of powers of access to files, keys and 'top dogs' (Pahl, 1977:130; Sparks, 1989:23), yet total powerlessness regarding any decision-making ability. Countless times, I was called upon to answer the questions;

• Who exactly are you?

- So, whose side are you on?
- What do *we* get out of it?
- What are you doing a job like this for?
  My explanations were followed by further questions:
- So, when are you going to get a proper job?
- Are you going to join the prison service, then?
  and last, but most frequent of all:
- When are you going to settle down and get married, like normal women?

Staff (and inmates) were impressed by long working hours, early starts, participation, good listening and low pay – so I did a lot of the first and occasionally mentioned the last. Staff did not like early finishes, any exclusive concern for the inmates, women in trousers, being left out, criticism, strangers with keys, demanding non-strangers without keys and strangers going for lunch with the governor grades. What everyone really wanted was someone who would just listen, and be supportive. Sparks (1989) sums up the prison researcher's role in his 'notes on a research process':

> the researcher, at least one coming into a particular prison for the first time, sets out with few natural advantages. He looks naive, 'green', uncomfortable, out of place. He has no uniform, no keys, no proper job or activity which at least at first, prisoners and staff are likely to recognise as such. He can expect to be routinely misidentified as one or other of the things he resembles which might have some reason to be there – a psychologist, a psychiatrist, a probation officer, a trainee-staff member, a reporter, a member of the Inspectorate, a new Governor, a CID man, a man come to fix the television. If he is always with staff he cannot expect to converse freely with prisoners. If he is alone, and unrecognized, he can expect to be challenged by staff.
>
> As a stranger and interloper he should expect to invite some suspicion and curiosity. How, after all, did he come to be there? He must have, people *correctly* infer, friends or contacts in high places. He must be 'reporting back' to somebody. He is in a private place, a place where people live and work, taking showers, going to the toilet, trying to have personal conversations, reading letters from home, trying to get some peace and quiet. His very presence is potentially intrusive and impolite – a reminder to prisoners and staff that they do not own their environment and that they can have people foisted on them whom they did not ask for. The researcher is in a doubly tricky position. He is an ignorant spy.
>
> (Sparks, 1989:16–17)

An ignorant spy who is eager to be educated, however, receives a great deal of support.

Role of gender

Never quite sure where 'role as self' should be thought of as 'role as woman', some soul-searching about class, race, culture and gender differences between myself and (many of) the research participants was undertaken, without really resolving the basic questions of bias these issues continually raise. Aware that I was not an invisible aspect of the research, I tried to be self-critical about the extent to which I might be shaping the findings, but also careful to seek ways of minimising my (unintended) influence in this respect, by cross-checking information and triangu-lating data sources around particular incidents. I remain confident that any dispassionate 'outsider' could have found what I found: a number of young inmates in serious distress. Many may not have drawn the same connections (or allowed them to emerge), but that is a question of methods rather than a question of truth.

The role of gender in prison research has been discussed before (Gelsthorpe and Morris, 1988; Sparks, 1989), but continues to elude satisfactory analysis. Gels-thorpe and Morris argue that there are a number of advantages relating to women researchers in both men's and women's prisons. Their style, assumptions, greater vulnerability and rather different interests add an important dimension to a male-dominated field. As indicated earlier, however, these insights are not necessarily unique to women, and it is clear that being female carries its own problems in the prison setting: Sparks reminds us of the predominantly conservative, 'masculine' officer who may express aspects of their feelings to women researchers (anxieties and problems) but not others (the use of violence, for example). Sparks concludes: 'Most of the interesting questions in the gender politics of prison research seem to me to be unresolved, and it seems likely that research by both men and women, together and separately, will continue to be necessary' (Sparks, 1989:24).

Being female (and young) may have encouraged participants to confide, relate and instruct, and may have facilitated access as a non-threatening outsider in a sensitive field (Foster, 1990:28). At times I was vulnerable, at other times assured that being female had numerous strengths and advantages, particularly in this area of research, and in all-male institutions. In women's establishments, there were also advantages, as many of the women had experienced abuse or differentials of power so marked that masculinity of any variety presented a threat. Could a man have carried out this research? I believe so; a particular type of man might have done it rather well. My only reservation is that few may have wanted to – most have tended to study riots!

Reflexivity

Researcher effects undeniably occur, and may interfere with the research findings. This is more significant in some types of research than others. The most direct effect of this project was – to some extent – probably to initiate a stricter adherence to Circular Instructions (and rather sooner) than might otherwise have been the case. Suicide Prevention Management Groups sprang up within weeks of the fieldwork starting date; training courses were arranged, copies of Circulars stuck on notice boards ... these features were occasionally pointed out as institutions competed to be the most conscientious followers of instructions. This Hawthorne effect was confirmed by the occasional comment from staff, usually in the context of a complaint about the difficulties of implementation, or the unpopularity of certain changes ('Of course, this was all stapled together for the benefit of this research'). Letting me into the secret was a way of accepting the validity of the research, as reality took precedence over reputation.

Personal involvement

The level of personal involvement that develops with the subjects of any research will vary according to many conditions, including personal style and accidents of the research setting. Methods of data collection also determine the likely range of involvement (McNeill, 1989:122). In the scale of events, record-based work and structured questionnaires tend to minimise the level of interaction between researcher and subject, whereas unstructured, discursive interviews and participant observation facilitate – and indeed depend on high levels of interaction. Large numbers also preclude personal involvement: 'If the researcher thinks personal involvement is important, the price to be paid is that fewer people can be studied. Where the survey researcher may claim reliability and representativeness, the ethnographer will claim validity' (McNeill, 1989:121). Without setting out to maximise personal involvement, the nature of the research topic, and my intention to understand the inner-life of the participants, determined where on the scale my own involvement with the subjects of the research would come to lie (see also Oakley, 1981:72). The record-based work, the demands of a tight fieldwork schedule, and the wish to include a continuous sample of inmates in the subject group placed (sometimes welcome) limits on the amount of time and energy that was spent in deep communication with inmates or staff. But there were at least two ways in which boundaries had to be negotiated, rather uncomfortably.

The first related to the relationships developed – quickly, but inevitably, during the interview. This had after-effects, as I continued to be present around the establishment, interviewing others, and maintaining informal contact. Two inmates (one male and one female) went on to injure themselves again, some time – days or weeks – after the interview. The young woman in particular expressed feelings of having 'let me down'. I could not deny the presence of feelings associated with their actions, that had *not* existed during the first interview. In other words, now that there was 'a relationship' between us, acts of self-injury became *experienced* also by myself in terms of that relationship. I began to understand the staff rather better at this point.

The second boundary concerned my increasing wish to intervene, where particular situations might have been improved, or where I felt a particular concern for the well-being of inmates still experiencing feelings of depression and hopelessness. It was impossible on one or two occasions to leave the interview without seeking some assurance that the inmate would be followed up, or helped in some way.

Ethical difficulties

As indicated above, there were several occasions where ethical dilemmas arose. The type of problem involved or encountered in this research can be discussed on two levels. First, the macro-level: is the research itself 'ethical' in its conceptualisation, design and implementation? On the micro-level, ethical and practical difficulties of actually carrying out the research often overlap, particularly during participant observation (Parker, 1974:220–21). What particular ethical problems arose, and how should these issues be (or have been) resolved?

To take the macro-questions first, how can one judge the integrity of research? 'The ethical values affected by contemporary social research are vague and difficult to formulate precisely. They refer mainly to human dignity, the autonomy of individual judgment and action, and the maintenance of privacy' (Shils, 1959:117). In the prison setting, questions of human dignity, autonomy and privacy are already pertinent, and present the 'problems of ponderable ethical significance' associated with social science research in an acute form. According to Shils, ethical problems arise from a confrontation of our liberal doctrine of free intellectual inquiry, and our quest for knowledge, with our equally strong (but fluid) adherence to the 'sacred values' of human autonomy and privacy. Ideal values in this case compete with the originally positivistic ideal of alleviating social imperfections or injustices by the application of knowledge: the original justification for social science: 'Why strive for knowledge of reality, if this knowledge cannot serve us in life?' (Durkheim, 1964:71).

Gouldner argued that social science 'must manifest both its relevance and concern for the contemporary human predicament' (Gouldner, 1973:13). If this is the underlying ethic of research, then this same concern should determine the researchers' approach to data collection, and its subsequent use. Professional ethics should flow from personal ethics. Any disjuncture between the two results in an 'impoverished profession' and an 'impoverished self' (Seeley, 1970:86). The motivation for the research was not dispassionate. A concern to understand and alleviate the problem drove the project, and the concern to communicate its results to those who want or need to (or should) know, was a further aim.

On a micro-level, incidents occurred which placed me in difficulties on more than one occasion. Staff and inmates both did and said things that I wished I had not seen or heard. What should the researcher do with such information? I filed it under 'pending', and said nothing. Only on one occasion was I tempted to break my own rule: a serious 'repeat cutter' I had interviewed in stripped conditions told me during the interview that she had smuggled a piece of glass into her cell, despite staff efforts to prevent this over a period of time. I asked her why she kept it – she told me it helped, just having it there ... just in case. She didn't want to use it, but she couldn't bear to be without it, to be 'controlled'. I said nothing to the staff, but found myself calling by her 'house' to make sure the worst did not happen. It didn't. Was that the right thing to do?

Constraints and limitations: negotiating access

One of the major obstacles to be negotiated at the outset of any prison research is the problem of access. For access to be granted, several conditions have to be met. The research project to be carried out must be at least acceptable, if not positively required by a customer in the Home Office. The 'customer–contractor' principle applied to this project, even though it was not funded by them, but by the Economic and Social Research Council (ESRC).

The formal access procedure requires a detailed application form (several pages long) to be completed, outlining full details of the research, its aims, its likely methodology, including materials and documents required, interviews planned and the eventual destination and purpose of the results. This process is time-consuming, difficult and entails the anxiety of uncertainty: the planned research may be refused, and the methodology has to be designed at the outset, before most of the reading and exploration has been carried out. Objections may be raised, or alterations requested (for example, to questionnaires) by members of DSRMU at any stage. Draft copies of all interview schedules must be submitted for comment, and any report or publication arising from the research is subject to prior Home Office approval or comment.

There were several serious constraints imposed on the research by this procedure. The field in which research could be carried out was restricted to particular YOIs accommodating sentenced inmates only, wherever possible. The major problems of suicide and self-injury exist amongst remand prisoners, which have a far faster turnover of inmates. Other institutions were excluded due to 'operational pressures'. This resulted in a possible bias towards the smooth end of the young offender spectrum: the worst problem areas were avoided. The implications of this constraint are discussed in the concluding chapter.

The process was time-consuming: time spent redrafting access forms had been originally allocated to consulting the literature and carrying out exploratory visits. One of the greatest shocks of the research process was the limited amount of time actually available to cover all desirable sources of information. The conflicting demands of the practicalities of the research versus the need to read more and more was a continuing tension.

The access procedure also had hidden advantages. Working in the institutions with fewest operational problems cleared the way for the research: co-operation was freely given, staff were happy to accommodate the project, and the problem was still sufficiently apparent to provide a ready supply of information. It was a confirmation of the original research interest to discover that suicide and self-injury was widespread even amongst sentenced young offenders in relatively smooth-running institutions. Many of the contributory factors were more subtle, but more universal aspects of imprisonment than 'overcrowding' or trial delays. The 'pains of imprisonment' were many and varied, but hidden. A second advantage of repeated contacts with Home Office researchers and policy-makers was the intense scrutiny of the research methods involved in the negotiation process; if the loopholes and hurdles can be penetrated, the research eventually receives the benefit of expert advice and comment throughout.

Quantification and qualification

One of the limitations of small-scale research is the restriction this inevitably places on the scope and range of the fieldwork. Ideally, fieldwork would have been arranged at perhaps half of all young offender institutions, drawing on a more representative group of inmates and staff (preferably over time) from which one could make confident generalisations. This luxury not being possible, it has to be said that the four establishments chosen had their own nature, and were studied at a particular time both in their own history, and the history of the young offender estate, as well as that of the prison service as a whole. Particularly significant at this time was the implementation of Fresh Start (see Introduction, note 4) – barely introduced, yet affecting every movement in the prison, as well as its mood. In addition, the time of year in which two of the placements occurred proved to be significant, as summer-leave periods left specialist departments depleted. These factors could be said to place certain limitations on the generalisability of the findings. However, what could not be achieved in breadth, was sought in depth.

A second limitation to interview-based research requiring some thought is the question of truth. For example, staff concern expressed verbally was not always consistent with their actions. One officer had been expressing to me the importance of respect and good relationships between staff and inmates, and how good these were in her establishment, when a female inmate came to the office door to ask whether her friend could come out of her cell to go to the toilet. It was the lunch-time lock-up period. Her period had started, and she had no means of sanitation. The officer gave a firm 'no', with no explanation, and returned to the interview, continuing to discuss the level of understanding and co-operation existing between staff and inmates. I offered to interrupt the interview, to allow her to let the inmate out of her cell (to go to the toilet and to find some means of sanitation), but the officer refused.

Prison staff themselves raised the question of truth on many occasions. It emerged in two contexts. First, and most often, they talked about the inmates, and how easily conned the other staff could be. Probation officers, medical staff and, of course, researchers were all too easily taken in by the sophisticated. Inmates are good at dissembling in their own interests, and they can put on a harmless image for the short periods of time they spend with non-uniformed staff. 'We see what they're really like – when they get out of bed, when they don't get their own way, when they're angry.'

How reliable are interviews and discussions with staff and inmates – particularly when the information is going to be used in some 'official' way? Older officers commented that they might be more honest and open than junior staff. Younger officers were still worried about their promotion prospects, and 'one sure way to lose promotion was to be seen stirring trouble for your seniors'. Staff wanted to impress, and might have performed for the research. Some evidence of this was apparent: staff performance in particular duties did not always correspond to inmates' reported experience of the relevant procedures (reception interviews, for example: when observed, they were thorough and long; inmate comments indicated that this was not normally the case, and that reception interviews were cursory and unpleasant. I could only assume that both sides were 'performing' on occasion, but that there was some truth in both accounts).

Other staff raised the question of truth. Doctors in particular saw themselves as mediating between officers and inmates, questioning the nature of the information that came to them:

> An officer tells us he's a baron. He tells us he's feeling suicidal – or he might tell us he's not, and the officers say he is. It is very difficult to get 'objective' information. We tend to go for the independent information.

By 'independent information', the doctor in question meant the inmate's record. As we saw in Chapter 4, information contained in records cannot unreservedly be given the status of 'objective truth'. It has no inherently superior status to the inmate's own verbal account.[5]

Information given in individual inmate interviews resisted all available 'lie-tests' (triangulation of sources, consistency throughout the interview and plausibility). Staff interviews had less alternative sources available for cross-checking attitudes expressed during interviews, but many would return to the spot throughout a placement, to continue discussions arising from the interviews; or they would become useful referral agents for the research, passing on information, or suggesting inmates who might be appropriate candidates to interview. Their support for the research indicated credibility in the interviews.

Finally, there were certain reservations which accompanied the refinement process, as each step in the data analysis took the information one step further away from the real, sometimes vague or contradictory, or uncategorisable material with which it had begun. It was satisfying to watch the data take shape, and appear so neat. It was less appealing to remember that this was an approximation to the absolute truth. As Parker noted in his *View From the Boys*: 'It has impressed upon me and I hope it will on others how easy it is for sociological research to do grievous bodily harm to reality' (Parker, 1974:224).

As each interview case approached its place in the organisation of the data, it lost layers of its actual nature: the visual contact with the inmate, his or her voice, as the interview was transcribed; the atmosphere in which the interview took place and the silences or struggles to find the right words. It is surprising that the research method of transcribing tape-recorded interviews receives so little attention in the literature. For one exception, see Kelly, 1988:

Whilst transcribing the taped interviews on which this book is based I became aware of problems involved in transposing the spoken to the written word. Meaning in the spoken word is often conveyed through gesture, tone of voice and emotional expression.

(Kelly, 1988: preface)

The 180 tape-recorded interviews on which this research is based took five months beyond the fieldwork schedule to transcribe, despite efforts to transcribe many of the interviews immediately after the interview, or during the evenings and week-ends away on attachments. I was tempted to look for help with this task, but had to concede that there is no substitute for transcribing interviews oneself, and in full, as the coding, writing and understanding of the research data requires an extensive familiarity with the material used. Listening to some of 'the best' interviews with both staff and inmates several times throughout the post-fieldwork stages of the research kept the information 'alive' and reminded me of the sound of distress, which was often lost on paper. These aspects of the data collection played an important part in my understanding of the words finally given, and inevitably contributed to the interpretation of the results, despite their absence from the 'analysis'.

Chapter 6

Understanding young prisoner suicides and suicide attempts

In their own words

In order to be sound and reasonable, the design and operation of prisons should be based not on any particular theory and ideology, but on some fundamental understanding of how imprisonment affects individuals. The clarification of the mission for the correctional system must begin with a valid and verifiable appreciation of how imprisonment impinges on human beings: whether it damages or leaves them intact; whether it affects some and not others; whether it affects people only in some ways or under particular circumstances.

(Zamble and Porporino, 1988:2).

We suicides have a special language.

(Diekstra and Hawton, 1987)

Les vrais appels au secours, les prisonniers ne les adressent par ecrit, ils les signent de leurs propre sang.
(Real cries for help, prisoners do not indicate in writing, they sign them in their own blood).

(Dr G. Fully, premier medecin, chef des prisons francais, cited in Bernheim, 1987:55)

INTRODUCTION

One of the limitations of previous prison suicide research has been that characteristics found to be associated with suicide in the community fail to distinguish prison suicides and suicide attempters from the rest of the prison population, who share many of these features. Most studies have lacked control groups, so it is impossible to know whether the alleged characteristics of suicides and suicide attempters are merely reflecting characteristics of the prison population group from which they are drawn. Prison suicides may in any case have a different profile from suicides in the community, on which the development of the prisoner suicide profile has been based. It is apparent from the previous chapters that criminal justice variables such as offence type, sentence length and so on, are of little help in the identification of inmates at risk of suicide. Other factors and characteristics should be explored.

It has been shown in the previous chapters that young prisoner suicides differ in significant respects from the general pool of prison suicides. Young inmates may be more susceptible to situational or environmental factors in the development of a suicidal crisis. They may also lack the coping resources and strategies necessary to avert such a crisis. In this chapter, an analysis of the notion of vulnerability to suicide is presented, illustrating how a particular group of young inmates may be especially at risk of suicide. The results presented in this chapter constitute a summary of the main findings of the research project just described, drawing selectively on those aspects of the larger study which are of most relevance to the arguments presented in the book. For the interested reader, further detail can be found in Liebling, 1991.

This chapter documents the major differences found between inmates who have made suicide attempts during their time in custody and those who have not.[1] These differences are illustrated with quotations from interviews, putting into their own words the experience of imprisonment in all its aspects. It is clear from the material presented here that we have paid too little attention to any understanding of how imprisonment 'feels'. The reader is asked to ponder: how can we argue about the possible positive or negative consequences of custody when questions have so rarely been asked of prisoners in this way?

It is shown that a group of young prisoners who show a marked vulnerability to suicide and suicide attempts can be differentiated from the general young prisoner population by the extent of the background deprivation they report, and by their inability to cope with or make any constructive use of their sentence. It is shown that the most vulnerable inmates can often be found in the worst situations, many having no job or activity in prison, and receiving very little contact from their families. They make few friends, experience more difficulties with other inmates and describe the prison experience as particularly distressing. It is the combined effects of hopelessness, their histories, their current situation, and their inability to generate any solution to their problems that propel the young prisoner towards suicide. Situational triggers may be decisive in a suicide attempt at different thresholds, depending on the inmate's vulnerability and the level of stress he or she experiences. Young prisoner suicide is much less of a psychiatric problem than is commonly supposed: it is also a problem of coping. The research summarised in this chapter raises wider questions concerning the ethos and regimes of establishments and their suicide prevention strategies. These issues are discussed in the last chapter. The chapter ends with a 'profile' of a group thought to be most vulnerable to thoughts or risk of suicide. This profile is *explanatory* – aiding us in our understanding of the causes of suicide in prison, rather than predictive. Predicting suicide remains an imperfect art – understanding it is more likely to provide guidance as to its prevention. The aim of this chapter is to distinguish young inmates who may present a serious risk of suicide from the general young-offender population, to explore characteristics and feelings they have in common, and to reach an understanding of their vulnerability.

SECTION I: SIMILARITIES BETWEEN YOUNG PRISONER SUICIDE ATTEMPTERS AND A COMPARISON GROUP

An important lesson to be learned from this research was that suicide attempters are not distinguishable from other young prisoners to any large degree by those factors traditionally expected to differentiate between them, that is, in terms of their criminal justice histories. To some extent there were differences of degree in their backgrounds rather than clear distinguishing features. There was no difference in age between the two groups; the inmates varied between 16 and 21 years of age. The average age of the subject ('suicide attempt') group was 19.1 years (males: 18.7, females: 19.9); the average age of the comparison group was 18.8 (males: 18.7, females: 19.1). No significant ethnic differences between the two groups were found: the comparison group comprised 44 UK white inmates, one Irish, four Afro-Caribbeans and one Asian. The subject group comprised 44 UK white inmates, three Irish and three Afro-Caribbeans. The proportion of Afro-Caribbean inmates amongst the women (in both groups) was higher than amongst the men, at 16 per cent, reflecting their greater proportion amongst the female prison population, but also in one particular establishment in the South East.

The most common offences for which sentence was passed were burglary and robbery. There was nothing distinguishing about their crimes as far as it is possible to know. What remains unknown is the extent to which their offences may have differed in terms of seriousness, the level of impulsivity or violence involved and so on. Most of the inmates (83 per cent) had previous convictions, the number ranging from one to 69.[2] As we shall see throughout, those inmates with numerous preconvictions and sentences are at least as vulnerable as those offenders coming into custody for the first time. Most previous convictions were again for offences of burglary and theft, including car theft, and taking and driving away (TDA). Fewer had previous (main) offences of violence (11 per cent), but several had a wide range of offences amongst those they had committed in the past, including violence (40 per cent), robbery (12 per cent), arson (6 per cent), criminal damage (30 per cent) and others (49 per cent) – including road traffic offences, public order offences, breaches of non-custodial sanctions, attempted offences and going equipped, conspiracy to commit, and assisting others. There were no significant differences between the groups in relation to type of previous offences committed.

As a group, then, the sentenced young offenders interviewed consisted largely of a group of criminally experienced prisoners who began offending early and who repeated their crimes, specialising in burglary and theft, interspersed with more violent or serious assaults. Few were newly received into custody, most having spent time on remand. This experience was described as being the worst part of the custodial experience in many ways. Far from being the end of uncertainty, however, the sentenced stage of custody brought equally harrowing uncertainties in its wake. Appeals, parole and outstanding charges, in addition to allocation arrangements and likely contacts with family were described as anxiety-arousing aspects of a sentence.

Many of the inmates interviewed had already received a wide range of alternative sanctions, some of which had been successfully completed. It was apparent that young offenders institutions contained a proportion of young men and women with little else in their lives than continuous offending and sanctions. The short time spent outside in the community between sentences confirmed this picture of the lack of integration into any meaningful 'law-abiding' life outside. This picture was true for all inmates, but as we shall see in the next section, the suicide attempt group were even less successful in their lives in the community.

Most of the inmates came from unstable or violent backgrounds, and were not involved in any permanent family-life situation of their own. Their own relationships were impermanent or uncertain, and their experience of family life was rarely happy. Many of the inmates had spent time in local authority care. Their living arrangements were impermanent, showing a pattern of frequent changes and stop-gaps once out of the parental home, within one area of the country. Despite this, a quarter of the inmates had a child or children. Their educational histories were poor, a great deal of truancy and no qualifications from school being the norm. This result was borne out by the number of inmates who had difficulty in reading and writing during the interview, and who preferred to have the (very basic) self-completion section of the questionnaires read out to them. This fact has serious implications for both letter-writing and the range of opportunities available for occupying themselves whilst locked in their cells. Again, as we shall see in the next section, the worst of all of these problems were found amongst the suicidal.

Suicide attempts were not uncommon in the families of all groups of inmates, and their own histories were chequered with behaviour problems, violence – both towards and from others – self-injury, suicide attempts, and alcohol and drug problems. Sexual abuse was not uncommon, almost invariably by a family member – although one inmate had been sexually abused by 'the only adult he had ever got close to' – his social worker. Comparisons with the general population on these variables or with other sections of the prison population were impossible to draw, due to the lack of any available data, but it is clear that taken by themselves, these young offenders have suffered multiple and extended deprivations, quickly translated into or exacerbated by behaviour problems. They have serious and identifiable unmet needs.

For all inmates, missing people or waiting for and receiving visits could be traumatic experiences, particularly where visits were late, unreliable or unhappy. It was clear that having nothing to do made these experiences harder to deal with. In a thematic review of regimes for young remand prisoners, the Chief Inspector of Prisons argued that inmates: 'should have the opportunity to engage in useful activity which would help him to cope more easily with the inevitable anxieties and frustrations of custody, and assist him in recovering and retaining his sense of perspective' (Home Office, 1990a:45).

It is not just remand prisoners who need these opportunities. Contrary to the implied assumption here and elsewhere that sentenced prisoners experience active and purposeful regimes by comparison with remand prisoners, young sentenced inmates may at times spend their sentences in idleness in their cells, dwelling on their own isolation and misery. Those with the least resources pondered on the least amount of family support.

The outside probation service did not always provide a supporting role for prisoners throughout the sentence; their function appeared to be primarily one of providing resettlement advice and post-sentence supervision and help, and this they did from a great distance, often towards the end of a sentence. Changes of probation officer, and lapses of contact were unhelpful. One of the major features of the young offender population, and the suicide attempt group to only a slightly greater extent, was that their release plans were vague, often unrealistic and, more often, demoralising. Inmates did not keep in touch with the outside, finding it difficult and upsetting to do so. Few read the papers or watched the news, so that the sentence became a hiatus between bouts of unplanned life in the community. If 'hope for the future' is a major insulator against suicidal thoughts (in addition to potentially reducing the risk of recidivism), some more systematic and realistic planning should be a primary function of any custodial sentence.

SECTION II: DIFFERENCES BETWEEN YOUNG PRISONER SUICIDE ATTEMPTERS AND A COMPARISON GROUP

As indicated above, few differences between the two groups of inmates emerged in relation to *criminal justice variables*. The subject group (that is, the 'suicide attempters') did have significantly more previous convictions (also found in Griffiths, 1990b). The subject group were slightly younger at the age of first conviction than the comparison group, but this figure did not reach a level of statistical significance. Many of the inmates in both groups had received multiple fines and alternatives to custody of all possible types for their previous offences. The subject group were significantly more likely to have spent *less than three months at liberty* before returning to prison (see Table 6.1). In some cases (seven) this was less than a week.

The social enquiry reports written for the subject group had significantly less positive recommendations. Sometimes recommendations were not made, often because custody was so likely. Of the reports for all inmates, 11 per cent ac-

Table 6.1   Time spent at liberty since last sentence

	Subject group No.	%	Comparison group No.	%
<3 mths	10	(36)	2	(9)
>3 mths <6 mths	5	(18)	3	(14)
>6 mths <12 mths	4	(14)	10	(48)
>12 mths	9	(32)	6	(29)
Totals	28	(100)	21	(100)

$$\chi^2 = 8.17 \ d.f. = 3 \ p < 0.05$$

knowledged that custody was inevitable, or in five cases, preferable. In six cases, SERs could not be found, nor had they been prepared, according to the inmates (and their records). The difference between 'positive' reports, recommending clear alternatives, suggesting specific specialist help (for example, with alcohol, drugs, gambling or psychiatric counselling) and giving good reasons, and the less positive, was marked. A poor social enquiry report, then, with less positive recommendations illustrates that poorer histories and poorer prospects may be an indication of vulnerability.

According to his social enquiry report, one inmate had made a serious attempt on his life just before coming into custody by taking a 'substantial overdose' and slashing his wrists. As a result of this, he was required to leave his lodgings.

Family backgrounds were unstable for both groups, but a higher level of family violence (particularly witnessed) and (psychiatric) pathology was reported by the subject group. A quarter of the subject group had witnessed violence severe enough to result in hospitalisation of one or other parent; 13 per cent of the subject group had themselves been hospitalised as a result of parental violence, according to their accounts (see Table 6.2). Many inmates related these incidents of violence at home to alcohol abuse. Some of the violence experienced was at the hands of step-parents.

When I was small my mum used to say he'd knock me out. I used to lose consciousness. I didn't like her telling me that. I told her not to tell me, I'd rather not know. He was drinking loads then. (SG)

My Dad has, yes. He was a bit of a drinker. He does it all the time when he's drunk, but it doesn't hurt me ... You get used to it. (SG)

The role of sexual abuse in childhood has been shown to be associated with future

Table 6.2 Parental violence

		Subject group[a]		Comparison group	
		No.	%	No.	%
Witnessed	None	17	(35)	24	(48)
violence between	Minor	9	(19)	17	(34)
parents?	Repeated	12	(25)	7	(14)
	Hospitalisation	10	(21)	2	(4)
	Totals	48	(100)	50	(100)
		$\chi^2 = 10.27$ d.f. $= 3$ p < 0.05			
Experienced	None	15	(31)	22	(44)
violence?	Minor	9	(19)	14	(28)
	Repeated	18	(37)	13	(26)
	Hospitalisation	6	(13)	1	(2)
	Totals	48	(100)	50	(100)
		$\chi^2 = 6.75$ d.f. $= 3$ p < 0.09			

Note: a for two subject group members, the information was not available.
For none/minor v. repeated/hospitalised – witnessed: $\chi^2 = 8.77$ d.f. $= 1$ p < 0.005; experienced: $\chi^2 = 4.99$ d.f. $= 1$ p < 0.05.

suicidal and self-destructive behaviour (Kelly, 1988; Widom, 1989). Few studies of male self-destructive behaviour consider the role of previous sexual abuse (however, see Mezey and King, 1987 and 1989). In the present research, 22 per cent of the subject group and 12 per cent of the comparison group reported or were found to have been sexually abused. In over two-thirds of both groups, the abuse was by a member of the family.[3]

Over a third of the subject group and 22 per cent of the comparison group reported a family member (that is, mother, father, siblings or more than one of these) with a history of psychiatric treatment so far as they were aware. Twenty per cent of the subject group and 30 per cent of the comparison group reported that one (or several) member(s) of their family had made a suicide attempt:

> I can't remember really ... I just woke up one morning and she'd cut her throat. It happened a couple of times. I can't remember anything else, I was 12. (CG)

Two inmates (one from each group) had experienced the suicide of a family member – in both cases this was the mother. In the community, suicide in a family member has been found to be associated with a greater risk of suicide. Shaffer found that 13 per cent of adolescents who died by suicide had experienced an attempt by a family member (Shaffer, 1974). Golombak and Garfinkle (1983) found that 8.3 per cent of adolescents had experienced a suicide attempt by a member of the family. Kreitman also found that having friends or acquaintances who had committed suicide was also associated with a slightly increased risk of suicide (Dyer and Kreitman, 1974). Explanations for this association have been genetic or psycho-social; the latter theories are usually expressed in terms of learning or imitation (Gillilend, 1990). Research has not investigated the psychological impact of a suicide or suicide attempt by a member of the family upon the young.

The subject group had fewer qualifications from school than the comparison group (84 per cent had none, see Table 6.3). This was particularly significant as few were able to read and write without difficulty. They were frequent truants (although only marginally more than the comparison group). For the subject group, the reasons given for truancy were slightly different, more of the subject group referring to particular problems, such as bullying, family or behaviour problems rather than 'boredom' or 'friends'.

The subject group were significantly more likely to have been the victims of bullying at school. Almost half (as opposed to a quarter of the comparison group) reported having been the victims of bullying:

> I had my nose fractured. I used to get punched around, teased – I was picked on because I was small. (SG)

Often inmates reported serious teasing about their parents, either their lifestyle, psychiatric problems or marriage breakdown; this was sometimes mentioned as a reason for not attending school.

More of the subject group had spent time in local authority care, and again the reasons given for placement with the local authority were different, more of the

Table 6.3   Schooling

		Subject group		Comparison group	
		No.	%	No.	%
Qualifications?	None	42	(84)	31	(62)
	CSE/O	5	(10)	13	(26)
	Other	3	(6)	6	(12)
	Totals	50	(100)	50	(100)
			χ^2=6.21 d.f.=2 p<0.02?		
Truancy?	None	4	(8)	8	(16)
	Less than 10 days	3	(6)	4	(8)
	Less than 4 weeks	3	(6)	9	(18)
	More than 4 weeks	40	(80)	29	(58)
	Totals	50	(100)	50	(100)
			χ^2=6.23 d.f = 3 p<0.6		
Reasons?	Bored	16	(36)	20	(50)
	Friends	6	(13)	4	(10)
	Both	2	(4)	3	(8)
	Problems	21	(47)	13	(32)
	Totals	45	(100)	40	(100)
			χ^2=2.64 d.f.=3 n.s.		

Note: For 'more than 4 weeks per year truancy' v. rest, χ^2=3.66 d.f.=1 p<0.05.

subject group referring to family and behaviour (civil) problems than criminal or offending activities alone. These differences in the reasons given for certain background events suggests that the incidence of these factors may be less significant than the reasons (given) for them. In a prison group, where the incidence of all deprivation variables is high, looking at both the scale of a problem and the reasons given for the various life events being studied, may improve our ability to differentiate between particular inmate groups.

The subject group were significantly more likely than the comparison group to have been treated, either as in-patients or out-patients, for a variety of psychiatric problems (see Table 6.4). Only 16 per cent had received no psychiatric treatment at all. Hawton found in his study of adolescent suicides that: 'estimates of the prevalence of psychiatric disorder are somewhat greater than those found in populations of adolescent suicide attempters, but far lower than reported for adult suicides' (Hawton, 1986:40).

For some inmates, their psychiatric contact was for a court report only. Some caution should be used in the interpretation of these figures as the level of treatment reported by the suicide attempt group could be related to other factors differentiating between the two groups (previous history of self-injury, higher number of sentences, referrals, etc.). A previous psychiatric history may indicate current

Table 6.4 Previous psychiatric history

| | Subject group | | Comparison group | |
	No.	(%)	No.	(%)
None	8	(16)	27	(54)
Reports only	7	(14)	8	(16)
Out-patient treatment	16	(32)	8	(16)
In-patient treatment	15	(30)	3	(6)
Other (prison treatment only)	4	(8)	4	(8)
Totals	50	(100)	50	(100)

$\chi^2=21.05$ d.f.$=4$ p<0.0005

vulnerability, but as we shall see, such a history does not constitute an explanation for the suicide attempt.

Half (15) of Backett's 33 prison suicides were recorded as having *alcohol or drug-related problems* (Backett, 1987), as we saw in Chapter 2. Topp (1979) found that 30 per cent of the 186 suicides in his study had a drink problem and 11 per cent a drug problem. The proportion found to have drug-related problems amongst prison suicides a decade later in Dooley's study was higher (23 per cent). Alcohol- and drug-related problems are important factors used to alert prison (e.g. reception) staff to potential suicide risk in inmates, although it has not been certain that the high level of alcohol and drug abuse are characteristics of prison suicides and suicide attempters alone (Hayes, 1983; McMurran, 1986; McMurran and Hollin, 1989). The importance of these factors in indicating suicide risk is confirmed by the present study.

The subject group had more major drink problems before coming into custody and were slightly more likely to have experimented with a wide range of drugs (see Table 6.5). Almost half (42 per cent) of all the inmates interviewed thought that alcohol had played some part in facilitating the offence ('I'd have never done what I did if I'd been sober'). 'Minor' alcohol problems were defined by the inmates

Table 6.5 Role of drugs and alcohol

| | | Subject group | | Comparison group | |
		No.	%	No.	%
Report alcohol problems?	None	17	(34)	19	(38)
	Minor	10	(20)	26	(52)
	Major	23	(46)	5	(10)
	Totals	50	(100)	50	(100)

$\chi^2=18.79$ d.f.$=2$ p<0.0002

Report drug problems?	None	21	(42)	20	(40)
	Minor	3	(6)	11	(22)
	Major	26	(52)	19	(38)
	Totals	50	(100)	50	(100)

$\chi^2=5.68$ d.f.$=2$ p<0.05

themselves, but had a minimum threshold of four units a day, and maximum of eight units a day. Most of those describing themselves as having minor drink problems drank more at weekends, and felt that this did contribute to their propensity to get into trouble (for example, causing them to lose accommodation, start fights, have arguments and so on (see McMurran, 1986; McMurran and Hollin, 1989)). 'Major' drink problems were defined as drinking more than eight units a day.

More of the suicide attempt group reported having experimented with a wide range of drugs. A small group (12 per cent of the subject group and 2 per cent of the comparison group) used glue or petrol.

More of the subject group had injured themselves before coming into custody: only a quarter had not injured themselves in any way before their sentence (see Table 6.6). Many of the inmates in both groups had in fact injured themselves deliberately before the custodial sentence: 28 per cent of the subject group and 10 per cent of the comparison group said that the injury had been a suicide attempt, some of these inmates having deliberately injured themselves in other ways at other times. Some did not describe their self-injury as a suicide attempt.

> I've taken an overdose once. I was depressed, down. I remember it, yes. I was 12. I think I felt I'd been shut out, and I was unwanted, like next to my brother and sisters. I felt rejected. I never talked about it, no – the problem just stayed there. I think more than anything I wanted to get revenge on them. I wouldn't say it was for attention – they never knew. (CG)

Others described the incident as attention-seeking:

> I just felt that no-one wanted me, and I felt really useless and all that.
> Did you get any help?
> No.
> Do you think you wanted to die?
> Not really just attention and all that. (SG)

Toch argues that attention may be the closest some inmates can get to receiving

Table 6.6   Previous self-injury

		Subject group No.	(%)	Comparison group No.	(%)
Previous self-inflicted injury?	None	12	(24)	35	(70)
	Yes	6	(12)	5	(10)
	Several	16	(32)	3	(6)
	S. attempt	6	(12)	4	(8)
	Both	8	(16)	1	(2)
	Other	2	(4)	2	(4)
	Totals	50	(100)	50	(100)

$\chi^2=26.09$ d.f.$=5$ p<0.0005

affection in their lives (Toch *et al.*, 1989:217). Some inmates had injured themselves several times, without wanting to describe what they did as a suicide attempt:

> Yes, I just cut my arm and my neck. I've done it quite a few times. The first time was when I was 15 I was in an approved school. I was depressed. It was too strict, I didn't like it. (SG)

An additional 4 per cent of each group had not actually injured themselves but had thought about it, or come close.

> I've cut myself. When I lost my temper I started smashing windows and that, then I thought of getting a razor. Sometimes I had the urge to jump in front of a car. In fact I was in a mess, and life wasn't worth living. (SG)

Amongst those who had deliberately injured themselves, there were no significant differences in the methods used between the two groups. In fact, the comparison group used cutting more than the subject group. Some had used 'other' methods such as hanging, arson, driving a car into a wall and burning with cigarettes.

On a range of background characteristics, then, the subject group could be differentiated from the comparison group. A dimensional approach to problem characteristics may be a more useful way of comparing groups within the prison population rather than looking for either the presence or absence of a range of events and attributes.

The current sentence

The subject group were more likely to have spent time on remand, 80 per cent as opposed to 62 per cent of the comparison group having been on remand before receiving the current sentence ($p<0.02$). A third of the subject group who had experienced remand at some time said they preferred being on remand to being at their current establishment either because visits were easier, it was closer to home or they had friends there. Forty-two per cent of the subject group and 68 per cent of the comparison group said that remand was worse than their current situation, either because of the amount of time spent locked up, the shock and uncertainty of the situation or the lack of any relationship with the staff.

Over half of the subject group felt that the sentence they had received was harder than they had expected, some describing it as a complete shock, having not expected a sentence at all. This was almost equally true of the comparison group, however, half of whom reported having found the sentence harder than expected. A relatively speedy emotional adjustment to imprisonment may be hindered by a sentence that is unexpected, thus exacerbating feelings of anxiety, depression and emotional disturbance associated with the early stages of custody (Zamble and Porporino, 1988). Just over a third of the comparison group thought the sentence was lenient – or 'fair' – which when probed, actually meant less than expected.

Many inmates – but more of the subject group – had been to more than one establishment before being allocated to the current one. Over half of the inmates went on to one, two or (in three cases) three further institutions before arriving at the current establishment, either for allocation, administrative reasons ('it was closed down'), or as a result of a transfer, usually for discipline or medical reasons. Some of the subject group had been transferred from open (or other) establishments because of their potential suicide risk. This was rarely appreciated by the inmate concerned as 'being in his own interests' – or in the 'interests of security'. Almost a third of the subject group had arrived at the present establishment as a result of a transfer (as opposed to 8 per cent of the comparison group, p<0.05).

Two-thirds of the inmates were eligible for parole (that is, had sentence lengths over 12 months and did not fall into any restricted category). Over a third of the subject group and a quarter of the comparison group were awaiting a reply, in some cases despite having passed their parole-eligibility date, sometimes by several months. Twenty per cent of both groups of inmates had outstanding charges at the time of the interview, many of which would involve a return to court during the sentence. Visits by the police to inmates in order to investigate futher offences or to arrange for charges to be 'written off' (assigned to the inmate) were more frequent than visits by probation officers.

An important finding to emerge from these questions about the sentence was that far from being the end of uncertainty, the post-sentence stage of custody may bring with it equally difficult problems. Appeals, parole procedures and outstanding charges, in addition to allocation and likely contacts with family, made the sentence difficult and unpredictable. High levels of anxiety were expressed by inmates about all of these issues. The reception and early stages appeared to be difficult and uncertain for all inmates. It is later during the sentence that significant and differentiating signs of vulnerability amongst inmates can be identified.

Life in prison

Toch *et al.* (1989:x) argue that the prison environment is a common one: that inmates' reactions are to a uniform world. This is not so. Where and how inmates spend their time can alter the experience objectively, both between but also within establishments. Differences in location, occupation, opportunities, relationships with others and time spent in cells can have a dramatic impact on the ability to cope with the sentence. The following section shows how inactivity can compound difficulties in coping, and that although coping ability differs, importantly – so do levels of inactivity.

Significantly more of the subject group said that they preferred to share a cell than to be on their own (see Toch, 1975:300–1 for a discussion of the effects of isolation in a cell upon the suicidal inmate). A third of the comparison group preferred a single cell – particularly if they were working, and needed to sleep well at night. Almost half of the comparison group were happy to share:

> I'd prefer to share a cell, because it gives you someone to, like, help you with writing letters and that. (CG)

The Prison Rules (29(1)) state that sentenced prisoners are required to work: 'A convicted prisoner shall be required to do useful work for not more than 10 hours a day.' The European Prison Rules adopted by the Council of Europe state: 'Sufficient work of a useful nature, or if appropriate other purposeful activities, should be provided to keep prisoners actively employed for a normal working day' (Rule 71 (3)). Only half of the inmates had regular work in their establishments. A further quarter worked sometimes, usually on cleaning duties, but this was sporadic, or only for a short period in each day. Over a third of the subject group were not working at the time of the interview. In only a third of these cases this was due to full-time education. Of those inmates who were working, half of the comparison group and just over a third of the subject group said they liked or enjoyed it:

> Yes, it's good. Lazing around all the time made me stiff and ratty. Having a job wakes me up. It's a trusted job, too – helps for your parole. I recently got my security clearance as well. (CG)

for whatever reason:

> Yes, I'm the hospital orderly. It's good – like last weekend we worked, and just sat around in the office drinking coffee. I enjoy it. I'm the only one on there, and the officers treat you different ... a little better. (CG)

Almost half of the subject group and 22 per cent of the comparison group however, disliked their work:

> I do wing cleaning. It gets really depressing doing it all the time. (CG)

> No, it's boring and monotonous. (SG)

The remainder were not enthusiastic, but recognised that it was better than the alternative:

> It passes the time. (SG)

> It's better than bang up. (CG)

> I'd rather be doing something, you know; I'd rather have things occupying my mind. While there's someone in my cell, it's no problem, but on my own, it's bad. I don't know why, they just haven't given us a job yet. (SG)

When asked if they got anything else out of their work besides passing the time, more of the comparison group thought they could. Only 37 per cent of the comparison group but 61 per cent of the subject group did not feel there was much point to the work they were doing. For those who did feel they got something out of their work (63 per cent of the comparison group and 39 per cent of the subject group) qualifications, experience and extra money were most frequently mentioned, but other benefits included getting out of their cells more, trust, better parole reports, better relationships with officers, exhaustion, having to concentrate on something and new interests. Negative responses usually referred to the nature of the work:

Not unless I want to go making cardboard boxes on the out. (SG)

Education and physical education

According to a report by the Education, Science and Arts Committee (*Prison Education*, 1990) education gives inmates a chance 'to find a new direction in life', to 'abandon criminal careers and settle down as honest and useful citizens' (ESA, 1990:vi). It can provide coping skills, basic literacy and vocational qualifications to inmates, acting as a counter-balance to the hopelessness and idleness of a prison sentence.

More than half of the inmates (54 per cent of the comparison group and 60 per cent of the subject group) were involved in education in some way, either full-time, part-time, periodically or in evening classes. A major problem regarding education, however, was its availability; summer holidays, fixed course dates and prison-staffed evening classes were difficult to reconcile with prison life:

They said I'd be starting in two week's time, when they come back from holiday. Till then I'm on bang-up. (SG)

No. By the time that starts, I'll be out. (CG)

I do classes, yes – when they have them. They're always cancelled. (CG)

Again, more of the comparison group than the subject group said that they enjoyed education (58 per cent and 39 per cent, respectively). A further third of each group thought education was 'OK':

I suppose so, because I'm out of my cell. (SG)

Some disliked education (18 per cent of the subject group and 16 per cent of the comparison group), or found the facilities limited, particularly if they did have a basic education from school. One problem in relation to education (as at work) was that disciplinary or 'other inmate' problems often secured removal:

I had to leave it because of the trouble I was getting. (SG)

I got kicked out for starting a fight. (CG)

Patterns reported outside seemed to be repeated inside – and the consequences were often the same. Impulsive behaviour or fights between inmates resulted in the permanent loss of many of the few privileges open to them. In addition, as argued by the ESA Committee Report (1990): 'Prison education suffers badly. Classes are closed or interrupted for prison officer shortage ... Education in numbers of prisons is curtailed, even closed, sometimes for long periods' (ESA, 1990:vi). They argue that this is because: 'There is no binding requirement on the prison service ... to conform to any pattern, standard or objective in its provision of educational opportunities or indeed of any other activities or aspects of the regimes' (ESA, 1990:vi).

Several of the inmates locked up for most of the day during the fieldwork period would normally have been involved in full-time education. The education departments, however, had closed for the summer holidays. These inmates in particular could rarely read and write sufficiently to continue their own studies alone.

Most of the inmates did PE. Only 4 per cent of the comparison group did not – usually for medical or disciplinary reasons. Almost a fifth of the subject group did not (see Table 6.7). Ninety-two per cent of the comparison group did PE and liked it:

That's the main thing that I enjoy in here really. (CG)

Yes, I do it as much as I can. (CG)

I like it; you get a shower. (CG)

Some would have liked to have done a lot more:

I love it. You don't get enough of it though. (CG)

As we can see in Table 6.7, a third (30 per cent) of the subject group disliked PE

Table 6.7   Activity in prison

		Subject group		Comparison group	
		No.	(%)	No.	(%)
Physical education?	Yes-Like	26	(52)	46	(92)
	None	9	(18)	2	(4)
	Yes-Dislike	15	(30)	2	(4)
	Totals	50	(100)	50	(100)
		$\chi^2=19.95$ d.f.$=2$ p<0.0001			
Time in cell?	Minimum	3	(6)	16	(32)
	Some	21	(42)	20	(40)
	Most day	26	(52)	14	(28)
	Totals	50	(100)	50	(100)
		$\chi^2=12.52$ d.f.$=2$ p<0.005			
Ever bored?	Often	41	(82)	25	(50)
	Sometimes	9	(18)	16	(32)
	Never	–	–	9	(18)
	Totals	50	(100)	50	(100)
		$\chi^2=14.84$ d.f.$=2$ p<0.001			
Get more bored through sentence?	More	27	(55)	22	(48)
	Same	16	(33)	10	(22)
	Less	6	(12)	14	(30)
	Totals	49	(100)	46	(100)
		$\chi^2=5.71$ d.f.$=2$ p<0.05			

compared with only 4 per cent of the comparison group, either because they felt they were pushed too hard, or because they had problems with the other inmates, or with staff:

> I do enjoy it, but I don't enjoy the staff, they push you too much. The hospital group, they try and treat us as if we're dumb. It gets on your nerves. (SG)

So how much time did inmates spend in their cells? Over half of the subject group spent most of the day there, either because of isolation (particularly as a result of suicide risk), or because the education department were on holiday or because they had no job.

> A fair bit. Like today, I'll spend 20 hours. Education are on holiday, and we're not on association tonight, we're on bang-up. (SG)

> A lot. Twenty-two hours a day at the moment. I've got a fortnight's bang up on the house, for fighting. (SG)

Only 6 per cent of the subject group, and 32 per cent of the comparison group spent the minimum possible time in their cells. This meant being unlocked at 8 a.m., for most of the day time, with a futher one and a half hours at lunch time and at teatime, then being locked up again at 8.30 p.m. Those who were locked up most of the day might well spend 23 hours there. How was this time in their cells spent?

Most of the comparison group could find things to do in their cells. They would either read, write (usually letters) draw or listen to the radio. Some would sleep; others might make matchstick models, do jigsaws, play cards, study, clean the cell, smoke or do exercises. Four per cent of the comparison group and 33 per cent of the subject group could find nothing at all to do:

> Just staring at the four walls ... there's nothing else to do. (SG)

> Lying on the bed, just trying to sleep. (CG)

> I just walk around, and lie on the bed. (SG)

> I just sit there and gaze out of the window, I can't read or write. Basically I just sit around, sometimes listening to the radio. (SG)

Many, but particularly the subject group reported feeling bored. Boredom some-times brimmed with other feelings, being an easy word to use, when anxiety, depression and emotional turmoil might have been more precise. The young men, in particular, resorted to the notion of boredom to describe the feelings they had just prior to a suicide attempt, where the word 'depression' was more readily used by the young women (see Chapter 7). It appeared that the same psychological state was being described (see also Gilligan, 1982 for a discussion of the differential use of language between men and women):

> Always ... though I'm more worried than bored. It takes some nerve to sit in a cell, two'd up with this geezer who gets on your nerves. I just ignore him. It's

Table 6.8   Inactivity in cells

		Subject group		Comparison group	
		No.	%	No.	%
Active in cell?	Active	23	(46)	45	(90)
	Bored	27	(54)	5	(10)
	Totals	50	(100)	50	(100)
			$\chi^2=22.24$ d.f.$=1$ p<0.0001		
What can you do	Nothing	28	(56)	25	(53)
when bored?	Positive	11	(22)	19	(40)
	Negative	11	(22)	3	(6)
	Totals	50	(100)	47	(100)
			$\chi^2=6.79$ d.f.$=2$ p<0.05		

very hard to sit around for 24 hours without going mad. Here, you get more worried than bored – about myself, whether I can cope. (SG)

When asked whether, during the sentence, they had become more or less bored, over half of the subject group, and 48 per cent of the comparison group said they got more bored:

More. I've read nearly all the books in the library. (CG)

More. It's getting to do my head in now. (SG)

A third of the comparison group became less so, often because they were given a job, or they just grew accustomed to life in prison. Many of the inmates reported having days when they just felt more bored than others, whatever the stage in the sentence:

You just get the occasional day in the week when you don't want to read, you don't want to listen to the radio, you're fed up with your tapes. (CG)

Coping with inactivity

A variable was devised based on the responses to these questions about what they did in their cells, dividing inmates into those who could find something active to do and those who could not (see Table 6.8). The 'active' group included any positive response, however limited:

I read, but you can get through all your books in a weekend. (CG)

This question evoked significantly different responses from the subject and comparison groups, less than half of the subject group describing themselves as 'active' in their cells. Ninety per cent of the comparison group could be described as 'active' in their cells, on the other hand. The inmates were asked if there were anything they could do to relieve feelings of boredom. Responses were coded into 'positive', 'nothing' and 'negative', as this was the range of answers given. 'Positive' responses included 'getting into a book', exercises and so on:

> If I get really bored, I just do press-ups, or sit ups, or something like that. (CG)

> I just strike up a fag really, just try to forget about it, or try to talk to people in the cell next to you. (CG)

The majority of the subject group (56 per cent) and the comparison group (53 per cent) said there was nothing they could do to relieve boredom:

> Nothing really, just put on my tape-recorder and fade away. (SG)

Twenty-two per cent of the subject group and 6 per cent of the comparison group spontaneously mentioned something negative, or slightly sarcastic when answering the question about finding some way of relieving their boredom:

> I don't know really – you can head-butt the wall. (CG)

> Commit suicide! The quick way out. (SG)

> Cut up. (SG)

So differences clearly appeared between copers and non-copers. It was becoming clear that inmates with the fewest opportunities to occupy themselves (for whatever reason, some self-induced) were those who were least able to cope with the isolation and boredom of confinement to a cell for long periods of time. This is consistent with the argument developed in Chapter 3. This particular group of responses relating to how time is spent in cells has important implications for suicide prevention procedures. It should be noted here that Johnson found a particularly marked need for activity amongst self-destructive imprisoned youths in 1978 (see Chapter 3).

> For some youths the need for activity reaches extremes. They describe a compulsive need for involvement to hold their feelings in check. They diagnose themselves as prone to tension, subject to outbursts, controlled by urges. In activity they find temporary release; in constant activity there is a kind of equilibrium.
>
> (Johnson, 1978:466)

The inmates were asked whether or not they could find rewarding things to do in the establishments they were in. Half of the comparison group and a quarter (significantly less, $p<0.05$) of the subject group said that they could, most mentioning education or work opportunities, and a small number (7 per cent of those responding positively) referred to personal achievements such as sporting activities or temporary release schemes. Most of the inmates thought that rewarding activities were limited, however, or unavailable, not just in terms of provision, but also in terms of timing, sentence length and clashes with other activities:

It's not too bad, I suppose, there's plenty of things going on, it's just getting on to them. (SG)

Only if they're not very bright really, like if they can't read or write very well. (CG)

Related to this, inmates were asked if they thought there were opportunities to improve themselves in their present establishment. Over half of the comparison group and 38 per cent of the subject group thought that there were, mentioning courses, drinking or drugs groups and work, but many inmates thought that opportunities were limited, or misdirected:

Yes, work, I suppose. Yes, getting qualifications. But as for not robbing again, I don't know.
• Did you expect help with that sort of thing?
No. I did the first couple of times, but I know better now. (SG)

It depends what you mean by improve. If you mean become a better burglar, then definitely. If you want to go straight, then it's no good. (CG)

The most significant point to emerge from the responses to these questions is the *consistency* with which the subject group are (and feel) worse off than their fellow inmates in terms of the availability and desirability of work, education, PE and other methods of occupation. They do not see as many opportunities for themselves in prison, nor do they seem able to make constructive use of their time. The combination of constraints and their own lethargy leaves them helpless and resourceless in the face of hours of unfilled time. It is their inability to occupy themselves constructively, combined with 'enforced idleness' (Home Office, 1990a) that increases their vulnerability to both impulsive acts of self-harm and suicidal thoughts.

Relationships inside

The subject group were slightly less likely to describe any of their fellow inmates as friends – and those they did, they were more likely to have met in prison than outside, unlike their contemporaries, who were almost as likely to know people from outside (see Table 6.9). The subject group described themselves as more isolated or alone in the prison, and were far more likely to report difficulties with other inmates. The stability of affiliation (Bondeson, 1989:68) is uncommon amongst the subject group.

It is important to note that still a third of the comparison group had no friends, and a further third were what Mathieson would have called 'wanderers', having few close ties, but floating amongst other inmates (Mathieson, 1965). The 'disrupted society' is evident, even amongst the general population.

Different patterns of friendships emerged between the two groups. The subject group were more likely to have met those friends they did have either on a current sentence or during a previous prison term. Almost half of the comparison group, on the other hand, knew their fellow inmates from outside. Almost two-thirds of the comparison group said they had no difficulties with other inmates. Thirty per cent of the comparison group and 43 per cent of the subject group had some problems:

> Sometimes there's a bit of hassle. There's always someone getting on to you. There's nothing you can do, just ignore them. (CG)

> They call you silly names ... I can get on with them, but they can make it hard for people – they tend to pick on particular inmates. (SG)

As seen in Table 6.9, a quarter of the subject group and 8 per cent of the comparison group said they had serious difficulties with the other inmates:

> Yes, that's why I came here on transfer. I was having a lot of problems at my last place. When I first came back here, it was alright, now it's all going down-hill, people keep picking on me. They used to beat me with sticks, every night, making me stand on a chair with a bowl on my head – stupid! That's what

Table 6.9 Relationships with inmates

		Subject group No.	%	Comparison group No.	%
Do you have any	None	27	(54)	15	(30)
friends in here?	Some	12	(24)	16	(32)
	Yes	11	(22)	18	(38)
	Totals	50	(100)	49	(100)
		$\chi^2=5.68$ d.f.$=2$ $p<0.06$			
Where did you	Here	16	(64)	19	(53)
meet them?	Previous prison	5	(20)	2	(6)
	Outside	4	(16)	15	(42)
	Totals	25	(100)	36	(100)
		$\chi^2=6.13$ d.f.$=2$ $p<0.05$			
How would you	On own	27	(54)	12	(24)
describe the way	One mate	9	(18)	7	(14)
you mix in here?	Few friends	3	(6)	13	(26)
	Group	3	(6)	2	(4)
	Float	8	(16)	16	(32)
	Totals	50	(100)	50	(100)
		$\chi^2=15.14$ d.f.$=4$ $p<0.006$			
Any difficulties	None	16	(33)	31	(62)
with inmates?	Some	21	(43)	15	(30)
	Yes	12	(24)	4	(8)
	Totals	49	(100)	50	(100)
		$\chi^2=9.78$ d.f.$=2$ $p<0.008$			

they did – happens to a lot of lads. You have to hold two buckets. They think it's funny. I don't think it's funny. (SG)

The role of bullying by inmates of each other is rarely investigated in relation to suicide attempts, but the fact of its prevalence amongst young offenders in custody in particular has been well-documented (McGurk and McDougal, 1986; Feld, 1977; Polsky, 1962). Some of the problem can be related to the inmate economy:

Yes, it's debt ... it happens by accident. (CG)

Several of the inmates explained how this came about:

Well yes, I have disagreements now and again ... it's stupid things really – like tobacco and biscuits, get nicked out of the cell. They weren't even my biscuits, but I got hassle over that. It doesn't bother me because I just keep myself to myself, apart from a couple of mates. There's always stuff going out of your cell ... people getting taxed and all that.
- Does it ever cause serious trouble?
Yes, it causes trouble, and it turns to bother and fighting and violence, or people gang up on you. If you go to the screws, you get called a 'grass' ... you can't win. It's not nice in here – you just get too much stick, it ain't worth it. The best way is to keep yourself to yourself.
- How do inmates get themselves into debt? Why does it happen so much?
Well, a new kid comes in, he's got no tobacco, so he borrows a quarter, he's got to pay a half back. He borrows to pay back – it just builds up ... he gets into a lot of debt. That's how I was to start with, I had no baccy and I was dying for a smoke, borrowed a quarter and had to pay back half. I wouldn't do it again, I got a lot of hassle over it. I'm paid up now ... You see, you get paid every Wednesday. If you come in on Thursday you get an advance on Friday. Time you get into debt is your first few days or if someone pinches your tobacco, you know what I mean? That starts it off as well. I always keep mine on me now ... or when I'm banged up, it's alright.

Some complained of severe beatings, threats and group 'blanking' (being ignored) – much of which was verified in the records. Some inmates seemed more vulnerable than others, and were (voluntarily) removed from ordinary location for their own protection, on Rule 43.[4] Teasing was often about personal disadvantage, families or outside relationships, and would be cruel, just as in school. Loyalties changed rapidly, regional clashes were voiced, and fights were frequent:

I had a bit of hassle, especially with one lad – that's how I lost my teeth! It was something stupid in PE, in the gym, and it ended up when we went to work in the afternoon having a fight. I ended up with a tooth missing and a nose-bleed. (CG)

The 'solidarity' between inmates described in some prison studies (Sykes, 1958; Sykes and Messinger, 1960; Bowker, 1977, Irwin and Cressey, 1962) may be true of small sub-groups of inmates: many remain in an 'atomized and depressed mass' (cf. Clemmer, 1940; Mathieson, 1965; Bondeson, 1989).

Relationships with staff

Relationships with the staff were less mixed: 14 per cent of the subject group and 10 per cent of the comparison group said relationships were good, and over two-thirds of the inmates thought they were 'OK' or some of their relationships were good:

> It's pretty good – you can have a laugh and a joke with them. (CG)

Some described the relationship as 'difficult', however, either because of a particular experience or because of particular frustrations:

> Well some staff stitch you up ... look for you to make a mistake once, to nick you for; petty things. It's their job, I suppose, they can't just let you off, but you still hate them for it. (CG)

Over a quarter of both groups of inmates thought the staff in their establishment were easy to get along with, however:

> Yes – as long as we're OK with them. (SG)

A small number of both groups found them difficult to get on with, sometimes because of particular incidents, or because of a personal feeling about prison officers *per se*:

> Well if you get too pally with the staff, you get called a cheat or a grass ... and they've got their keys, and you have to do as they say or it's tough, you get put down the block, or you lose association, you know, as if to say, 'I can control them'. (CG)

Over three-quarters of the inmates thought that the staff could be helpful, generally or some of the time:

> They sort out your problems for you, help you feel your way. (SG)

Only 22 per cent of the subject group and 14 per cent of the comparison group felt that the staff were not helpful:

> Half the time, they don't want to listen, they're too rushed – they're always pressed for time. Half the time they've got enough to cope with without thinking what's going off on the unit. There's never enough screws, man! (SG)

Of those inmates who thought the staff were helpful, almost half felt that this was mainly in practical ways:

> They let you ring your mother ... they help you out with your problems, they can find out things. (SG)

Other positive areas were arranging job changes, home leave, discussing possible work opportunities on release, parole procedures and psychiatric referrals. A further third (and slightly more of the subject group) thought they were helpful in personal ways:

> They cheer you up. (CG)

> Just in the way they speak to you and take time to speak to you. I mean, I get very depressed easy, especially waiting for this answer, and there has been a few times when I'm going, you know, mad. A few of them take time to sit with me and talk to me and help me and that, and I think that is something that you need. (CG)

It would appear that *relationships with inmates* are more significant (and more difficult) than relationships with staff in relation to the ability to cope with the sentence. (For a discussion of previous research on prison staff as helping agents and their potentially central role in the prevention (or aversion) of suicide attempts, see Johnson, 1977.) Bondeson showed that inmates are more sensitive to both negative and positive feedback from other inmates, particularly to criticism, than they are to the staff (Bondeson, 1989:59). They spend far more time with other inmates (Ibid.:46) and 'group affiliation' is thought to be more common amongst the young (Ibid.:65). Staff have a facilitating role, however, in their ability to grant letters, phone calls, or solve other problems – including those between inmates. Inmates do find staff helpful, in both personal and practical ways – but wish they could be more (or more consistently) so, particularly in personal ways.

Half of both groups felt that the staff could be more helpful in personal ways:

> They could sit down and understand – you know what I'm saying? – what you're going through. (SG)

Disciplinary procedures

Over two-thirds of the inmates had been punished during the sentence for at least one disciplinary offence. Most accumulated up to four punishments (41 per cent), some receiving more than 50. Of those who committed disciplinary offences, slightly more of the subject group had been adjudicated upon for offences of violence (fighting, or smashing up the cell, for example), more had also been found guilty of disruptive activities (causing a disturbance, or barricading, for example). Almost half of the subject group's offences and two-thirds of those of the comparison group were for more ordinary breaches of the prison rules (not shaving, swinging a line, staying in bed, being out of bed, shouting through cell doors, wearing somebody else's clothes, eating when shouldn't, being absent without prior leave or refusing any order).

The subject group had more complaints about the disciplinary system, feeling it to be less fair, and – perhaps related to this – they were far more likely to have spent time in seclusion or protective custody (which may involve varying levels of isolation or association during the day) for a variety of reasons including both punishment and suicide risk. 'Most experts on the subject of inmate suicide agree that placing the detainee in isolation greatly increases the chances of him or her attempting or committing suicide' (Massachusetts Special Commission, 1984:20).

The longest time spent in seclusion was 94 days. Many of the inmates interviewed were afraid to admit their suicidal feelings to institutional staff for fear of being re-admitted to the hospital (or the punishment block, where hospital accommodation was not available or adequately staffed) in stripped conditions. Seclusion was often used in response to the observation needs of inmates at risk. They were placed in single or protected cells, and observed at 15-minute intervals. Ironically, this procedure actually reduces the level of observation possible: inmates are left out of visual contact with one another and with staff:

> This accomplished two things: the detainee is denied human contact, which could intensify an already traumatic situation and hence lead to a suicidal crisis, and it prohibits other detainees from witnessing a suicide attempt, and possibly alerting duty officers.
>
> (Massachusetts Special Commission, 1984:20)

A separate variable was introduced after the interview, based on whether or not the inmate could be described as a 'disciplinary problem' or not, in the light of the available evidence. The number, type and frequency of offences were noted, and comments made by staff taken into account. However, the classification remains subjective. Significantly more of the subject group presented serious disciplinary problems than the comparison group. The view of inmates being either internal or external expressors of disturbance was thus disconfirmed, as more than half of the subject group were also a 'disciplinary problem' within the institution. Toch's thesis of 'maladaptive' inmates, moving between the medical and disciplinary services may have some support here (Toch et al., 1989). Where misbehaviour is perceived as volitional, the institutional response is punitive. Only if a problem is seen as wholly 'psychiatric' is the appropriate response thought to be therapeutic. Most self-inflicted injury occurs in the context of a range of maladaptive behaviour, some of which may be seen as deliberate, manipulative or disruptive (cf. Toch et al., 1989). The dichotomy between discipline and medical problems is, according to Toch, false.

Referrals to the doctor and psychiatrist

Not surprisingly, significantly more of the subject group had been referred to the doctor since coming in on reception, and more had been referred to, or were currently seeing, the visiting psychiatrist. Far more of the subject group reported having current problems, and these were more likely to be prison problems or a combination of inside and outside problems (see Table 6.10):

It ain't just the lads ... it's being locked up all the time, hearing keys rattling, not being contacted from home ... and just being here (SG).

Problems inside included other inmates, waiting for decisions, losing confidence and worrying about going mad; outside problems were invariably, contacts with family, or not being able to go home on release. It is important to note here that inmates are willing to admit and identify their own problems, that the problems themselves are frequently of a practical and solvable nature, and that those with the skills and contacts necessary to help are the prison staff. They have often emerged as inmates with difficulties during the sentence, not necessarily as a result of their suicide risk, but for other reasons. The point is that psychiatric training is not necessary to identify or resolve many of their problems and concerns.

Outside support and contacts

An uncomfortable irony of statements issued by the Prison Department about the importance of family ties throughout a sentence, is the extent to which imprisonment puts serious constraints on the amount of contact inmates will have with their family and community. The severance of family and other outside ties is known to make resettlement prospects worse; it also contributes to suicides and suicide attempts in custody (Home Office, 1986a). Considerable emphasis has been placed on the maintenance of family and outside ties by the Prison and Probation Departments, with throughcare (CI 40/1988), home leave, the prospect of phone

Table 6.10 Referrals to doctor and psychiatrist

		Subject group No.	%	Comparison group No.	%
Referral to doctor?	None	9	(18)	30	(60)
	Some	32	(64)	18	(36)
	Often	9	(18)	2	(4)
	Totals	50	(100)	50	(100)
		$\chi^2=19.68$ d.f.$=2$ p<0.0002			
Referral to psychiatrist?	None	22	(44)	38	(76)
	Yes	9	(18)	5	(10)
	Current	19	(38)	7	(14)
	Totals	50	(100)	50	(100)
		$\chi^2=10.49$ d.f.$=2$ p<0.006			
Current problems?	None	10	(20)	31	(62)
	Inside	10	(20)	4	(8)
	Outside	8	(16)	12	(24)
	Both	22	(44)	3	(6)
	Totals	50	(100)	50	(100)
		$\chi^2=28.57$ d.f.$=3$ p<0.0001			

cards (Home Office, 1990a), and the concept of prison as a pre-release course (CI 40/1988) all attempting to combat the unintended and negative impact of imprisonment on life outside. The likely and eventual extent of family ties is one of the major 'risk factors' guiding staff in their identification of potential suicide risks.

The subject group received significantly fewer visits, wrote fewer letters and missed specific people (family members, or mates) more than the comparison group (see Table 6.11). A third of the subject group were not receiving visits at all. A further 16 per cent received them rarely:

> When I first came in, she was coming up once a fortnight, then it went to once a month, then less. It went downhill then. (SG)

> I used to, but not here, no. It's too far for anyone to come. (SG)

> I'm not sending them VOs any more. I can't be bothered, it's a waste of time. (SG)

Only a third of either group of inmates received the maximum allowed fortnightly visit. Many of the subject group received less, or varying frequencies of visits:

Table 6.11 Contacts with family

		Subject group		Comparison group	
		No.	%	No.	%
Frequency of	Every 2 weeks	9	(18)	17	(34)
visits?	Once a month	5	(10)	14	(28)
	Few months	12	(24)	10	(20)
	Rare	8	(16)	5	(10)
	None	16	(32)	4	(8)
	Totals	50	(100)	50	(100)

For once a month or more v. every few months v. rare or none
$\chi^2 = 13.42$ d.f.$= 2$ p< 0.005

Letters out per	None	15	(30)	4	(8)
week?	One	18	(36)	9	(18)
	Two	7	(14)	15	(30)
	Three	6	(12)	7	(14)
	Four+	4	(8)	15	(30)
	Totals	50	(100)	50	(100)

$\chi^2 = 18.72$ d.f.$= 4$ p< 0.001

When was last	1–3 days	9	(18)	6	(12)
visit?	4–7 days	1	(2)	9	(18)
	8–14 days	8	(16)	12	(24)
	15–28 days	4	(8)	10	(20)
	29 days+	28	(56)	13	(26)
	Totals	50	(100)	50	(100)

$\chi^2 = 15.86$ d.f.$= 4$ p< 0.004

Note: For 'no letters' v. '1 letter out' v. 'more than1', $\chi^2 = 16.78$ d.f.$= 3$ p< 0.005.

Sometimes they come every two weeks or so, and then they lapse a bit. (SG)

Three-quarters of the subject group and two-thirds of the comparison group reported some problems regarding visits: either distance, transport, domestic, financial, or work arrangements, several of these, or other problems such as health, tension between family members or other difficulties in relationships. Several inmates commented that these practical difficulties were often used as an 'excuse':

Transport mostly – and they just can't be bothered to turn up. (SG)

A third of the subject group as opposed to 8 per cent of the comparison group were not writing letters out, sometimes because they could not write, or find anyone to help them, or because they were not receiving letters back:

Things went downhill then. I didn't write for a few months ... it gets harder to think of things to say. Now I only write in reply to ones I get. When I first got sentenced, I'd send out both each week ... but I didn't get many replies. (SG)

Most of the inmates would have liked to have been receiving more letters, visits or both during the sentence. Some found letters difficult ('I'm not too clever at writing'). Others, however, found other difficulties:

I've only just had my private cash – it took three weeks to come through, so I'm writing lots now. (CG)

Did visits and letters help them get through the sentence? Most of the inmates who received them said they did:

Yes, because you come in and you see a letter on your light switch after dinner or after tea, and you feel really excited. (CG)

Yes, you know there's someone out there thinking about you. (SG)

Some thought that letters did, but visits did not:

Letters do ... visits don't – it upsets you when you get back to your pad. (SG)

It depends. Sometimes you feel really gutted – depends how it goes. (CG)

Cohen and Taylor argued that some inmates find prison less stressful when they cut off contact with the outside world (Cohen and Taylor, 1972). As we shall see, this may be the case, but it is a difficult state to achieve.

In order to further explore the question of visits, and the possible effects of both receiving *and* not receiving them, further more specific questions were asked. Each inmate was asked to remember his or her last visit: How long ago was it? Who had visited them? and How had they felt just before the visit was due? Over half of all those receiving visits had felt excited beforehand:

Buzzed up – on a high! (CG)

I always get butterflies! (SG)

I get so happy that I think I'm going to cry when they come in! (CG)

A third of the subject group and a quarter of the comparison group however, felt nervous, or anxious before the visit:

Edgy. I didn't know how it would be. (SG)

Panicky – getting ready, hoping they'd show up. They often couldn't come, for about two months, they just don't show up. One day you'd just give up and you don't get ready, then they come! (CG)

A small number felt depressed before the visit:

I didn't know whether they were coming or not. (SG)

A small group felt 'the same as normal', often because they didn't know they were getting a visit:

I wasn't expecting them. I was expecting them on Sunday and they didn't turn up. (CG)

The inmates were also asked how they felt just after the visit was over. This time, 67 per cent of the subject group and 72 per cent of the comparison group (of those receiving visits) said they felt depressed:

Down ... I don't know why. It happens all the time. (CG)

I feel pretty sad and lonely. (SG)

Gutted ... you know, I feel like shutting myself away and just forgetting. (SG)

Words like 'gutted', 'choked', 'on a downer', sad, nostalgic, lonely, low and miserable came up over and over again. About a quarter of those receiving visits still felt excited after a visit, but even some of these inmates had to fend off troubled sentiments:

For a while, you're still on a high, but then you come down a bit ... you have to start looking forward to the next one. They slowly go out of your mind – it turns to here. If you get bad news, then you feel really fed up. (CG)

Other feelings were mentioned too:

I felt happy that I'd seen them, but angry that it was such a short time ... it's nowhere near enough. You get so mad. You just want out. (CG)

Both absconds and suicides were mentioned in the context of family contacts:

My cell mate's thinking of breaking out because he wants to see his parents ... he's thought of hanging himself, you know. (CG)

This link between absconding and suicide attempts had been mentioned during interviews before. A theory that absconds were an alternative to suicidal gestures and attempts gained considerable support throughout the research, particularly as both were usually motivated by either domestic or prison-related worries.[5]

How long did these feelings last after the visit – of either depression, anger, excitement or anxiety? Almost half of both groups of inmates experiencing such feelings said they lasted until the next day:

> About a day. When you wake up in the morning, you're still thinking about your visit, but you're not so depressed. (CG)

Over a third of both groups of inmates said the feelings lasted for several hours:

> Until after tea – or longer sometimes, it depends how bored you are. (CG)

Sixteen per cent of the comparison group, and 21 per cent of the subject group reported that the feelings lasted for several days:

> You feel depressed ... just run down again, I'd say the first couple of days afterwards drags, and then you just have to black it out of your mind – it's awful. (SG)

As is clear from the above account, having nothing to do makes these experiences harder to deal with. In a thematic review of regimes for young remand prisoners, the Chief Inspector of Prisons argued that inmates: 'should have the opportunity to engage in useful activity which would help him to cope more easily with the inevitable anxieties and frustrations of custody, and assist him in recovering and retaining his sense of perspective' (Home Office, 1990a:45). It is not just remand prisoners who need these opportunities.

Contacts with the probation service

All young offenders sentenced to custody are statutorily required to undergo a period of supervision by the probation service on their release, as part of the throughcare intended to maintain their links with the community and encourage their resettlement after the sentence. A probation officer is responsible for this part of an inmate's throughcare, maintaining contact with him throughout the sentence, providing a source of contact between him and the outside world and linking any positive efforts and changes he might make during the sentence to his plans for release. Organisational and resource constraints, and variations in the way that probation teams specialise, affect the extent to which probation officers are able to fulfil this task.

Sadly, the subject group had less contact from the probation service, fewer finding their contacts useful:

> He's not very useful. He's alright, but when he comes to visit me, he just sits there, and I have to do the talking. (SG)

Almost a third of those inmates in the subject group had received no contact from the probation service at the time of the interview (which could be at any stage during a sentence). Contacts with the probation service were useful for a variety of reasons: in practical ways, solving problems or contributing to parole or release arrangements, maintaining contact, for welfare or counselling purposes, for help with particular problems or for a mixture of these reasons. Many inmates simply appreciated the contact:

> Just that she is there. She is someone that is not involved with the prison I can talk to. She comes from outside, and I know that when I eventually am released she is going to be there to help me. (CG)

Well over half of both groups of inmates had recently been designated a new probation officer, either because they had no previous contact with the probation service (this was rare), or more likely, because the probation officer had moved, left the service or changed roles. Sometimes several changes of probation officer during one sentence was reported:

> I've had three changes ... I'd only just met the other one! (CG)

> I don't know whether I've got a probation officer or not – it all changed. Mine was really good, but he left. I've seen no-one for four months. I've had letters from all sorts – one just said they're not recommending parole. (SG)

It is significant that the subject group are amongst those least likely to be receiving regular contact and support from the outside probation service. They are also less likely to perceive this contact as useful. Their needs and problems may be distinct in their nature as well as in their extent.

Thinking about outside

The subject group kept in touch with the outside slightly less and found it marginally harder to keep in touch with the world outside, preferring to forget it, even if in the end, they could not. Some of the subject group said they tried not to think about people outside, they found it too depressing. Despite (or because of) the lack of contact with their families, the subject group thought about their families a lot, and missed them a great deal.

Over two-thirds of both groups of inmates found that thinking about people on the outside made the sentence harder. Only 4 per cent of both groups thought it made the sentence easier. Some missed people less as the sentence went on:

> Not as often as I did – rarely now. As you progress through your sentence, you stop missing them. (SG)

For some inmates, particular times were more difficult than others – night-times, weekends or special occasions, such as birthdays or Christmas. A third of both groups, however, just said 'all the time'. Others included 'when I'm not busy', 'when I'm banged up', or:

> Yes, like something triggers it off – you hear a song on the radio, or something like that. (SG)

> When I've got a letter, or I look at the pictures in my cell. (CG)

> Yes, every night! The only time I really think about them is when I'm on my own. Like, in a strip cell ... They say it helps you in the end, but I don't reckon it does, anyway. I mean, the state you can get yourself into ... if you're out there with the rest, you just forget it, you just get out there on the landing. In here you've just got these two blankets. (SG)

Over half of the comparison group either tried, or did manage to keep in touch with life outside, usually through letters to and from family and friends. Sometimes the family or probation service would send in local newspapers, and local radio was popular, or inmates would see newspapers occasionally. Over half of the subject group did not read the newspapers or watch the news on television:

> No, I've given up totally. You don't hear about things, like Fergie having a baby, I had no idea. I don't really know what's going on – I haven't kept in touch ... it doesn't really bother me. (CG)

Less than a quarter of both groups kept in touch with the national news. Restrictions were mentioned:

> You can't have papers down the block. (SG)

> I used to, but I had my radio took off me. (CG)

> I can't spend money on papers, me – I need it for my baccy. (CG)

But like family contacts, keeping in touch with the outside world could sometimes be troubling:

> I used to have our local paper sent in, but it sort of gutted me up, reading that all the time, seeing what everyone else was doing. (CG)

In accordance with Cohen and Taylor's description of the 'emotional relief' experienced by reducing reliance upon the outside world (Cohen and Taylor, 1972), over 40 per cent of both groups of inmates said it was easier to forget the world outside, and just get on with the sentence:

> Trying to forget it, because if you're always worrying and thinking about what people outside are doing, it seems to drag. I'd rather just forget about it and get on with my time. (CG)

Few of either group of inmates had release plans for when they got out. Many of the inmates said they did not know what they wanted, felt confused or had no idea how they were going to achieve their aims. Life outside was not much better than life in prison.

Coping with custody

Bondeson showed that over 80 per cent of inmates in all types of penal establishments in Sweden reported feeling more irritable, more anxious, more depressed and more apathetic in prison than they do outside (Bondeson, 1989:175). The prison experience may be differentially perceived, however. The level of significance of some of the differences to emerge between the subject and comparison groups in relation to the experience of imprisonment were both surprising and instructive.

There were few differences between the subject and the comparison groups in their description of the worst aspects of imprisonment. Most inmates felt that losing their freedom or being away from the family were the worst things about being in prison:

> I don't really know – it's all bad really. I think the worst thing is being away from your family and friends. (CG)

Being told what to do was a frequent response, and a small group thought that coping with other inmates was particularly difficult:

> Other inmates. It's not just sex offenders who get trouble. If you're slow, or a bit stupid ... or you're a grass, or you tax ... The worst thing is when no-one wants to talk to you – they say, 'don't sit next to him', 'don't talk to him', you know? (SG)

Other 'worst things' included boredom, being banged up, slop out, the food, being lonely; some could not specify any one item:

> There's the hospital, the food, not being able to wear your own clothes, having to use a pot for a toilet, being locked up like an animal, lack of contact with outside, or the opposite sex, missing family and friends. (CG)

> Actually getting adapted to the prison environment, associating with other inmates ... it depends what kind of person you are.
> • Does it get easier?
> It gets worse, that's my personal experience ... I don't know why. (SG)

Using time or doing time

Toch *et al.* (1989) argue that the expression 'doing time' implies that survival is an occupation:

> with a concomitant suspension of development. This feature of prison life is unfortunate, given the relative youthfulness of most prison inmates, and the fact

that much of the conduct for which offenders are imprisoned suggests that they could usefully acknowledge that there is room for personal improvement.

(Toch *et al.*, 1989:xi-xii)

Likewise, the Chief Inspector of Prisons (Home Office, 1990a) argues that inmates should be encouraged to *use* time, not just to *do* it, and that constructive occupation may relieve some of the frustration common to young anxious prisoners. Most inmates, however, 'do' their time – finding little to occupy themselves with fully. Neither group planned the sentence, or the time they had to serve, both taking each day as it came. Only 10 per cent of the subject group and 14 per cent of the comparison group planned their sentence, or set themselves goals:

It's all pretty routine, you can't tell one day from another, it all just goes by. (CG)

Less than half of the inmates thought they were using the sentence to achieve something constructive for themselves. Almost half of both groups of inmates said that they were just getting through the sentence, not achieving anything:

I'm just getting through it – no option. (SG)

Inmates wanted to get fitter, become more intelligent and 'wise', and better qualified; they wanted to give up drugs, reorganise their lives, change their personalities and 'sort their heads out'. Significantly more of the subject group wanted to change personal things about themselves:

I want to stop cutting up. (SG)

I want to change the way I'm living.
• How are you going to do that?
I don't know. (SG)

The most important things they had done during the sentence were education, work, vocational courses and PE, although over half of both groups of inmates said that nothing they had done in prison was important. Some mentioned visits, association, illicit drugs and the television, and two said that having time to think and reflect had been important.

Coping with problems

Staying in one's cell during association is sometimes mentioned as a possible sign of depression or even suicide risk. However, only a quarter of the inmates would ever vary whether or not they came out for association according to their mood. The majority (slightly more of the comparison group) would always come out: an indication that restricted hours out of cell alters this pattern:

No, everyone's quite glad to get out of their cell, I think. (SG)

When asked what they would do if they had a problem or were feeling down almost three-quarters of the subject group said they would just keep it to themselves. A fifth of both groups would discuss the problem with someone; more of the comparison group would find something to do to take their minds off it. Others would write a letter, did not foresee having any problems, or had other coping strategies:

> I'd just smoke loads of dope! (CG)

> I pray. Yes, that helps. (CG)

> I sleep – or try to. (SG)

> I don't know what to do ... that's why I get uptight and why I try to slash myself. (SG)

Who would they turn to for help? Over half of both groups would turn to no-one:

> No-one really. Like I said, its just a job to the screws, innit? They've been doing it for years – you know, they've seen it all before, you know what I mean? (SG)

> It's not worth turning to other inmates, they just take the piss. On something that's not too important to you, or don't mean a lot to you, then you can. But anything that means too much, you can't – you have to try and sort it out yourself, and if you can't, then you have to learn to forget about it. (SG)

Some would turn to another inmate. Some (slightly more of the subject group) would turn to staff; a small group might turn to either, others would either write a letter, turn to the probation officer, the chaplain or a psychologist, or in one case:

> Just the razor blade – it's more help than anything else. (SG)

Thoughts of past and future

The subject group were significantly more likely to day-dream: 80 per cent said they spent a great deal of time day-dreaming – some all the time:

> All the time – I prefer my world. (SG)

Almost all of the inmates spent time thinking about the past:

> All the time ... I think about how stupid I've been. (SG)

> A lot actually ... a lot of things I'd like to change, a lot of wishing I could turn the clock back. (CG)

Slightly less inmates spent time thinking about the future. Over a third of the subject group never thought about the future:

> I try not to think about it – it scares me. (SG)

> You try not to think about it.
• Why?

I don't know – like, it does your head in ... you've 18 months left, your probation officer comes up and asks you what you are going to do when you get out and that – it does your head in. (SG)

It's still in the dark – it's just like being in the deep end. I just can't see what I'm going to do in the future. (SG)

There's nothing to think about. (SG)

The subject group were significantly less hopeful about their release. A third did not feel at all hopeful about their release:

No it scares me. (SG)

I don't know ... I don't know about keeping out of trouble. (SG)

Most of these inmates were worried about gate arrests, getting into trouble again, unsolved problems awaiting them and a future void of plans.

Nights

The subject group had far more problems sleeping at night (see Table 6.12). Almost two-thirds, serious problems. They complained of nightmares, worries, feeling restless and not being able to stop thinking:

Yes, even if I'm tired, I just don't get to sleep straight away, like – I just lie there awake, thinking. (SG)

Much of the sleep problem was related to sleeping during the day, whiling away hours locked in cells:

Yes, going to sleep at night – everyone sleeps over dinner – you see them on parades, all sleepy eyed ... we all do. (CG)

Yes – sometimes I get bad-tempered with my room mate because I can't get to sleep. Then by the time I get to sleep its time to wake up, so I wake up in a bad mood – and that's the *beginning* of the day! I sleep mostly in the day, you know – that's the main problem because that's all you can do if you're banged up. (SG)

Table 6.12 Sleeping problems

| | Subject group | | Comparison group | |
	No.	%	No.	%
A lot	30	(60)	10	(20)
Sometimes	12	(24)	14	(28)
Never	8	(16)	26	(52)
Totals	50	(100)	50	(100)
			$\chi^2 = 19.68$ d.f.$=2$ p<0.0002	

Those who didn't have sleeping problems at the time of the interview often had at some stage – a job may have solved the problem:

Not since I've worked in the servery, no. (CG)

The prison experience

The subject group reported having found the prison experience more difficult. Almost two-thirds of the subject group thought the experience was difficult, a bit of a struggle – or negative:

It's bloody awful. I'll never come back again never in my life. (SG)

Gruelling, I don't like prison. (SG)

It's bad, it's no good for no-one. If I didn't keep my head together, I'd come out of here a nutter, a fruitcake. (SG)

Over half of the comparison group, on the other hand, thought it was indifferent – or a roughly even mixture of good and bad:

It depends, like – how you get on. Sometimes it's been a crack up. Apart from that it's been boring. One day it really does your head in, other days it's OK. (CG)

It's a strange mixture ... funny I enjoyed myself in Cardiff at Christmas, we had all the OAPs in and that, but it's not nice. It's difficult. (CG)

An eye-opener into a side of life that you wouldn't normally see. You can mature a lot, you can learn through it. You learn to understand people better, because you live in such close proximity. I think it's also depressing. It can be a real struggle. (CG)

Only 2 per cent of either group thought the experience was positive:

Well, you learn quite a lot in here, I'll say that ... and that's the main thing. You're doing all different jobs, so that when you get out, you know what to do, you've got some experience. (CG)

When asked specifically what the prison experience had been like *for them*, far more of the subject group thought that it had been difficult (see Table 6.13). Three-quarters of the subject group reported that the prison experience was difficult; almost half of the comparison group said they had found it, or were finding it difficult.

So what were the main problems inmates faced during a sentence? The subject group were significantly more likely to have found 'being banged up' the main problem of imprisonment (see Table 6.14). Lack of freedom, lack of contact and bang up were mentioned most frequently. Other problems included other inmates, uncertainty, the length of time, boredom, not sleeping, slop out, transfers, feeling

Table 6.13 The prison experience – for you

	Subject group No.	Subject group %	Comparison group No.	Comparison group %
Difficult	38	(78)	23	(46)
Indifferent	1	(2)	13	(26)
Positive	1	(2)	1	(2)
Other/both	9	(18)	13	(26)
Totals	49	(100)	50	(100)

$\chi^2 = 14.69$ d.f. $= 3$ p< 0.003

Table 6.14 Main problems faced

	Subject group No.	Subject group %	Comparison group No.	Comparison group %
Lack of freedom	16	(33)	20	(41)
Lack of contact	8	(16)	15	(31)
Bang up	15	(31)	4	(8)
Other	10	(20)	10	(20)
Totals	49	(100)	49	(100)

$\chi^2 = 8.94$ d.f. $= 3$ p< 0.02

helpless in the face of problems outside, fitting in, getting into debt and physical deprivations such as ill-fitting clothes, not enough tobacco and the food.

Hopelessness

Finally, the subject group scored higher on the Hopelessness Scale (Beck *et al.*, 1974; 1989). On this scale based on the responses to 20 questions (self-completed, usually), half of the comparison group scored three or less on the Hopelessness Scale, indicating that they were not feeling hopeless (see Table 6.15). Over a third of both groups scored between four and eight (some hopelessness); 36 per cent of the subject group scored between nine and 14; 8 per cent of the subject group scored

Table 6.15 Hopelessness score

	Subject group No.	Subject group %	Comparison group No.	Comparison group %
0 – 3	9	(18)	25	(50)
4 – 8	19	(38)	20	(40)
9 – 14	18	(36)	5	(10)
15 – 18	4	(8)	–	
Totals	50	(100)	50	(100)

$\chi^2 = 18.90$ d.f. $= 3$ p< 0.0005

15 or over, indicating extreme feelings of hopelessness. A score of nine or over has been found to be associated with suicide risk (Williams, 1986; Beck *et al.*, 1989).

To summarise, inmates who are feeling short of coping resources, say so, and show signs, both indirect and direct, indicating that they are at a loss. The most significant point to emerge from the responses to questions about the experience of imprisonment was the *consistency* with which the subject group were (and felt) worse off than their fellow inmates in terms of the availability and desirability of work, education, PE and other methods of occupation. They did not see as many opportunities for themselves in prison, nor did they seem able to make constructive use of their time. The combination of practical constraints and their own lethargy left them helpless and resourceless in the face of hours of unfilled time. Inmates in the subject group appeared to be *less able to occupy themselves constructively when locked in their cells*. They felt more bored, did less, got more bored as the sentence went on and yet spent more time there. If there is a 'vulnerability factor' not yet explored in prison suicide research, this must be one of the most significant. If these inmates cannot read or write, and so spend so much time staring at four walls, the inability to relieve this prison pressure could contribute directly to the crossing of a threshold that otherwise may never have been reached. It was their inability to occupy themselves constructively, combined with enforced idleness (Home Office, 1990a) that increased their vulnerability to both impulsive acts of self-harm and suicidal thoughts. Still, it should be remembered that the actual numbers showing positive indications of these adverse variables – even amongst the subject group – are small, often less than half of the group (= 25 inmates). The 'profile' towards which this analysis is moving provides an *understanding* of vulnerability. It may precede many young prisoner suicides. It does not claim to predict them. Their vulnerability constitutes part of a suicidal process. Of equal relevance to policy and understanding are the situational factors provoking such distress. Inactivity is a central variable in this context.

The hopelessness of a sentence, doing time, living day by day, with no plans, no thoughts of the future and nothing meaningful or interesting to do; long nights with little sleep, inmates dwelling on the past, or day-dreaming about inaccessible people outside, having few people to turn to for help – it is not the conditions of imprisonment we have to understand, but the *experience*:

> The point is that segregation hurts, not so much because of its objective deprivations, though these are admittedly unpleasant, but because it exposes men to special environmental challenges, and calls for special psychological resources. Those unable to marshall appropriate resources are abandoned to defeat and left to ponder, alone and unaided, the nature and import of their failure.
>
> (Johnson, 1978:469)

In hopeless young people, with the least available skills and resources for coping with adversity and stress, confinement, isolation and boredom – particularly if combined with conflict and pressure from other inmates – can be the last straw.

This is one unintended consequence of imprisonment no society should knowingly or willingly inflict on its law-breakers. 'Looking after with humanity' should exclude boring people to death.

> La solitude, répetons-le, ne corrige pas l'homme.., l'expérience nous l'a prouvé; elle le rend ou insensé, ou furieux, ou brute, ou bien elle le pousse au suicide par le deséspoir.
> [Solitude, let me repeat, does not reform men, ... experience has proved this; it makes him insane, or furious, or brutal, or else it pushes him to suicide via despair.]
>
> (Leon Vidal, Inspecteur général des prisons, 1853).

Discussion

An exploration of the prison experience offers a variety of significant questions for both suicide prevention policy and for future research. These are exactly the sort of questions that personal officers (or other prison officers) could pursue, without having to concern themselves exclusively with the question of suicide ('So, what do you do with yourself when you're banged up in your cell?'). The proportion of the subject group who disliked PE, for example, may have been expressing difficulties with other inmates, or an inability to achieve the level of activity expected of other inmates. It is interesting to note how an attitude towards an everyday (sic) prison feature may indicate other important feelings. Prison officers could be encouraged to make these sorts of enquiries as part of their general 'welfare' role, taking an interest in all inmates without 'homing in' on the suicidal. As part of a series of related questions, officers could look for signs and symptoms at least, of stress, or an inability to cope. Lack of contacts with outside, or lack of interest in the outside world, are already well-established indicators of risk. Visits and contacts are evidently an important area for inmates, whether they are receiving them or not. Lack of socialisation within the prison may be another indicator of risk, particularly if the inmate has few friends inside, spends a lot of time on his own, has difficulties with other inmates or knows few other inmates from his own area. Importantly, inmates who present disciplinary problems to the staff cannot be assumed to be (just) manipulative, or obvious trouble-makers (cp. Toch et al., 1989). Their disciplinary problems may be another feature of the difficulties they are experiencing in coping with prison.

Clearly, frequent or current referrals to the doctor or psychiatrist indicate possible problems, but far more significant is the finding that, when asked, inmates in the sample group *report far more problems* than their contemporaries, often relating to the prison situation, or a combination of inside and outside problems. This suggests that, given a willing ear, inmates will indicate their own vulnerability. The only other requirement is that the listening ear recognises and acknowledges these signs as signs of risk – or valid cries for help.

Having serious problems sleeping at night, day-dreaming, signs of hopelessness and viewing others' self-injury as serious and genuine, could all be indicators of the risk of 'the onset of a suicidal crisis', particularly if these immediate responses have a context of poor release plans (and hopes), few outside contacts and disappointments in relationships. A profile of 'vulnerability', based on the material in this section is included below. See also Figure 9.1, p.235.

SECTION III: SUICIDE ATTEMPTS – IN THEIR OWN WORDS

All inmates were asked if they had ever had serious thoughts of suicide during the sentence. Eighty-six per cent of the subject group and a surprising 14 per cent of the comparison group said they had.

The proportion of inmates who knew others who had attempted or committed suicide in prison was high: two-thirds of both groups. Even if the actual events are infrequent, the attempts and suicides were known about and discussed: the problem has a high profile within prison life. Almost half of the subject group thought that the reason why inmates attempted or committed suicide during a sentence was because they couldn't handle their sentence. This vague and largely unhelpful statement was used frequently by both inmates and staff to explain suicide and self-injury in prison, without further elaboration. A small number of the subject group said it was because these inmates were depressed, others said it was because of particular problems they were experiencing. A small number in each group thought it was for attention.

This question proved to be particularly instructive in the case of those inmates who had felt suicidal themselves. They often found it easier to find reasons why *other* inmates might have felt that way, when they had been unable to articulate their own reasons a few moments earlier. Their explanations of others' attempts illustrated a plausible explanation of their own:

> Being banged up, and cut off in the dead of night ... it's more than just being banged up ... you lose your head. (SG)

> They do it because it's too much pressures on them, it gets to them and that, and they're sick of being locked up, and they're sick of taking orders, and they're sick of no-one caring. (SG)

Not being able to cope was the most frequent explanation for suicide attempts: they were 'inadequate', 'weak', resourceless. Other inmates' attitudes were divided into sympathy for the 'genuine' and disdain for the 'attention-seeking'. Surviving prison without self-inflicted scars was mentioned as a sign of being able to do your time.

Two-thirds of the subject group and half of the comparison group thought that either most or at least some of the attempts were serious. A quarter of the subject group and 40 per cent of the comparison group thought that most were not. Many referred to incidents they knew.

It was a surprise to discover how many inmates from the comparison group had thought about or even attempted suicide at some stage during their sentence. The subject group tended to be more 'understanding' of the problem – and were more likely to relate suicide attempts to the sentence.

The topics of suicide and suicide attempts were not unusual subjects for discussion amongst young prisoners. There existed a series of explanations for and opinions about these activities, which all inmates shared. A language (argot) was perceptible: 'he's slashed up', she's 'cut-up' again, he's got 'tram-lines', they 'topped themselves'. More of the subject group saw self-inflicted injuries as 'serious', many of which could be described as a suicide attempt.

When asked about specific triggers or events which might have provoked their attempts or injuries, almost a third of the subject group inmates (30 per cent) said there had been some problem with other inmates before the incident: either threats, bullying, teasing or arguments. Prison pressures were most often chosen from a list of alternative problems that might have precipitated the suicide attempt: 22 per cent said they had recently received a long or unexpected sentence, 24 per cent had recently been punished or segregated, 12 per cent had received (or were expecting) a 'Dear John' letter, 4 per cent had received a parole refusal and 8 per cent had either been transferred or moved from one location in the prison to another. Most of the inmates reported what had happened fluently and clearly, appearing not to find the question in any way delicate. Many expressed relief to finally be given an opportunity to talk about what they had done.

Almost half of the group had cut their arms – although these cuts could vary between single cuts requiring simple stitches, and deep or multiple lacerations that in two cases had resulted in nerve injury, causing the permanent loss of feeling in the forearm. Other deep cuts were on the inside of the top half of the arm, where serious loss of blood was likely. These latter injuries were dangerous. It was generally known that 'scratches across the wrists' would not result in death – only 16 per cent of the group had cut their wrists. The injuries were rarely as 'superficial' as staff comment and discussion might have indicated. The inmates often showed their scars, some of which were over 18 inches long, or so raised as to permanently disfigure the skin. Twenty per cent of the subject group had attempted to hang themselves and 4 per cent had swallowed razor blades; 4 per cent had cut their throat – again, scars showed the evidence of serious intent. Others had not carried out their intentions, or had been unable to find anything to injure themselves with. Of the three inmates in the comparison group who reported having made an attempt at suicide without having been discovered, one had tried to hang himself, one had cut his arms and one had cut his wrist.

Most of the inmates had been in a single cell at the time of the incident: 6 per cent had been in double cells or 'two'd up', 6 per cent had been in dormitories, one on a landing, one in the hospital and one in the punishment block. Another had injured himself in a variety of places on several occasions, attempting to hang himself, cutting himself and setting fire to his cell. Others' threats had been prevented.

The attempts or thoughts were usually brought about by identifiable problems:

10 per cent of the subject group said that the major motivation was an outside problem, usually to do with family or girl/boyfriend. Almost a third said it was a prison problem:

> Being padded up on my own, it was a bit hard, I felt depressed and all that, there was no-one there to talk to, and I was scared, I just didn't want to be on my own.

Over half mentioned motivations that were a combination of inside and outside problems:

> I just couldn't do any more time in prison, and I didn't know if my girlfriend would visit on Saturday, and ... you know, I'd just had it.

Many of their own explanations for the injury differed from those found in their records. It was not unusual for inmates to express feelings during the interview of having been under pressure to 'tell the doctor what he wanted to know':

> I had to say that, you know? It's what they want you to say ... I couldn't answer their questions ... I didn't know what to say.

Six inmates left a note, indicating their intention, and usually referring to the main reasons for the attempt. These notes were usually expressing anger and resignation, and were concerned with lack of contact and concern from both outside and inside. 'I've had enough', was the most frequent sentiment indicated.

Towards the end of the interview, all inmates were asked: 'Would you say, then, that you had ever had serious thoughts of suicide on this sentence? Have you ever actually attempted suicide on this sentence, and if so why?' At this stage, the end of a long and sometimes difficult interview, responses were much more fluent and forthcoming:

> It was everything – my brother's death, the sentence, my family, worrying if everything was going to be alright, prison – it was everything – even being in prison.

> Loneliness ... it's a very lonely place.

> You just feel that there's no hope, when you're banged up just looking at four walls.

Many mentioned not being able to turn to anyone, or not feeling like anyone cared:

> People just haven't got time for me.

> It was the sentence ... how long it was, feeling down ...
> • Did you tell anyone?
> I thought the screws or probation might laugh at me – they're not really concerned, they're just collecting their pay cheques.

As indicated above, on several occasions the reason given during the interview was different to that recorded in the file, or it became clearer as the whole picture was painted:

> It's so hard to talk about 'the real problem' in case you end up being locked up even more. No-one will talk to you, it's mad, it was doing my head in. No-one asked me about it – they did ask me why I'd done it, I didn't want to say 'owt because, you know, I didn't want to tell them the reasons because I knew they'd just shove me back in the strip cells, like.

Most of the inmates gave several reasons – a build up, followed by a closed door:

> in your cell you have these razor blades ... I was just thinking all about what I had left and things like that, thinking about my girlfriend and daughter, and I don't know ... and that's what I done (shows several severe cuts and scars) ... that was about 8.30 p.m.
> • Did you ring your cell bell?
> I didn't ring my cell bell until 11.30 p.m. – I thought I'd be dead by then. I was cold, shivering. I didn't know it'd be so hard to die.

The reasons were varied, sometimes specific, and sometimes undefinable:

> I don't know ... I was just fed up at the time, just a build-up of things. I didn't think, I just did it.

But the feelings were common:

> I just felt so helpless.

> I just felt that there was nothing.

> There was no-one to talk to.

> All sorts ... missing my girlfriend ... I just don't like it here.

The young suicide attempter is 'a lonely child without friends and without firm ties with his parents' (Rood de Boer, 1978). He or she does not feel safe or loved (Bowlby, 1965; Diekstra, 1987). Difficulties in communication and isolation expose their resourcelessness. In prison, this vulnerability is crucial. As shown in Figure 9.1 (p. 235), the trigger for a suicide attempt might consist of something apparently 'trivial': a threat by other inmates, a bad letter, a visit which does not materialise, too much time alone, a sleepless night – but the context for this precipitant is an emotional state of despair. The threshold at which prison-induced distress becomes unbearable varies, and the pains of imprisonment may vary according to the inmate's situation as well as his or her resources.

Discussion

Amongst adolescent and young children, it is thought that external (exogenic) factors play a greater role in the development of suicidal behaviours than the internal (endogenic).

(Rood de Boer, 1978:451)

Several questions were asked about the reasons behind each incident: 'What was going on at the time, why do you think you did it, was there anything you were intending to do, or achieve?' Inmates found these questions difficult, and often responded indirectly at first, building up to a 'real reason' only in stages, unable to articulate the 'cause' immediately or in one go. The story is better told whole, looking for more than a single precipitating cause. There were also predisposing causes, and several precipitants before the most immediate (Rood de Boer, 1978). Reasons given during the interview can be seen as divisible into two separate levels of explanation: the first (superficial) level refers to practical or *outcome-explanations*, and comprises the accepted rationale for such acts ('he was attention-seeking'; 'he just wanted out'). Notions of escape, crisis, panic, avoidance and sanctuary search (articulated by Toch, 1975) best describe these accounts. These were the types of explanation most often found in inmates' records. Often the second-layer (underlying) explanation consists of an emotional or *appeal-explanation*, and this sometimes contradicts the first response, being more compelled than instrumental. This group of 'reasons' has the common denominator of despair: the 'ingredients of despair' are hopelessness, isolation, fear and breakdown (Toch, 1975). The first- and second-layer explanations have one common theme: *the last straw*:

> 'Why does someone kill himself?' asked Klaus Mann in his autobiographical novel, *Turning Point*, and then gave the answer: 'Because one will not, cannot go through the next half hour, the next five minutes. Suddenly one comes to a dead end, the point of death. The limit has been reached.'
>
> (Diekstra and Hawton, 1987:43)

The trigger might consist of something apparently 'trivial': a threat by other inmates, a bad letter, a visit which does not materialise, too much time alone, a sleepless night – but the context for this precipitant is an emotional state of despair. Maltsberger articulates this subjective experience of despair, and wish for release amongst suicides outside: 'First, the patient finds himself in an intolerable affective state, flooded with emotional pain so intense and so unrelenting that it can no longer be endured. Second, the patient recognizes his condition, and gives up on himself' (Maltsberger, 1986:2–3).

The threshold at which prison-induced distress becomes unbearable varies, and as we have seen, the level of pain experienced during the sentence may vary according to the inmate's situation as well as his or her resources. This pathway to young prisoner suicide is summarised in Chapter 9. If there are those who still argue that the level of stress and unhappiness involved in prison life is unremarkable because long-term deterioration has not been shown to occur, it should be remembered that those who die by suicide in prison have never had a voice in those studies.

The concept of motivation, where it has been considered at all, has implied that these acts are carried out with their likely consequences in mind. This operant/behaviourist view of (particularly destructive) conduct is misleading and inadequate for the purpose of understanding self-inflicted injury, which is often impulsive rather than 'purposive'. It can be seen instead as a respondent behaviour (more like a reflex), a cry of pain, not just a cry for help (Williams and Hassanyeh, 1983).

There is an element of instrumentalism in some of these injuries: inmates do injure themselves in order to escape from a situation they find threatening or unbearable. Sometimes the 'threat' is a result of their own behaviour or misjudgment – borrowing, failing to repay debts, being seen as a 'grass', or just being seen as 'weak'. Avoiding these traps requires considerable skills and resolve – skills many inmates do not have. In trying to escape they are acknowledging (and communicating) their own resourcelessness; their failure to cope.

From the material outlined above, it can be argued that inmates injuring themselves in custody share certain characteristics which distinguish them to some extent from the rest of the inmate population. However, it must be reiterated that these characteristics are shared by only a proportion of those who injure themselves, and they may also be shared by many inmates who do not. A 'profile' of the vulnerable inmate can be constructed (see below). The profile should not be regarded as a predictive tool, but as an aid to understanding.[6] The lack of coping resources and ability provides a useful way of conceptualising this cluster of variables.

A vulnerability profile

1   CJS History

pessimistic SER*
many previous convictions*
less than 3 (–6) months at liberty*
current transfer*

2   Background

no qualifications*
frequent truancy
bullied at school*
local authority care*
family/behaviour problems
previous psychiatric treatment****
major drink problems****
experimentation with drugs*
parental violence*
previous self-injury****

3   Current Sentence

prefers to share cell*
dislikes PE****

inactive in cell*****
spends more time in cell**
bored***
getting more bored*
cannot relieve boredom*
few friends inside*
met only mates in prison*
sticks to himself**
difficulties with other inmates*
disciplinary problem*
feels discipline system unfair*
been in solitary (long time)***
frequent/recent referral to doctor****/psychiatrist*
reports current problems (esp. including inside*****)

4   Family and Outside Support

few visits*
writes few letters***
long time since last visit*
misses family*
little contact from probation*
finds thinking of outside difficult

5   Coping with Custody

wants to change self*
day-dreams*
not hopeful about release*
problems sleeping****
finds prison difficult**
finds bang-up difficult*
feelings of hopelessness****
suicidal thoughts/attempts*****
thinks others' attempts are serious*

Note: * $p < 0.05$, ** $p < 0.005$, *** $p < 0.001$, **** $p < 0.0005$, ***** $p < 0.0001$

It is the resourcelessness and emptiness of their lives that distinguishes the vulnerable from the less vulnerable: the degree of deprivation and the scale of their destructiveness.[7] They show a 'psychological anomie'. Unable to help themselves, and receiving little support from elsewhere, their actions are 'desperate expressions of unhappiness' (Rood de Boer, 1978). The suicide attempt, and all that comes before it, is a declaration of bankruptcy; of 'psychic collapse and hopelessness or impotence' (Diekstra and Hawton, 1987; Toch et al., 1989). The vulnerability may have been in evidence in their behaviour for some time: 'Young people often express their feelings in their behaviour rather than in their speech; they become impatient and impulsive in their speech and actions' (Diekstra and Hawton, 1987:44).

The 'cognitive triad' (Beck, 1976) of self, the future and the environment are all negative. The contribution of isolation in stripped conditions, or the boredom and inactivity of a stagnant regime is certainly not in the direction of the reconstruction of either the self, the future or this environment.

SECTION IV: THE SEARCH FOR A 'SERIOUS SUICIDE GROUP'

Still problematic is the heterogeneous nature of the subject group, containing as it does a variety of cases, some more clearly related to suicide than others. There are a series of unanswered questions in this research: the following brief account explores some of these questions, without being able to provide conclusive or satisfactory answers. Their further exploration may be a task for future research.

Variables were sought which could best identify the most 'serious suicide group' for a separate analysis, selecting those incidents most likely to have been the most dangerous suicide attempts to see whether they differed in any significant respects from both the other inmates in the subject and the comparison groups. The 'less clearly serious' cases were put into a second group (this time including any respondents from the comparison group, where appropriate), and these two groups were compared separately with each other, and with the 'non-suicidal group'. Any inmate not showing some clear indication of suicide risk was excluded from either of the first two groups.

The first variable selected was severity of injury, originally divided into four categories: superficial, some concern, serious and nearly fatal (see Liebling, 1991 for elaboration). Consistent with the literature, severity of injury did not correlate with other combined measures of suicidal activity, such as reported thoughts of suicide or describing one's own actions in terms of a suicide attempt. In accordance with the literature in the field, it was concluded that severity of injury alone did not necessarily indicate the severity of intent affordable to the attempt.

Two other variables were possible selectors of the 'most seriously at risk' group. The first of these was the response to the question: 'Have you ever seriously thought about suicide during this sentence?' that is, suicidal ideation. However, suicidal ideation is differentiated from suicide attempts in the literature (Hawton, 1986; Williams, 1989, pers. comm.), in part to distinguish the translation of ideation into action, from the 'mere' contemplation of suicide. This variable was therefore also felt to be inadequate for the purposes of any further analysis. A suicide attempt translated into action is one further step in the direction of self-inflicted death. Therefore the variable chosen to select out the most serious group of cases, was the question asked of the subject group towards the end of the interview: 'Would you say, then, that you would describe your injury during this sentence as an attempted suicide?' Responses were coded into three categories: 'yes', 'could have' and 'no'.'No' included those (few) members of the subject group and those members of the comparison group who had either not injured themselves at all, or who did not describe their self-injury as a suicide attempt. An example of an inmate in the subject group falling into this category said, for instance: 'I wouldn't call it a suicide attempt, no. I really just had to get off the unit. If I'd wanted to kill myself, I'd have done it.' There is a possibility of denial, so some selection was imposed if the researcher felt that all other information in the interview did after all indicate a suicide attempt. These cases were included in the next category, 'could have', which also comprised those inmates who were not sure whether they intended to kill themselves or not:

> Not seriously. I felt like it, I really did. But it's hard. I don't know, I was going to do it, and then I just thought. 'No!', and pressed the buzzer.

Finally, 'yes' included all those inmates who said they had made a serious and genuine suicide attempt during the sentence:

> I did mean to, yes. You just feel that there's no hope, when you're banged up looking at four walls; people just haven't got time for you. You think, 'what's the point?'. I tried to hang myself; I used my shoe laces – they snapped.

The inmates were then divided into three groups: those who had, in their own view, made a suicide attempt, those who had either made an ambivalent attempt, or who thought that they had come very close, and those who did not describe their actions as suicidal at all, or who had not injured themselves. The results were complex, and showed the middle-range group to have rather more significant differences from the non-attempters than the attempters did on some variables. Certain important differences did remain, however, leaving the basic hypothesis intact. The numbers are too small for statistical tests to be reliable. This exercise is especially tentative given the finding that most suicide attempts are 'ambivalent' to some degree. These explorations are presented as a warning to the reader not to assume that the answers to the prison suicide problem are clear, or known. Our search for understanding begins but cannot end here.

The 'serious suicide attempt' group

This group (n = 21) comprised those who described their own actions as a serious and unambivalent suicide attempt, in the light of the discussion of the incident, their feelings precipitating the attempt, and their reflections about it. They comprised 16 males and five females. This group were compared with all the other inmates, to see whether clear differences were apparent. What emerged was that the ambivalent group were in some areas found to show more significant differences from the comparison group than the 'serious suicide group'. Crudely, the distinctions between groups seemed to follow an inverted 'U'-curve, so that the ambivalent (middle) group scored more highly on a range of significance tests. This seemed important, as it was possible that two slightly different groups of suicide risks were appearing: the first, a clearly serious group of suicide attempters, individually and perhaps more personally disposed for a variety of reasons. This group were still affected by immediate or institutional variables, but had a less readily identifiable pattern to them as a group. This group could comprise (or contain) the most difficult group to identify or prevent: the determined suicide. The 'ambivalent' group may be those more directly affected by the prison situation:

less individually disposed (and therefore more preventable). A tabulated summary of the pattern that emerged looked as follows:

Significant differences between 'clear' and 'ambivalent' suicide attempters

Serious attempt group (n = 21)	Ambivalent attempt group (n = 11)
more offences of arson	more transfers
less affected by alcohol	less likely to know probation
more affected by drugs	officer
more time on remand	poor SER recommendation
(and for longer)	major drink problem
lived further from establishment	
time in care for behaviour problems	
more depressed after a visit	
less likely to report missing family	not keeping in touch with outside
miss people at night/weekend	
more serious difficulties with inmates	current problems with inmates
	made only friends in prison
more difficulties with staff	does nothing in cell
more disciplinary offences	least active
(of a more violent nature)	spends most time in cell
more of a disciplinary problem	spends more time as sentence
referred to doctor/psychiatrist	goes on
more injuries in custody	more previous injuries outside
attempt by hanging	many disciplinary offences

unstable accommodation plans
psychiatric treatment
lost more remission

The middle-range or ambivalent group may be less committed to the notion of suicide, still at risk, but on the edge, driven by circumstances, unable to cope with the immediate environment. This group: struggling with the sentence, and perhaps slightly less resourceful than most, could be easier to identify, and prevent. Closer to the threshold, their risk may be shorter-term, more environmentally dependent, and easier to reduce. Their attempts may be easier to interpret as 'attention-seeking', reflecting the ambivalence characteristic of their actions, but if denied rescue, the balance could just be tipped ('you try crying for help, and nothing happens – or you get shoved in strips. That just about finishes you off!').

What the above account shows, however cursorily, is that any simple or total theory of prison suicides is yet to be developed. As indicated in earlier chapters, it may be that other explanations besides the model outlined here must be sought for some groups of young prisoner suicides, for suicides occurring during the remand period, early in custody or amongst adult prisoners. This book presents a first model of the prison suicide process, a model which applies readily to the young sentenced prisoner not suffering from mental illness. The model requires testing, supplementing and adapting in the future by further research.[8] It represents the beginnings of a theory, not a general or conclusive model. What we can conclude is that listening to prisoners moves us further forwards in our endeavour to understand. In Chapter 8 we shall see that listening to staff is also a step which could have been usefully taken many years ago.

Chapter 7

In different words?

The gender factor

I was one of them ... I'd never seen anyone cut-up before, but I went and did it.
I felt helpless, I wasn't attention-seeking. It was all there was left to do ... hit in.
I was warned, told to hide it: 'They'll wash their hands of you!'. They saw it;
they said: 'People like you make me sick.' They screamed at me, then ignored
me. No-one ever asked me, 'how do you feel?'.

(Self-harmer, CMH Conference, 1988)

Throughout the nineteenth and into the twentieth century women reacted
differently from men to the pains of confinement in terms of physical self-injury
and psychological introspection ... Such individualized responses generated
further medical intervention into their lives reinforcing the view that it was they
rather than the pressurized structures and policies of the prisons that were at
fault.

(Sim, 1990:178)

You feel relief – and then disgust. It's like the blood from the injury is doing the
crying for me, 'letting' out the pain.

(Consumers of Mental Health Services, 1988)

At first, I was repulsed by the very *idea*, when I saw other inmates who'd done
it. Then one day I'd been locked in strips, everything was getting on top of me.
I'd had a bad letter from home, I wasn't getting any visits; I'd been thinking
about the consequences of what I'd done – I was depressed. I hit out at the
window – smashed it. I was shocked – but felt, for the *first time*, an *inner peace*,
as though I was released from all the strain.

(Ibid.)

INTRODUCTION

This book set out to explore and understand the problem of suicide and self-injury
amongst young offenders in custody. As such, the research upon which it is based
has considered males and females. Possible differences between male and female
patterns of and explanations for self-injury were expected, although the scale and
complexity of these differences was not anticipated. The naivity of the author's

approach to her subject now better understood, I would with hindsight advocate a more systematic and informed consideration of the gender issues raised in this chapter. As it is, they are raised but not resolved. In retrospect, as will be seen from the discussion, it would appear that gender differences are strong enough to make research on prison suicide attempts amongst both males and females too complex for a single enterprise. On the other hand, restricting the research to one or other gender blinds us to features of the individual, their situation and the prison experience which are more significant for one gender than for the other. Without comparative research, the two fields of male and female imprisonment will have nothing to teach each other. It will be for future research to explore in more depth and with greater expertise the complexities of male–female differences in prison life. This chapter sets out with some humility to express those differences that were found in the research. It considers possible explanations for these differences and sets them in a context of literature and research on women's imprisonment and women's self-harm.

SECTION I: SUICIDE AND SELF-INJURY IN WOMEN'S PRISONS

Few women have committed suicide in prison. According to official figures, seven women have died by suicide in prisons in England and Wales between 1973 and 1986 (Dooley, 1990a; Home Office, 1986a). Two more recent deaths by suicide occurred at Risley remand centre in Cheshire, in 1989 and at Durham, in 1990. Backett's study of suicide in Scottish prisons found that of 33 deaths recorded as suicide between 1970 and 1982, all were male (Backett, 1987). Dooley's study of prison suicides in England and Wales between 1972 and 1987 found that five females had been classified as suicides. The suicide rate for women in prison is slightly lower than for men (Dooley, 1990a). Of all prison suicides between 1972 and 1987, 1.7 per cent were female; women constituted 3.5 per cent of the total prison population during that time. Dooley's study of 'probable suicides' not classified as such showed that deaths by women in custody were significantly less likely to receive a verdict of suicide than men: of 52 consciously self-inflicted deaths occurring in prisons between 1972 and 1987, 7.8 per cent were by women (Dooley, 1990b:231). Dooley argues that this finding could be explained by chance, but that equally likely is the possibility that 'it may be related to the fact that deliberate self-injury is more commonly seen in females, both in the general population and in prison, again bringing into question the intent' (Dooley, 1990b:232). In women, suicidal intent is not expected: other explanations for their self-inflicted injuries are found.

   Most of the recent studies or reports on suicides in prison do not refer to women (Home Office 1984, 1986a; 1990d; Backett, 1987; see Chapter 2). Those that do point out that one of the factors associated with 'risk' in inmates is being male. Studies assessing factors associated with suicide in inmate populations are based on information collected only for the male population. A recent Home Office Report argued, for example: 'it is known that remand status, a history of previous suicide attempt and a history of psychiatric treatment are all associated with higher than average risk'(Home Office, 1986a:8). Women are not mentioned in this report, despite the fact that a high proportion of female inmates are on remand (4.8 per cent: higher than their percentage of the prison population (Casale, 1989)), they are more likely to have a history of psychiatric treatment, and indeed, many have a history of suicide attempts. It could be argued that more female than male receptions into custody present risk factors associated with suicide. The only studies of female deaths in custody in the UK have been published in association with campaigning groups or organisations with gender interests at heart (Scraton and Chadwick, 1986; Women's Equality Group, 1987; Gibbons, 1990). They are deliberately non-empirical, and unrelated to the literature on imprisonment or prison suicide for men.

The pattern of relative neglect is reversed when self-injury is considered: 'One need more prevalent in the female prison population than among male prisoners manifests itself in the phenomenon of self-injury' (Casale, 1989:89). Women far outnumber men in terms of the number of incidents of self-injury per head of population. Cookson found that self-injury occurred in individual women's prisons at a rate of at least 1.5 incidents per week (Cookson, 1977:335). This is a cautious estimate at best. There may be a core group of women in one institution who account for most of the incidents that occur. Twenty or thirty episodes of cutting during one sentence is not unusual for particular female inmates. Wilkins and Coid found that 7.5 per cent of women received into Holloway had a previous history of self-mutilation (Wilkins and Coid, 1990). An earlier study by Turner and Tofler found that 21 per cent of the women remanded into Holloway had 'attempted suicide' (Turner and Tofler, 1986).

In England and Wales there were 734 recorded incidents of female inmates injuring themselves over a 15-month period (1984/85 Prisons Report (Home Office, 1986b)). This represents 0.1 per cent of the average daily prison population. Baldwin compares this with the incidence amongst males (Baldwin, 1988). In the same period, 983 incidents were recorded, a rate of 0.005 per cent of the average daily population. Baldwin argues that 'self-injury is probably the most common form of behavioural disturbance in women's prisons'. Although it may be part of an illness, 'it can occur in other situations as a manifestation of personality difficulties, or more commonly, a response to environmental stress' (Baldwin, 1988:63). The problem with Baldwin's analysis is that the frequency of repeat injuries (that is, many injuries by relatively few women) makes these comparisons of limited value. She does not refer to recording practices either, assuming that recorded self-injury is a consistent and valid reflection of its prevalence.

Cookson studied self-injury in a closed prison for women (Holloway) during a six-month period from the beginning of 1974 (Cookson, 1977). She found that the self-mutilating women were younger than the average age of the general inmate population of Holloway; they had longer sentences, more previous custodial sentences, more psychiatric treatment, more violent offences and higher hostility scores. Details of 48 self-mutilating incidents by 39 women were collected. Most of the women (27) had injured themselves before; just over half (20) were sentenced, 18 were on remand; there was a tendency for self-injury to occur near the beginning of the sentence. The largest proportion of the incidents occurred on the hospital wing (13), but episodes occurred on seven of the eight wings of the prison; only the mother and baby unit had no incidents to report. Of those for whom the information was available, about half (17) the incidents appeared to have a precipitating 'cause', such as disciplinary action, bad news or a quarrel with another inmate. Over half of the women were given extra medicine or other treatment as a result of the incident. Nineteen out of thirty women for whom the information was available had been in-patients in psychiatric hospitals. None of the incidents could be described as attempted suicide, according to the author; instead, it appeared that overall, 'tension relief' was the aim of the behaviour. Precipitating events included the cancellation of parole (disappointing young children to whom no explanation could be given); unwanted transfers; cancellation of home leave; changing court appearances; custody action; distressing (or incomplete) news; and removal of a cell-mate. According to Cookson: 'It can be seen from these examples that helplessness and uncertainty may precipitate self-injury' (Cookson, 1977:345).

Cullen compared 50 young female trainees who did not injure themselves with 45 who had, during six months of a period of Borstal training at Bullwood Hall (Cullen, 1981). The self-injurers included 11 who had also attempted suicide. The self-injurers were more likely to have had regular psychiatric treatment, to have made previous suicide attempts, and to have received governors' reports for serious institutional rule violations. The training house that had a 'therapeutic regime' with group counselling as the central element of its programme had by far the lowest rate of self-injury during the study period, 'and both staff and trainees described it in overwhelmingly favourable terms': 'Staff and trainees rated support, expression, involvement, and personal-problem orientation as the most important aspects of this injury-free environment' (Cullen, 1981:139). Most of the incidents occurred between 6 p.m. and midnight, while the trainee was alone in her cell. The main reasons given were depression (25), homesickness (12), escape or avoiding a problem (eight), desire for sympathy (five) and feelings of guilt (five).

According to Cullen, self-injury was an operant (instrumental) behaviour, occurring in an environment in which other 'escape' responses were limited. It was intended to reduce tension, attract sympathy and comfort, to punish oneself or to manipulate a change. A reduction in self-injury occurred when staff were encouraged to reward injury-free periods with attention and practical help. During this experimental period (only) it was found that trainees were less likely to repeat an attempt, once one incident had occurred. This therapeutic response has been found to reduce levels of self-injury in other studies (Ross et al., 1978).

Cullen also found that suicide attempters were discernibly different from those who only injured themselves; self-injurers had more custodial experience. Suicide attempters were less likely to have children. He also distinguished between two types of self-injurer in his study. The first and largest group comprised those who injured themselves once or twice within a few weeks of their arrival, relatively superficially. This group responded well to practical intervention and advice. The second (small) group committed numerous injuries and appeared immune to efforts at positive intervention.

Three unpublished papers by Coid and his associates comprise the largest and most recent study of self-mutilation amongst female prisoners (Coid *et al.*, 1990a; 1990b; Wilkins and Coid, 1990). Their study consisted of structured interviews carried out with 974 women remanded into Holloway over an eight-week period. Seventy-four (7.5 per cent) were found to have a history of self-mutilation. Overdoses and hanging attempts alone were excluded from the study. Only five of the women were injuring themselves for the first time on reception into custody. Fifteen (20 per cent) of the women had cut themselves for a second (third, etc.) time within the short period between their reception and the interview (Wilkins and Coid, 1990:7). Most of the women described a progressive build-up of symptoms of anxiety, dysphoria, irritability and feelings of emptiness prior to the injury. Nine of the women (12 per cent) said they were intending to kill themselves. Others described wanting to relieve tension, anger and feelings of depression. The subject group were more likely to have been convicted of violence or property damage than the controls and were more likely to have received psychiatric treatment, usually receiving diagnoses confined to the categories of (borderline) personality disorder. The subject group were significantly more likely to have a history of alcohol abuse, disorders of appetite and other 'impulse disorders' (Wilkins and Coid, 1990:11). The extent of family disruption, physical and sexual abuse in their histories was 'depressingly high'. Most of the incidents occurred in the evening. Low self-esteem and a failure to comply with treatment also characterised the self-injuring women.

Coid and his team carried out a cluster analysis based on the profiles of the self-injuring women, and concluded that a sub-group could be identified, 'with an endogenous disorder of mood who injured themselves as a symptom-relieving mechanism' (Coid *et al.*, 1990a). The second, more heterogeneous cluster were more likely to have injured themselves as a reaction to life events, psychotic illness or as a suicide attempt. The first group were younger at the age of onset of the behaviour, had injured themselves more often, in a variety of ways, and they could not explain their injuries in terms of external events. The authors argue that the 'endogenous' group manifest a complex syndrome with a multi-factorial aetiology and a poor outcome. The form and content of this syndrome requires further research. The 'reactive' group may have injured themselves more severely, and were likely to have carried it out as a 'symbolic gesture of distress' (Coid *et al.*, 1990a:9). Coid and colleagues conclude that the 'reactive' group have more in common with the control group of prisoners, and may be reacting to both external life events and environmental pressures. Despite the large sample size and the frequency of incidents of self-injury included in this collection of studies, little is learned about the pathway to self-injury amongst women either as prisoners, or earlier in their lives.

An important final study of relevance to a consideration of self-injury in women's prisons was carried out by Mandaraka-Sheppherd in six women's prisons in England and Wales. The study is concerned with aggression in prison, and omits to consider self-injury (for example, as one possible manifestation of aggressive impulses, or as an example of 'misbehaviour'), but the approach of the study and its conclusions provide some additional insight into the possible contribution of environmental factors to self-destructive behaviour in women's prisons:

> A review of the existing literature on residential institutions for young offenders, mental hospitals and schools, suggests that institutional processes are, on the whole, more important than individual differences in determining when and how misbehaviour takes place. However, existing studies of *prisons* have not paid sufficient attention to the importance of institutional variables.
>
> (Mandaraka-Sheppherd, 1986:xi)

This book also constitutes one of the best and most detailed studies of women's imprisonment. Based on the extensive use of attitude scales and questionnaires, Mandaraka-Sheppherd found that when differences in individual characteristics were controlled, it appeared that the prison and the nature of its organisation bore an independent relationship to both minor and serious misbehaviour. Misbehaviour, she concludes, is 'a product of the interactions between the individual entering prison and the various pressures encountered there' (Mandaraka-Sheppherd, 1986:xi).

Mandaraka-Sheppherd's study was primarily concerned with the nature and extent of rule violations in women's prisons, in order to understand the context in which such behaviour occurs, and with finding ways in which it could be counteracted and prevented. Perhaps her most important conclusion is that: 'we can more successfully predict situations in which violence will occur than to predict those persons who will act violently' (Mandaraka-Sheppherd, 1986:104). She found that friction among inmates was caused by trivial things which (according to the inmates) would not have caused problems outside the prison. Boredom and provocation, and unreasonable or unfair treatment by the staff were thought to contribute to arguments and fights. The denial of rights, favouritism and constant security checks were also found to contribute to friction. For both minor and serious misbehaviour, the younger age groups (18–23, 23–29) misbehaved more frequently than the older groups. It was also found that single women and those without children tended to misbehave more frequently: 'The fact that the young and single inmates are more troublesome than the older and married ones, has been pointed out by all the studies dealing with misbehaviour in prison' (Mandaraka-Sheppherd, 1986:104).

In contrast to the adaptation 'types' suggested in much of the sociological literature, it seemed that in (women's) prisons the inmates did not organise themselves into a cohesive and anti-institutional group but rather, '*anomie* prevailed in their social system' (Mandaraka-Sheppherd, 1986:129). She found that although inmates in the more coercive regimes appeared to be more defiant towards the institution, they did not seem to adhere to friendships of a cohesive social system. A coercive regime did not bind female inmates together, but contained rather individualistic inmates who mistrusted each other as well as the staff. Younger inmates were found to be more defiant and hostile towards other inmates, especially if single; this defiance increased with higher levels of reported victimisation. Younger inmates were found to have a more negative self-esteem, and to identify less with the staff. They were more likely to be victimised by other inmates. Inmates increased in confidence, 'hardness' and stability as the months of a sentence went by: the longer the exposure of inmates to the institution, the worse their behaviour became. Those inmates who imagined themselves more negatively in the eyes of the staff were more likely to score highly on the misbehaviour scale. Inmates who were unstable and unsure of themselves were more likely to be victims in prison than stable and confident inmates (Mandaraka-Sheppherd, 1986). The author concludes: 'it seems that to a very large extent serious misbehaviour of women in prisons is directly a function of their responses to the particular negative aspects of institutions' (Mandaraka-Sheppherd, 1986:189).

Institutional features found to be conducive to bad behaviour were: severe methods of punishment, a lack of incentives for good behaviour, variations in the quality of staff/inmate relations and the composition of the staff. Mandaraka-Sheppherd concludes that the functional and importation models of prison behaviour are useful, but should be supplemented by a consideration of inmates' perceptions and expectations. This conclusion is supported by the results of the research reported in Chapters 6 and 7. It is clear from this and other studies that the experience of imprisonment for both males and females is not a uniform one, and that perceptions and expectations constitute an important element in our understanding of the development of suicidal feelings in prison and the extent to which they are brought about by aspects of imprisonment itself.

Two clear omissions in the studies outlined above are: first, any consideration of women's experiences of the distress leading to self-injury, or any adequate theoretical explanation for it. The presence of 'low self-esteem' is documented without any analysis of what the 'lack of self-esteem *feels like*' (self-harmer, Consumers of Mental Health Services, 1989). Secondly, the application of previous research on suicides in prison, or on any aspect of imprisonment – research which is normally about men – is omitted, so that comparisons, refutations or adaptations based on this material cannot be made.

In the community, it has been suggested that important differences exist between men and women in relation to suicide and suicide attempts (Birtchnell and Alacron, 1971; Lester and Gatto, 1989; Stephens, 1987). Women are thought to show less suicide intent than men, the ratio on unsuccessful attempts to suicide being much higher amongst women. They appear more concerned with present feelings (for example, feeling lonely or unwanted) than with feelings about the past (for example, feeling ashamed of something, or that they had failed in life), which are more often reported by male suicide attempters (Birtchnell and Alacron, 1971). According to this study: 'men are more reluctant to attempt suicide; they think about it longer; they need to be more depressed; and when they do it they are more determined and consequently more often they succeed' (Birtchnell and Alacron, 1971:51).

Other studies, however, show that women are more likely to suffer from depression (Vrandenberg et al., 1986; Stoppard and Paisley, 1987; Brown and Harris, 1978), that they are increasingly likely to both attempt and commit suicide (McClure, 1984a), and that a verdict of suicide is less likely to be brought in the care of a women, in part because of assumptions about their low suicide intent (Dooley, 1990b). Many of the differences reported in research in relation to male–female suicide are subject to challenge: perhaps the gap is closing (Anderson, 1987:45).

The experience of imprisonment: a different world?

Most studies of women's imprisonment look at women in isolation from men (Carlen, 1983; Morris, 1987; Dobash et al., 1986; Women's Equality Group, 1987). Comparisons between men's and women's imprisonment are therefore weak or unfounded, based on a separate analysis of the prison experience informed by particular conceptions of women's socialisation patterns or sexuality (Mandaraka-Sheppherd, 1986; Dobash et al., 1986). Any complete dichotomy between male and female experiences of imprisonment is misleading, despite the many differences existing between male and female penal establishments and their organisation. One of the important findings of the research reported in this book, as we shall see below, has been the consistency of the pains of imprisonment, regardless of gender. Isolation and boredom are gender-neutral, to a large extent, as are their remedies. A missing feature of penal discourse is any sophisticated or empirically tested dialogue about the differences and similarities between males and females in the prison experience, and in prison behaviour.

The next section will discuss differences found between the males and the females in the research. This will be followed by an examination of the differences related to their suicide attempts and self-injury. It should be remembered throughout these accounts that the numbers in each group are rather small, and that the numbers of women are not equal to the numbers of men. This will place limitations on the validity of the results reported. As indicated earlier, this section is exploratory, raising more questions than it can answer.

SECTION II: DIFFERENCES BETWEEN THE YOUNG MALES AND YOUNG FEMALES

In the research carried out by the author, the women prisoners as a group were slightly older than the young men. This was due to their accommodation in adult establishments, which often resulted in a slight delay in reclassification as adult on reaching 21, since no geographical move was required. Many of the 'young offenders' referred to me during the course of the fieldwork were therefore 21. The proportion of Afro-Caribbean inmates amongst the women was higher, at 16 per cent, reflecting their greater proportion amongst the female prison population, but also in one particular establishment in the South East. The young women were significantly more likely to have been convicted of violent or drug-related offences, robbery and arson; the men were more frequently convicted of burglary. The only two homicide cases in the research were female. The women tended to be older than the men at first conviction (often 16–18), and they had slightly less previous convictions. Previous sentences received were different, reflecting differences in provision (no attendance centre orders, detention centre sentences for women, etc.), as well as differences in offending behaviour.

The women were slightly less likely to have been living with their parents before coming into custody. They were more likely to be living on their own or with friends. They were also more likely to be going out to a different address on release from that given on reception, if they had anywhere to go at all. They were less likely to be in touch with their parents. More of the women (37 per cent) had children.

The two suicides of family members were amongst the male groups. A previous psychiatric history was equally common between them, but the women were slightly more likely to have received in-patient care (28 per cent compared to 13 per cent). *Far more of the women reported having been sexually abused (31 per cent, almost exclusively by male members of the family). They were also more likely to have experienced violence at home (see Table 7.1). Their educational histories showed no differences, the women being equally poorly qualified, having truanted frequently from school. The women were more likely to blame particular problems at home and school for their truancy. Fewer of the women had been bullied, but more had been involved in fighting at school. More of the women (63 per cent) reported having used a wide range of drugs on the outside.

The experience of imprisonment

The women were more likely to spend their sentence in dormitory conditions, and preferred to share a cell or room. They spent less of their daytime locked up, but suffered only slightly less from increasing boredom. It appeared that women found it easier to make friends in prison, and that their friendships originated from prison, rather than being part of any outside life. The young women reported slightly fewer difficulties with other inmates. More of the women received between four and ten disciplinary punishments, often for minor offences, but also for disruptive behaviour. The young men, on the other hand, could be divided into those who received few punishments and those who were in constant trouble in the institution. Fewer of the women believed the disciplinary system to be fair, and slightly more of the women presented as a 'disciplinary problem' within the establishment. Accordingly, the young women were more likely to have spent more time in solitary confinement for a mixture of reasons, with those isolated as a result of potential suicide risk often having been punished for their behaviour at other times, and a small group having been isolated for rather long periods.

Table 7.1   Parental violence and sexual abuse

	Male No. (%)	Female No. (%)	Male SG No. (%)	Male CG No. (%)	Female SG No. (%)	Female CG No. (%)
Witnessed:						
between parents						
none	29 (44)	12 (38)	12 (37)	17 (50)	5 (31)	7 (44)
minor	17 (26)	9 (28)	6 (19)	11 (32)	3 (19)	6 (38)
repeated	12 (18)	7 (22)	7 (22)	5 (15)	5 (31)	2 (12)
hospitalisation	8 (12)	4 (12)	7 (22)	1 (3)	3 (19)	1 (6)
Totals	66(100)	32(100)	32(100)	34(100)	16(100)	16(100)
		n.s.		$p<0.05$		n.s.
Experienced:						
none	24 (36)	13 (41)	8 (25)	16 (47)	7 (44)	6 (37)
minor	20 (30)	3 (9)	8 (25)	12 (35)	1 (6)	2 (13)
repeated	18 (27)	13 (41)	13 (41)	5 (15)	5 (31)	8 (50)
hospitalisation	4 (6)	3 (9)	3 (9)	1 (3)	3 (19)	-- --
Totals	66(100)	32(100)	32(100)	36(100)	16(100)	16(100)
	$p<0.08$			$p<0.02$		n.s.

	Male No. (%)	Female No. (%)	Male SG No. (%)	Male CG No. (%)	Female SG No. (%)	Female CG No. (%)
Sex abuse:						
None	62 (91)	21 (66)	30 (88)	32 (94)	9 (56)	12 (75)
yes family	2 (3)	10 (31)	2 (6)	-- --	6 (38)	4 (25)
yes other	4 (6)	1 (3)	2 (6)	2 (6)	1 (6)	-- --
Totals	68(100)	32(100)	34(100)	34(100)	16(100)	16(100)
	$p<0.005$			n.s.		n.s.

The women were more likely to have been referred regularly to the doctor and to the psychiatrist, and they were more likely to report current outside problems (see Table 7.2). They reported more problems relating to visits, and were more likely to report wanting both more letters and more visits. The women were much more likely to see visits and letters as helping them through the sentence, although they were more likely to feel anxious about them, to spend time thinking about their families, and to feel depressed after visits. Fewer of the women had had a recent change of probation officer (although this was still 47 per cent), so that more of the women knew their probation officer. They more often wanted to change something personal about themselves, and were more likely to talk to someone in prison about their problems if they had any, and were especially more likely to turn to staff when they needed help (29 per cent compared to 12 per cent of the men;

Table 7.2   Referrals to doctor and psychiatrist

			Male		Female	
	Male No. *(%)*	*Female* No. *(%)*	*SG* No. *(%)*	*CG* No. *(%)*	*SG* No. *(%)*	*CG* No. *(%)*
Referral to doctor?						
none	32 (47)	7 (22)	8 (23)	24 (71)	1 (6)	6 (38)
some	30 (44)	20 (62)	21 (62)	9 (26)	11 (69)	9 (56)
often	6 (9)	5 (16)	5 (15)	1 (3)	4 (25)	1 (6)
Totals	68(100)	32(100)	34(100)	34(100)	16(100)	16(100)
	$p<0.05$		$p<0.005$		$p<0.05$	
Referral to psychiatrist?						
none	46 (68)	14 (44)	17 (50)	29 (85)	5 (31)	9 (56)
yes	4 (6)	10 (31)	4 (12)	– –	5 (31)	5 (31)
current	18 (26)	8 (25)	13 (38)	5 (15)	6 (38)	2 (13)
Totals	68(100)	32(100)	34(100)	34(100)	16(100)	16(100)
	$p<0.005$		$p<0.01$		$p<0.08$	
Current problems?						
none	34 (51)	7 (22)	9 (26)	25 (73)	1 (6)	6 (38)
inside	9 (13)	5 (16)	6 (18)	3 (9)	4 (25)	1 (6)
outside	6 (9)	14 (44)	2 (6)	4 (12)	6 (38)	8 (50)
both	19 (28)	6 (19)	17 (50)	2 (6)	5 (31)	1 (6)
Totals	68(100)	32(100)	34(100)	34(100)	16(100)	16(100)
	$p<0.005$		$p<0.005$		$p<0.02$	

more of the young men said they would keep the problem to themselves (64 per cent), or said they would find themselves something to do to take their minds off it. The women were far more likely to day-dream. Finally, the young men were more likely to report 'bang up' as being one of the main problems of imprisonment than the women, who found the lack of freedom and lack of access to their families more difficult (see Table 7.3).

Thoughts and experience of suicide

Slightly more of the male subject group reported having had serious thoughts of suicide whilst in prison (92 per cent). A quarter of the female subject group would not describe their injury (or threat) as a 'real' suicide attempt. On the other hand, more of the female comparison group had thought about suicide at some stage during the sentence, or during a past sentence (37 per cent). As we shall see throughout, this variable (having thought about suicide during the sentence), and most other measures of current suicide risk, cannot clearly differentiate the two female groups from each other, whereas the young males can be differentiated more easily according to a range of variables relating to suicide risk. The women were more likely to report knowing someone who had committed or attempted suicide. The smaller size of the female estate could account for this difference. Slightly

Table 7.3 Contacts with family

	Male No. (%)	Female No. (%)	Male SG No. (%)	Male CG No. (%)	Female SG No. (%)	Female CG No. (%)
Frequency of visits?						
every 2 wks	18 (27)	8 (25)	7 (21)	11 (32)	2 (12)	6 (38)
once a month	11 (16)	8 (25)	3 (9)	8 (24)	2 (12)	6 (38)
few months	19 (28)	4 (12)	11 (32)	8 (24)	1 (6)	3 (19)
rare	6 (9)	6 (19)	3 (9)	3 (9)	5 (32)	1 (6)
none	14 (21)	6 (19)	10 (29)	4 (12)	6 (38)	– –
Totals	68(100)	32(100)	34(100)	34(100)	16(100)	16(100)
		n.s.	$p<0.09$		$p<0.005$	
Problems with visits?						
none	24 (36)	4 (13)	10 (29)	14 (42)	2 (14)	2 (13)
some	30 (45)	15 (50)	17 (50)	13 (40)	6 (43)	9 (56)
several	13 (19)	11 (37)	7 (21)	6 (18)	6 (43)	5 (31)
Totals	67(100)	30(100)	34(100)	33(100)	14(100)	16(100)
	$p<0.02$		n.s.		n.s.	
Letters out per week?						
none	13 (19)	6 (19)	9 (27)	4 (12)	6 (38)	– –
1	20 (29)	7 (22)	13 (38)	7 (21)	5 (31)	2 (12)
2	13 (19)	9 (28)	4 (12)	9 (27)	3 (19)	6 (38)
3	8 (12)	5 (16)	5 (15)	3 (9)	1 (6)	4 (25)
4+	14 (21)	5 (16)	3 (9)	11 (32)	1 (6)	4 (25)
Totals	68(100)	32(100)	34(100)	34(100)	16(100)	16(100)
For 'none' v. '2+'		n.s.	$p<0.02$		$p<0.005$	
More letters or visits wanted?						
both	23 (34)	17 (57)	14 (41)	9 (27)	8 (57)	9 (56)
visits	20 (29)	5 (17)	9 (27)	11 (32)	3 (21)	2 (13)
letters	4 (6)	5 (17)	2 (6)	2 (6)	2 (14)	3 (19)
no	21 (31)	3 (10)	9 (26)	12 (35)	1 (7)	2 (12)
Totals	68(100)	30(100)	34(100)	34(100)	14(100)	16(100)
	$p<0.01$		n.s.		n.s	
Do visits and letters help through sentence?						
yes	45 (67)	28 (93)	21 (64)	24 (71)	13 (93)	15 (94)
no	20 (30)	2 (7)	11 (33)	9 (26)	1 (7)	1 (6)
other	2 (3)	– –	1 (3)	1 (3)	– –	– –
Totals	67(100)	32(100)	33(100)	34(100)	14(100)	16(100)
	$p<0.02$		n.s.		n.a.	
When was last visit?						
1–3 days	8 (12)	7 (22)	5 (15)	3 (9)	4 (25)	3 (19)
4–7 days	8 (12)	2 (6)	1 (3)	7 (21)	– –	2 (12)
8–14 days	16 (23)	4 (12)	8 (23)	8 (23)	– –	4 (25)
15–28 days	10 (15)	4 (12)	2 (6)	8 (23)	2 (12)	2 (12)
29 days+	26 (38)	15 (47)	18 (53)	8 (23)	10 (63)	5 (31)
Totals	68(100)	32(100)	34(100)	34(100)	16(100)	16(100)
		n.s.	$p<0.01$		$p<0.05$	

more of the women thought that depression was the main cause of suicides in prison. More of the male groups thought that being unable to handle the prison sentence was a major cause.

On some variables (e.g. family breakdown, suicide attempts in the family, feeling anxious before a visit, depressed afterwards and missing people) the female comparison group were significantly worse off than the subject group. The pattern reported in Chapter 6 of finding a whole range of variables which can distinguish the subject group from the comparison group in the expected direction does emerge, and these variables are summarised on p.190 (Young Female Prisoner Vulnerability Profile). The female subject group were more likely to do something negative, such as injuring themselves, banging their heads, being disruptive or getting depressed when bored than the male groups. The women were more likely to use the word 'depressed' in talking about their injuries than the men, who often said they were 'bored' and 'couldn't take any more'. Often the various groups appeared to be describing the same feelings, and the same outcome, but they used a slightly different language (see Lester and Gatto, 1989; Gilligan, 1982).

Gender differences in relation to suicide attempts and deliberate self-harm

There were several important differences between the suicide attempts and self-injury incidents carried out by the males and the females. Most of the women (56 per cent) cut their arms, although many also cut their legs and faces. It is significant that many of the women made several cuts, one of which may have required stitches, but the rest would be superficial or requiring only a plaster or steri-strip. None of the males cut their faces. In addition to cuts on their faces (which two of the women interviewed bitterly regretted), two of the women had also scarred their faces with scouring pads. Two of the three women to have cut their faces asked during the interview whether I thought the scars would heal, and whether it spoilt their appearance. Another woman cut herself all over her body, including her face, when she caught sight of herself in a mirror after a visit with her daughter and a male friend. She had been in the segregation block for several weeks, her hair had dried and showed dye growing out, and her legs were 'shapeless' after so long without proper exercise.

More of the women carried out their injuries in a dormitory, sometimes in the company of others. 'Mutual self-cutting' was not unusual. Two of the women injured themselves in the hospital and in the segregation unit – glass would be smuggled in from a period of exercise, or laces concealed about their person. The battle to eliminate such articles (which could also include plaster from the walls, rings from strip-clothing, plastic cups, fingernails and so on) between inmates and staff could become quite fierce. Far more of the males carried out their attempts or injuries at the weekend (38 per cent). None of the women injured themselves at the weekend, although many injured themselves on several different days. All of the female incidents occurred between 4 p.m. and 1 a.m. Fewer of their injuries were nearly fatal, although a similar proportion to those of the male group were serious enough to require prompt hospital treatment. All of the women who had carried out their injury or had tried to injure themselves reported that they occurred impulsively. Birtchnell and Alacron reported that males and females differed significantly in their periods of contemplation of suicide attempts, and that women were far more likely to act impulsively. Impulsivity, they argue, is significantly associated with low suicidal intent (Birtchnell and Alacron, 1971:47). Slightly more of the women felt that they would repeat their injuries (44 per cent).

The following profile summarises those variables found to distinguish the female subject group from the female comparison group to a level of statistical significance. As we can see, background factors of a slightly more 'pathological' nature, and aspects of imprisonment related to outside such as family contacts, dominate the profile. Having spent time on remand may be associated with the nature of the offence, the previous histories of these women and the requirement of a psychiatric report (see Allen, 1987).

Young female prisoner vulnerability profile

1 CJS History

Offence of arson or violence*

2 Background

Less than 3 months at previous address
Witnessing violence at home requiring hospitalisation*
Parental separation before 16
Truancy as a result of particular problems*
Previous (in- or out-patient) psychiatric treatment**
Major alcohol problems**
Multiple previous self-inflicted injuries*

3 Current sentence

Time spent on remand
Location (and solitary confinement) in hospital*
Not working in prison*
Dislike PE*
Spending more than minimum time in cell**
Inactive in cell*
Do something negative when bored*
Few friends or on own in prison
Difficulties with other inmates
Disciplinary offences for violence or disruption*
Disciplinary problem*
Long time spent in isolation**
Frequent referrals to doctor*/psychiatrist
Report current (especially outside) problems*

4 Family and outside support

Few visits**

Writes few letters**
Long time since last visit*
No contact with probation*
Missing people less
Missing people on special occasions
Not keeping in touch with outside*
Wants to forget outside (but cannot)*

5 Coping with custody

Finds being told what to do worst aspect of prison
Stays in room/cell when feeling down
Sleeping problems
Finds prison difficult (or both positive and negative)*
Suicidal thoughts/attempts*
Know others who have attempted/committed suicide in prison*
Thinks reason is unable to handle sentence**

Note:* p<0.05, ** p<0.005

Two conclusions can be drawn from this profile (with the same cautionary note as in Chapter 6: that this profile is a pattern only, and that many inmates at risk of suicide will not show these characteristics). First, women in prison suffer relatively more often than males from the problems associated with families and outside contacts. Problems in this area are a major cause of distress, and may contribute to the development of suicidal feelings. Decreasing contact with (and decreasing interest in) the outside world may be an indication of risk. Secondly, it appears that women in the subject group show more of the 'pathology model' characteristics associated with suicide, particularly in their violent histories (see Coid et al., 1990a, 1990b; Wilkins and Coid, 1990; also Smart, 1977). The 'importation' components of prison suicide may be more significant in the development of female prisoner suicides, where 'deprivation' variables contribute more to male suicidal crises (see Zingraff, 1980; and also Figure 9.1 (p.235), showing how these components may vary in individual cases). Some of the differences between the male and female 'vulnerability profile' may be confounded by differences in the content of their records and reports, and in the readiness of women to talk in terms of 'depression' and 'problems'. It is possible that psychiatric treatment is more readily available both outside and in prison and that all 'problem' variables (such as the abuse of alcohol) are more readily recorded or interpreted as 'problems' for women (see Allen, 1987; Gilligan, 1982; Vrandenberg et al., 1986). These are the dangers of comparative research.

DISCUSSION

There is no profile of the female suicide attempter in the literature. Studies of self-injury amongst females in custody tend to focus on the pathological and psychiatric aspects of the behaviour (Coid *et al.*, 1990a; Wilkins and Coid, 1990; see also Allen, 1987). This can be explained in part by the tendency to 'medicalise' women's problems and their criminality (see Sim, 1990; Women's Equality Group, 1987; Dobash *et al.*, 1986; Carlen, 1983; Smart, 1977), but this also represents apparent differences between vulnerable males and vulnerable females in custody. Few studies seek to understand female deliberate self-harm as a response to pain. Even fewer studies understand both male and female self-harm as a very real expression of their distress: a distress which may well emanate from within the boundaries of ordinary mental health. A conference organised by 'Consumers of Mental Health Services' in 1988 provided a forum for (mainly) women in the community, some of whom were ex-prisoners, to seek an understanding of this behaviour in their own language:

> Self-harm is a way of *controlling* anger and pain ... You *can* feel physical pain, it is easier to cope with than emotional pain.

> Self-harm is a way of expressing that *hurt* ... How else do you say: 'Inside, I feel like my *soul* is dying?'

One speaker told how her current label was 'schizophrenia: in remission ... an interesting case with a poor prognosis':

> My life was reduced to a history of symptoms ... *objectifying behaviour is dehumanizing!* ... You get this medical examination, an IQ test, questions about who the Prime Minister is ... what does that reveal about *a person's inner world*? Labels don't alleviate distress. Being a patient (prisoner) means being 'invalid', *if* you are listened to at all.

One of the oversights of any comparative analysis between males and females has been committed throughout this account: 'gender' has been interpreted as 'sex'. It was apparent during the research that many of the males (particularly the 'repeat-cutters', and some of the bullied) resembled the female subject group: they described the same histories and the same feelings. Amongst the males were a small number displaying the same 'self-cutting syndrome' identified by Coid and his associates in relation to female self-injury. Amongst the women were several suicidal inmates without previous injuries, and without the 'tension-relieving' aspect to their attempts. There is no exclusive difference between the males and the females in this research. Areas of overlap and similarity cannot be ignored. Some consideration of the notion of 'masculinity' and 'femininity' may be a more helpful route towards the understanding of gender differences in suicidal and self-injurious behaviour (see Stoppard and Paisley, 1987; Feather, 1985 and Lester and Gatto, 1989). Aspects of femininity (such as 'learned helplessness') contribute to the relatively greater vulnerability to depression shown by many women in the community. The prison population contains many males and females whose vulnerability is expressed as 'learned helplessness'. Learned constructiveness and increased self-esteem would ameliorate the depressive effects of such tendencies (Stoppard and Paisley, 1987).

Because of the small numbers involved in this analysis, it would be misleading to give too much weight to each variable. An overall pattern based on gender differences and found in the research reported here can be summarised as follows:

1 Slightly fewer clear differences between the subject and comparison groups can be found amongst the women, the comparison group showing many of the characteristics associated with adversity and poor coping ability found amongst the male subject group only.
2 Visits and contacts with the outside are more significant indications of (and causes of) suicide risk amongst women.
3 If the small number (32) of females in the two groups is removed from the analysis, the differences between the male groups *increase*: the extent of some of these differences had been masked by the presence of the women.
4 The concept of gender as 'sex' may be insufficient on its own for any explanation of vulnerability in prison. A notion of 'masculinity' and 'femininity' may be a useful supplement.

The female groups were less clearly differentiated from each other, appearing at extremes on many variables, but not necessarily in relation to their membership of the suicide attempt group. For the young males, other inmates and time spent in cells with nothing to do were major causes of distress, and the ability to cope with these difficulties clearly distinguished the subject group from the comparison group. For the young women, family contact (particularly regarding children) was more distressing, and slightly fewer clear and consistent differences between the female subject and comparison groups emerged (this will be in part due to the smaller number of women in the two groups). The basic hypothesis of the research outlined in this book: that many signs of vulnerability are consistently available for detection, and that imprisonment contributes disproportionately to the distress of such inmates, is confirmed. It applies more clearly, however, to the young males. Almost all of those variables found to distinguish the subject from the comparison group amongst the young males remained statistically significant when the female group were removed to be analysed separately. Some of the variables found to differentiate between the two female groups were different from those distinguishing the men. More of the young female comparison group reported having thought about suicide, for example, having problems sleeping at night, and so on. Those problems associated primarily with the subject group amongst the males, were simply more widespread amongst both groups of women. Both groups of women wanted to change themselves, both groups day-dreamed a lot, and expressed feelings of hopelessness.

Because the numbers were so small, and did not equal the numbers in the male groups, the conclusions relating to male–female differences are tentative. These results suggest that distinguishing the vulnerable from the less vulnerable young male is a more realistic prospect than distinguishing one group of female young prisoners from another. Too little is known about the characteristics and experiences of females in custody. The differential role of psychiatric morbidity should be considered. It is possible to see much of the female self-injurious behaviour as wholly self-destructive, without it being clearly related to suicide (in all cases). Much of the self-destructive behaviour by the male groups on the other hand, *can* be seen as instrumental, strategic or determined to achieve some outcome, either death, or the avoidance of present distress (see Elpern and Kemp, 1984 on this point). This difference is a matter of degree, however, and many similarities between these behaviours and the feelings and motivations associated with them, exist. Comparative research on all aspects of imprisonment is urgently needed. Other significant differences indicating the potential value of future research are that the women use *different words to describe their pain*, and that women offenders in custody as a group share a common background involving a level of violence, abuse, use of drugs and self-injury characteristic of only a sub-group of the males. What both groups wanted in response to their 'cries for help' and 'cries of pain' was the same:

> We want *nurturing* ... we want to *talk* ... we want to take the pain away ... we want to feel clean, and lovable. We want to believe in love ... we want to be mothered ... we want carers who may not understand, but who can *accept*.
>
> a chance to scream, to shout ... to cry ...
>
> We just want to be listened to ... by another human being.

Chapter 8

Managing to prevent suicide

Staff attitudes and perspectives

It's devastating to the staff. I'd feel that we haven't done our job properly. I suppose the word is inadequate. We feel inadequate. (Senior Officer)

I think everyone feels a certain amount of guilt and self-recrimination. Could we have done something about it? Should we have seen this coming? Should we have done more? (Governor)

You don't get so much your depressives.. it's more a case of people who are pressured. On the adult side it's different, you do get those who are going through a depression. Kids are different, it might happen out of the blue, it's more – immediate. Either way, the staff are in trouble. We're told we can spot the signs. Kids don't show those sort of signs. As for adults, those that are determined make a pretty good job of hiding the signs. So we're done for, really. You're told you can spot them, so you feel you haven't done your job properly if you don't. But you know, *we* don't want to lose them, either! (Prison Officer)

INTRODUCTION

Very little has been written about staff attitudes towards and opinions of suicides, suicide attempts and self-injury in prisons. Where they are mentioned, reference is usually made in the context of prevention procedures, outlining the various roles and responsibilities expected of them, and making some suggestion about training, often without any further detail about the content and feasibility of this training. Staff attitudes, experiences and problems are usually overlooked (Lloyd, 1990:46–47; Home Office, 1986a); neither is there likely to be any discussion of where suicide prevention fits amongst the many other varied tasks expected of a prison officer. Prison staff are, however, an essential component in the exploration of suicide and deliberate self-harm in prison. It is important to discover how this behaviour is understood by those who most often discover and deal with it, and how far prison officers are able (and willing) to identify or seek out possible risk factors.

Much of the material in this chapter is based on the combined results of the 80 formal interviews carried out with all grades of staff. In addition to these formal interviews, material from a substantial number of lengthy informal discussions is included in the account. The chapter begins by outlining the position of prison officers in young offender institutions, and presenting the major themes emerging from the interviews. Section I discusses staff views about the suicide problem in prison. What causes it, is it distinct from the problem of self-injury, and is it related to the experience of imprisonment in any way? Section II outlines the Circular Instruction issued to prison department establishments on suicide prevention, and discusses staff views about these instructions, about the way they work in practice, and the various problems relating to their implementation. Section III concerns staff attitudes towards their own role, and discusses the extent to which the identification and management of suicide risk fits into the more general work carried out by prison officers. Finally, Section IV presents the various problems identified by staff which may interfere with the successful implementation of the Circular and the acceptance by prison staff of their central role in the prevention of suicide.

THE PRISON OFFICER IN YOUNG OFFENDER INSTITUTIONS

On 1 July 1989, there were 31,271 members of the Prison Service, including those working in headquarters and regional offices (Home Office, 1989a). Of these, 22,832 are uniformed grades. Approximately 1,200 of this number are women. The average ratio of inmates to officers is 2.3 inmates per officer (NACRO, 1990).

Prison officers who work in young offender institutions may differ in several respects from staff in adult and/or local and remand prisons. Many of the officers interviewed expressed a preference for working with young inmates, commenting that there was more 'hope' with the youngsters, that they were still amenable to change. It was not unusual to find officers who had only worked with young offenders, or who, once transferred to a YOI, had remained in young offender establishments. One of their most significant shared characteristics was having a working knowledge of 'the old Borstal system', with its reformative regime, its non-uniformed style and its indeterminate sentence. This (now defunct) regime had enabled staff to influence a young inmate's release date, and great emphasis was placed on the relationship between housemasters, staff and 'trainees'. Even if staff were too young to have tasted this still savoured stage of prison service history themselves, older officers made sure that they knew 'it was better', and that life had never been quite the same since its abolition in 1983. Three of the four host establishments had in fact been (or at Styal, had contained) Borstals before the implementation of Criminal Justice Act, 1982, and all had retained a high proportion of their staff. Several features of the Borstal regime (such as the personal officer scheme) had been retained to some extent in the new Youth Custody Centres, or Young Offender Institutions, as they became in 1988. However, other more drastic changes, in the prison service as a whole (such as the implementation of Fresh Start, see note 4 in Introduction (p.246)), and in the young offender system, made retention of 'the best of the Borstal system' an uneven process.

It is likely then, that a core of the prison staff working in YOIs share some enthusiasm – if recently jaded – for notions of welfare and reform (Bottomley and Liebling, 1987; 1988). They are encouraged to get to know their charges, and this is facilitated in principle as YOIs do not have the constant throughput of locals and remand centres. They may have inherited a history of shared working with the probation service (O'Connor, 1984; MacAllister, 1990), having played a clear welfare role themselves in the past.

What the uniformed staff in young offender institutions share with other prison officers, however, is also important. They share the same job, the same training, the same career structure, the same working practices; they share a common history, and crucially, the same professional association. Many will have worked in several different types of establishment. Prison officers are a strong culturally bound body; they share a language. Like many highly structured (and uniformed) services, they share an ideology. Above all, at the time of this research, they shared in the effects of the recent implementation of Fresh Start.

Despite recent changes in recruitment policy and preference (McGurk and Fludger, 1987; Bagshaw and Baxter, 1987), a high proportion of (particularly senior) staff have a background in the uniformed services, or in other similar jobs. They are confident in action, in communication with others and in the exercise and receipt of well-defined and regulated authority. They are less confident at 'reaching for their pens'. The male side of the service is composed largely of middle-aged family men (Jones et al., 1977:171; OPCS, 1985:22; Stern, 1989a). They are better paid than their probation service colleagues, but have slipped behind their closest allies, the police, in recent years. Most of their daily work involves strict routines – unlocking, slopping out, feeding, escorting, counting, observing, receiving, discharging, searching and censoring, taking applications and locking up. Simply getting through the day according to the strict requirements of the prison routine is quite an achievement. Within and between the formal routines, there is the constant and inevitable 'relationship with inmates': firm, and sometimes troubled, but often committed. Individual efforts made to solve particular problems, or to develop an interest, or help inmates through times of crisis, must be one of the most under-estimated activities of the prison service staff. As a routine, however, the relationship is constrained by multiple other requirements. Prison officers deal daily with inmates' welfare – from providing them with their basic entitlements, through teaching them how to wash and dress, to saving their lives. This they do from the moment the inmates wake up, throughout every part of their day, and to some extent, their night. With the assistance of various specialists within establishments, a prison officer's job is to 'look after' inmates. What they do without specialist assistance is to keep them securely inside. Security is their specialism. Custody, care and control (Dunbar, 1985:30; Vinson, 1982:10) are the key features of a prison officer's job. How far they share this role with others is one of the central determinants of the priority and skills attributed to each.

Four major areas of enquiry were covered by the interviews and discussions with staff, that were thought to affect directly and indirectly how effectively and smoothly suicide prevention procedures operated in each establishment:

1 What do staff think are the main contributory factors to suicide in prison? What links do they see between suicide, attempted suicide and self-injury?
2 What problems do they experience in carrying out official prevention procedures?
3 How do these views and tasks fit into their overall perception of their role?
4 What problems do staff themselves face, that may interfere with the successful implementation of suicide prevention procedures?

In the account that follows, as with the inmate interviews, the categories into which responses fell emerged from the interviews and discussions; very few of the questions were pre-coded. Staff are talking, in so far as this was possible, in their own words.

SECTION I: THE NATURE OF THE PROBLEM

An important aim of the staff interviews was to elicit their views and understanding of the problems of suicide and self-injury in prison. How far were the causes personal and individual – or related to the situation in which inmates found themselves in prison? Staff views about suicide prevention procedures were inevitably informed by these opinions, and it seemed an important part of any meaningful exploration of suicide and self-injury in prison to consider how far, if at all, staff and inmate explanations of these problems differed.

Explanations offered for suicide in prison varied from hopelessness about the future, to experiencing particular problems inside prison:

> Insecurity, and a lack of future. Lack of future is one of the biggest problems here. (SO)[1]

> I think mainly it's peer pressure. (BGO)

> The main one is girlfriends – sometimes they're the only one that cares about them. Parents don't care for them, the schools don't care for them. (PO)

> I think a big motivator in that way is self-pity ... some can take it better than others. (SO)

> Frustration ... a sense that nothing can ever change for the better. (BGO)

> It must be a complete feeling of inadequacy – of failure. (BGO)

Some of the staff were less ready to suggest possible causes;

> I don't know. It's got me completely stumped. (SO)

> I don't know ... you're going into psychiatry now, which is not my field. (BGO)

Other staff referred to 'places like Risley', where suicide figures were high, arguing that the high rate was caused by bad conditions and overcrowding. This was not a typical response, however. Most of the staff located the causes of prison suicide in the individual – domestic problems, weakness or 'inadequacy' and psychiatric illness were the main causes of suicide in prison.

When given a choice of possibilities to rate on a three-point scale ('very important', 'quite important' and 'not very important' as factors causing suicides in prison), 'depression' was seen as the most common factor (see Table 8.1).

Table 8.1   Staff perceptions of main factors in prison suicide

	Staff indicating			
	V. imp. No. (%)	Q. imp. No. (%)	Not v. imp. No. (%))	Totals No. (%)
Depression	60 (77)	17 (22)	1 (1)	78 (100)
Lack of communication	51 (65)	21 (27)	6 (8)	78 (100)
Bad news or Dear John letter	45 (57)	31 (39)	3 (4)	79 (100)
Prison pressures	44 (56)	27 (34)	8 (10)	79 (100)
Mental illness/breakdown	40 (53)	29 (38)	7 (9)	76 (100)
Temper/anger	19 (24)	34 (44)	25 (32)	78 (100)
Boredom	17 (22)	33 (42)	28 (36)	78 (100)
Guilt (at the offence)	16 (21)	33 (42)	29 (37)	78 (100)

Depression and lack of communication from the outside were chosen as very important factors by the largest group of staff. Receiving bad news or a 'Dear John' letter from loved ones, prison pressures and mental illness or breakdown are seen as very important factors by over half of the staff. Boredom, guilt and anger were not seen as very important factors by many of the staff. Inmates in the subject group had rated prison pressures first, and had chosen boredom as a factor more often than the staff did (see Chapter 6, p.162). Two-thirds of the inmates had chosen depression as a factor in their attempts or injuries. Most of the staff commented that they rarely saw any evidence of guilt in their young inmates: those that did suffer, suffered badly. Significant differences were apparent in the various staff groups' ratings of the items given as possible factors.

Perhaps most interesting were the differences relating to mental illness, guilt and prison pressures. Hospital staff clearly ranked mental illness as one of the most common factors in prison suicide, with only depression ranking as high. Discipline officers also rated depression as the highest factor, putting lack of communication and prison pressures next. Guilt for the offence was thought to be a very important factor by only 9 per cent of the uniformed officers. The hospital staff (perhaps because they accommodate all receptions thought to be at risk of suicide due to the nature of the offence for their first few days in custody) were more likely to see guilt as a very important factor. Two factors could account for these differences.

First, levels of training, and working notions of 'the client' may differ between staff groups. Secondly, the level and type of communication between inmates and staff groups will differ, with discipline staff seeing inmates more frequently – some would argue more naturally – and over time, more diversely.

It is important to note that four of the five factors most highly rated as causes of suicide in prison are factors unrelated directly to the internal prison context. However, most of the categories given were 'non-prison' related. Lack of communication, and receipt of bad news could arguably be seen as indirectly relating to the prison situation, as a break-up in a relationship, or being unable to make contact with a relative at the time of death, may be two of the unintended consequences of imprisonment. These are factors that the prison officers see themselves as having no control over – bad news comes independently to the inmate from outside. Depression is projected onto the individual, and is rarely seen as relating (either directly or indirectly) to the prison situation. This location of the causes of depression occurred despite reports by inmates that (for example) bullying by other inmates is often a major factor in their current misery. There are difficulties inherent in assigning a 'problem' to the 'inside' or the 'outside': most are a combination (e.g. lack of communication from outside). It can be seen from the above findings, however, that staff were aware of many of the major problems facing inmates.

The tendency to locate the causes of the problem in the individual was borne out in the following responses: a view prevailed amongst uniformed and hospital staff that the causes of suicide in prison were personal and individual, rather than situational. Only 3 per cent of the uniformed officers thought that the causes were mainly situational:

> Yes, if an inmate feels there is a lack of understanding on the part of the staff; if she feels she's been discarded by society outside, and by the prison staff as well, then I would suspect that this can bring out grave feelings of wanting to end it all, which is why it is so important to show people who are in danger that they do have support and that there is someone who wants to help. (SO)

None of the hospital staff thought that the causes of suicide in prison were mainly situational. The majority of the discipline staff (63 per cent) felt that the causes of suicide in prison were largely personal and individual. The governor and specialist grades on the whole preferred a dual set of explanations, assuming that both personal and situational factors played a part (76 per cent).

An important question relating to these findings is, to what extent the prison situation might be (or be seen as) important in the understanding and prevention of suicide in prison? When given a list of possible factors to rate on a scale of importance, prison officers rated 'prison pressures' as amongst the most important factors contributing to suicide. This concept is rather vague, however, and difficult to define in an interview. When asked where they would locate the main causes of prison suicide: inside or outside, most felt that personal and individual factors were to blame, although only a third of the prison officers suggested that both situational

and personal factors might be responsible. Factors relating to the prison environment, or pressures directly or indirectly brought on by the prison situation were
less likely to be recognised as being important when given a choice. This perception
is consistent with the widespread assumption expressed by prison staff that suicides
in prison cannot be prevented or averted – as staff assume that most of the
significant factors are beyond their control. This does not altogether correspond to
the explanations offered by inmates, summarised earlier. On the contrary, many of
the final triggers precipitating suicidal thoughts and gestures were apparently
'trivial' or practical matters over which officers (or others) had considerable
influence. Many of the major factors relating to the prison situation (such as
transfers, parole delays and allocation decisions) were not in the hands of the
uniformed officers, but were part of a larger system that staff argued they had little
influence over. In this they were justified – their own lack of power to influence or
improve the lot of their charges was often manifested as resignation or detachment.
Those with the power to improve life for inmates were seen as distant and
unconcerned – about inmates or staff.

Few of the staff of any group had not experienced prisoner suicide or suicide
attempts at some stage in their career. The groups most likely to have experience
of an inmate suicide were the hospital staff and the governor grades, as they would
often be the first to be called to the scene. Over a quarter of the uniformed staff had
personally experienced the suicide of an inmate. Many of those having experienced
a suicide had also known several serious suicide attempts:

> I was a young lad – that upset me, actually. It would if any of these did. They
> must be really desperate to go that far. (PO)

Several staff members had been called upon to attend inquests, none of whom found
the experience an easy one. A third of the staff said they had felt shock, they had
felt upset and, in many cases, devastated when a suicide had occurred. Words like
'sad', 'powerless' and 'inadequate' came up often:

> It's devastating to the staff. I'd feel we haven't done our job properly. (Governor
> grade)

> You feel shattered – afterwards. (BGO)

> It was a big shock to me. I was frightened, and felt very down and depressed for
> a while. (PO)

Twenty-nine per cent of the staff (but 43 per cent of the uniformed grades) said that
they could cope with the situation as they would any other part of their job:

> I don't think now after 14 years that it would affect me personally – it might
> have at the beginning. I would want to look into whether there was anything
> more we could have done. (PO)

Twenty-one per cent of the staff (but 38 per cent of the hospital staff) said that they
would feel guilt or a sense of failure:

It's quite upsetting, actually. Guilt is one of the main problems, because we tend to be the recipient of a lot of the family's guilt as well, especially at coroners' inquests. (HSO)

Seventeen per cent of the staff said that they would feel a mixture of guilt, shock and in some cases, anger or frustration:

I feel angry at times because the lad has let himself get in such a state without communicating with anyone. I also feel angry because it could have been avoided if the lad had been in a therapeutic community or something similar. I guess I do feel angry with all these self-injurers, too, when they've come inside and got into debt, they're irresponsible. Also towards parents. It's often their fault. (HSO)

Officers frequently expressed the need for some staff counselling provision – one of the major oversights of current procedures (as they were at the time of this research). Everyone else's needs are taken into account – even on occasion, the cell-mate – if there is one. Officers and other staff felt they were just expected to cope.

Suicide and self-injury

Most of the staff – particularly the prison officers (74 per cent) – saw suicide and self-injury as being separate and distinct problems, with their own causes and motivating factors. The hospital officers and specialists saw some overlap or connection between them. Even so, most preferred to perceive the two behaviours separately.

I think the motives are very, very different. Most of the self-injury is in order to get something, or to get somewhere, or stop something. (BGO)

I think they are two separate problems. One is an attention-seeking action, the other is a despairing act. (Specialist – psychiatrist)

I think anyone who really wants to commit suicide will just do it and succeed. Most lads, I feel, are just doing it for a cry for help – they can't survive in here amongst the lads, they're weak, or they borrow money ... and then they'll do all sorts of things as a way of getting out of trouble – a transfer. (PO)

The view that self-injurers and suicide attempters have different profiles and motivations was common, despite some evidence, both in staff experience and training, that the two behaviours may be linked. Some saw a connection:

Yes, they're related. I would think that self-mutilation is the first stage, it is a cry for help, but a suicide attempt can be too. (HPO)

Well, they're separate problems, but the one can go over into the other, if they don't get the attention. (BGO)

They were asked how they would distinguish between a 'genuine' and a 'non-genuine' attempt or injury. Twenty per cent of the staff replied that this was difficult, and they could not answer. Most of those who would make a distinction would do so on the basis of method used (48 per cent of the total but over half of the uniformed officers), or factors relating to method, such as the extent of the injury, or its timing:

> Self-injury, he will bring to your attention, either by pressing his bell, or telling you that he's going to do it, and the injuries tend to be fairly superficial; whereas the genuine ones I have come across, there's no inkling at all. (PO)

> I think the first 12–24 hours in the Unfurnished Rooms is the way to tell the difference – some will very quickly start to talk once you get them there. This is if he is attention-seeking, or if he's under a little bit of pressure on the unit – he probably owes a bit of tobacco to the bigger lads ... they use it as a means of escape. With these ones, as soon as you lighten things up for them, they begin to talk. The genuine ones – the one's who've really attempted suicide, are probably in a bit of a pit. He'll stay there for quite a while, and he needs quite a bit of help to get him out of it. (Specialist – psychiatrist)

Others said they could not put their thoughts into words, but that they could tell the difference – it was intuition:

> That's the million-dollar question ... I don't know. I defy anyone to really know. Sometimes you have a gut feeling. (PO)

A remaining 24 per cent (but almost half of the hospital staff) replied that they could only tell after talking to the inmate concerned:

> I think there are indicators, but some of these you can only discover in relationship with the person, in talking and listening – how far is everything hopeless, or seen as hopeless? Where people use terms like, 'there's nothing there' ... 'emptiness', I think that is distinguishing. (Specialist – psychiatrist)

The experience of imprisonment

As we saw earlier, when asked directly about the causes of suicide in prison, staff were likely to blame the problem on personal and individual factors, sometimes seeing the causes as exacerbated by situational variants. However, staff (particularly uniformed officers) did say some telling things about prison-related factors, without actually expressing or acknowledging their significance in relation to suicide when faced with a choice between individual and situational factors. Life in the establishments as a whole – the regime, staff–inmate relationships, the inmate culture and the experience of imprisonment as a whole, were all identified as potential stressors or sources of problems.

Perhaps most significant, in the light of inmates' responses in the previous chapter, was the issue of bullying. The level of reported bullying and intimidation of inmates by each other was very high in the interviews. Few of the staff were able to say that inmates did not have to worry about their physical safety from each other. Uniformed officers were the least likely to report major problems when asked (still 54 per cent), without expressing some reservation or qualification, many suggesting that only a particular type of inmate was really at risk (40 per cent). This difference between uniformed staff and others might be explained by two factors. First, officers may be concerned about their own self-image, feeling reluctant to appear inadequate in their (primary) role as safe custodians. Alternatively, uniformed staff, who see more of the 'life' of the establishment may be expressing the realistic view that some but not all inmates have reason to worry about being physically attacked, or may have a more realistic appraisal of the actual levels of inmate victimisation apparent on the wings. Either way, reported levels were high.

Many of the staff added that the inmates' fears were justified, and that often quite serious violence occurred between inmates. Unexplained bruises and cuts were frequent, inmates often refusing to admit the pressure they were under, for fear of reprisals. The staff reporting 'some' problems either restricted their response to particular (groups of) inmates – such as the 'weak' or 'inadequate', or the 'Rule 43s' (those segregated for their own protection, because of the nature of their offence, or debts and so on; see Chapter 6). Others replied that most inmates had problems during particular phases of their sentences. Only 6 per cent of uniformed officers, and none of the other staff thought that inmates had little or nothing to worry about.

Bullying was seen as a major cause of self-injury, as inmates resorted to cutting themselves as a way of getting moved from a wing, or achieving a brief respite in the hospital. It was acknowledged by one or two of the staff that if the problem remained unresolved, this could lead to suicide, but often this was thought to be an accidental outcome resulting from a gesture or 'cry for help'. Hanging 'gestures' were more effective methods of removal from a wing, as they were taken more seriously. Inmates might progress from superficial scratching to 'staging a hanging', in order to force the staff to remove them to the hospital. Again and again, the example of an inmate listening for footsteps and keys before jumping from a chair or bed was given. He or she wanted to be rescued – inevitably, staff were delayed for some reason, and on occasion, the 'gesture' would go wrong. Alternatively, inmates would squeeze blood from their veins, trying to make the injuries look more serious than they were – or mix the blood with water, to increase the visual effect. Staff could be scathing about these 'gestures' – 'attention-seeking', 'manipulative' gestures, which forced the staff to respond. If the bullying or pressure the inmate was under was 'his own fault' – that is, if, for example, he owed tobacco – officers were all the more reluctant to give in to the pressure. Many of the more superficial of these incidents never led to an appearance in the hospital.

Generally, self-injury was not a successful method of achieving given ends. It was often seen as antagonistic towards the staff, particularly if it occurred (as it often did) at mealtimes or late at night. Particular officers might feel that an inmate had deliberately injured him or herself whilst they were on duty. These activities put the staff 'at risk', as they were obliged to follow precautionary procedures, and prevent any escalation of the behaviour. It was often seen as deliberate and calculated, with the degree of injury corresponding inversely with the degree of sympathy it received. Only one officer said:

I suppose they're telling us we're not paying them enough attention. (BGO)

Few of the staff moved beyond the 'attention-seeking' explanation, suggesting possible reasons why inmates might feel the need to demand attention in this way, or elaborating on the type of attention wanted from the staff. Their comments about suicide and self-injury tended to remain simple and pragmatic, unrelated to the features of prison life they identified later as problem areas.

Uniformed officers were slightly more likely than other staff groups to describe staff–inmate relationships at their establishment as good (54 per cent). Some of the staff reported difficulties – usually between individuals, or with particular members of staff. On the whole it was not felt that staff–inmate relationships were a major problem, and most of the officers liked to show how their wing surpassed others in this respect. This was a feature of most of the YOIs visited during the course of the research. Some pride in officers' ability to relate to inmates was apparent, particularly in individuals, or on particular wings. As we saw in Chapter 6, inmates' description of staff–inmate relationships were sometimes less generous.

The prison experience

The experience of imprisonment as described by staff is rather indifferent. It was said to have no impact on the majority of inmates, who simply accepted the fact of imprisonment as 'an occupational hazard'. Over half of the staff thought that inmates could find rewarding things to do at their establishment. Examples included work and educational opportunities, training and vocational courses, and sport. Just less than half of the staff said that inmates probably could find rewarding things to do, but that their opportunities were limited, either by the short amount of time they could spend out of their cells, or by the facilities on offer, and their suitability for the inmates. Only 3 per cent of the staff (uniformed and hospital officers only) thought that it was impossible to find anything rewarding to do at their establishment.

Not all inmates were willing to make use of these opportunities, however. Fourteen per cent of the staff said that inmates found nothing useful or interesting to do in prison, despite the opportunities (however limited) for them to do so. Sixty-two per cent thought that education, work and training were interesting and important activities for inmates and gave examples of programmes and courses that were popular and of direct benefit to the inmates. Other interesting activities included sport and gym (12 per cent), visits (4 per cent), and association (6 per cent). Many of the (particularly non-uniformed) staff said that they did not know what inmates found interesting or useful in prison, or commented that their own response was no more than an assumption about inmates' preferences, because they had never asked them.

Almost two-thirds of the staff thought that most inmates did not try to use their sentences constructively, but were just getting through it, 'keeping their heads down' and 'doing their time quietly'. Over a third thought that some inmates tried to use their sentence and many commented that these individuals 'stood out' in many respects from the average pool of inmates, often having more stable backgrounds outside. Only 2 per cent of the staff thought that inmates did try to use their sentences, on the whole.

The major problem faced by inmates, according to almost half of the staff, was lack of contact with their families (also chosen as one of the major factors causing prison suicides). Loss of freedom, and all that entailed was a second major problem (29 per cent): losing control of their lives, and having to rely on others for every contact, every movement and never having any privacy, or an outlet for frustrations. Other inmates were the main problem according to 15 per cent of the staff, mainly because of bullying, taxing,[2] and teasing:

> Anybody who's different will suffer ... snooty accent, or bad eyes, or a bit weak. (BGO)

Twelve per cent of the staff mentioned several of these problems. Others included boredom, the physical environment, parole and anxiety about what they will face when they get out. As we saw in Chapter 6, staff descriptions of the problems faced by inmates during a sentence are very close to their own. The only omission in the staff account of the problems faced by inmates is the problem of 'bang up'.

So what sort of experience was imprisonment, on the whole, or for the average inmate, if there was such a thing? Perhaps predictably, 41 per cent of the staff thought that it varied greatly, depending on the inmate, and often on his circumstances (e.g. family); for some, it was endurable, or even positive, for most just boring:

> It's not a good thing. It doesn't touch them ... it's just one of containment and boredom. (PO)

or it might vary throughout the sentence;

> Frightening to start with, then quite a bit of fun. As time goes on it becomes quite serious and sometimes boring. Then, they might do something with it towards the end, or they might just heave a great sigh of relief that it's all over. (PO)

For a few it was devastating:

> It's confusing, lonely and isolating. (PO)

SECTION II: SUICIDE PREVENTION PROCEDURES IN PRISON

Staff explanations of suicide, suicide attempts and self-injury in prison were related to their views about its management and prevention. It was an important aspect of this study to elicit staff views about the suicide prevention procedures laid down by the Home Office. How far did they help or inform staff about the problem; how relevant were they to the actual problems faced by those seeking to prevent suicide in prison; and how easy were the instructions to implement and follow?

With the implementation of Circular Instructions 3/1987 and 20/1989, suicide prevention was given a new emphasis within prison department establishments (see Introduction, this volume). Responsibilities were more clearly defined, and communication was facilitated between departments, and between wing staff themselves.

The Prison Service strategy for the prevention of suicide is set out clearly in Circular Instruction 20/1989 (hereafter, CI 20/89):

> The Prison Service has a duty to do everything it can to prevent inmates from committing suicide. Its strategy is based on the report of the Prison Department's Working Group on Suicide Prevention, which defined the Service's task as 'to take all reasonable steps to identify prisoners who are developing suicidal feelings; to treat and manage them in ways that are humane and are most likely to prevent suicide; and to promote recovery from suicidal crisis.'
>
> (CI 20/89:1)

The Prison Service's strategy for carrying out this task is to:

1 *Identify inmates who may be suicidal*, by means of
- systematic assessment by the Medical Officer on reception, assisted as necessary by Hospital Officers; and
- vigilance on the part of all staff throughout the inmate's time in custody.
2 *Help suicidal inmates to recover from crisis*
- by appropriate location in the hospital or elsewhere in the establishment; and
- through systematic and supportive contact with other inmates, with people outside the establishment, and above all with staff.
3 *Reduce the opportunities for suicide* without reducing the quality of life for inmates.
4 *Ensure that all staff are aware of the problem* of inmate suicide and how to prevent it by
- regular overviews by senior management, through the Suicide Prevention Management Group and its annual review;
- good communication with staff; and
- training.

(CI 20/89:1–2)

Prison officers are assigned the responsibility for the detection and referral of potentially suicidal inmates to the Medical Officer; they are required to 'offer maximum contact and support to any inmate thought to be at risk of suicide', and they are expected to carry out special supervision procedures, as instructed by the Medical Officer. The tasks of risk assessment and of the issuing of specific instructions for the management of potentially suicidal inmates rests with the

Medical Officer at each establishment, within clear guidelines provided by the Circular. Interim measures are to be carried out by hospital officers and nurses (CI 20/89:5). What the Circular makes clear is that the risk assessment 'is a matter for the Medical Officer' (CI 20/89:21). Prison officers are responsible for noticing 'signs of being at risk', and referring the inmate quickly and effectively to the hospital, 'for example if an inmate becomes upset or withdrawn after receiving a 'Dear John' letter, or talks of or threatens suicide' (CI 20/89:21).

After referral, and following assessment by the Medical Officer, instructions should return with the inmate to the staff on the wings, indicating that special watch procedures, or shared accommodation, should be initiated, until a further review is carried out. If the inmate is considered to be a serious enough risk to warrant immediate location on the hospital, the Wing Manager (Principal Officer) should be informed of such a decision, and this should be related to the originator of the referral form (F1997). Staff should then 'consider any further action which can be taken to assist the inmate' (CI 20/89:27).

The Circular stresses support, communication (both with the inmate and between departments) and contact with the inmate, suggesting that officers play a 'vital role' and stressing that the 'relationship between staff and suicidal inmates should be maintained, and wherever possible, enhanced'.

Attempts at suicide are to be managed or prevented in a similar way, so as to avert any further attempt:

> As a general rule any inmate who attempts suicide should be admitted to hospital immediately for at least 24 hours and the Medical Officer should attempt to probe the reasons behind the attempt and to deal with the underlying problem. The inmate should only be returned to normal location on the written authority of the Medical Officer, who should advise staff how he or she should be treated. The inmate should not be placed on a disciplinary report for his or her action and chaplains should be notified.
>
> (CI 20/89:39)

Unfortunately, the Circular gives no indication of what an 'attempt at suicide' includes. This leaves hospital and other staff with so much scope for discretion, and so little guidance for judgment, that individual establishments (and personnel) complete forms and follow rules inconsistently (see Chapter 4).

Procedures at all four of the host establishments had been overhauled to take account of the new instructions relating to suicide prevention. The introduction of two new forms – the F1996 (Reception Screening Form) and the F1997 (Suicide Risk Referral Form) had necessitated some training and reinforcement to persuade staff to use the new paperwork appropriately. All four centres had a recently formed suicide prevention management group; the chair of this group was normally given responsibility for the oversight of the new procedures. Problems emerged, however, and staff were eager to discuss these issues.

Prison staff training

Prison officers' initial training comprises a nine-week course at one of two national training centres (Newbold Revel and Wakefield), or at one of the emergency centres opened to cater for a surge in recruitment of new entrant officers, e.g. at Hull University. The course covers security, regime-related procedures, assertiveness training and, more recently, suicide prevention.

McGurk and Fludger (1987) argued recently that the selection criteria used for the last 25 years in selecting prison officers for training 'were not sufficiently related to those thought necessary to carry out the job of a modern Prison Officer' (McGurk and Fludger, 1987:154). It is evident from the account presented by McGurk and Fludger that the range of tasks performed and skills required as a prison officer is broad: 'Overall there is a great deal of personal contact, alertness, working irregular schedules and performing structured work in personally demanding situations' (McGurk and Fludger, 1987:158). As principal officers emphasised in McGurk and Fludger's study, it requires:

> reliability ... drive, enthusiasm and determination and the use of initiative, anticipation of problems and the ability to make decisions. Mixing easily with others, using common sense and intelligence, confidence, willingness and being able to handle discipline and authority ... Interpersonal skills ... being considerate and helpful to others, being consistent and fair, *showing understanding of others' problems* and functioning well as a member of a team.
>
> (McGurk and Fludger, 1987:160; my italics)

Understanding the problems of inmates (as well as each other's problems, both within and between ranks) is already meant to be an established aspect of the prison officer's job. Arguably, this can be seen as incorporating suicide prevention, explicitly or otherwise.

In 1988 suicide prevention was incorporated into the officer training course, to ensure that all new entrant prison officers were familiar with the Circular Instruction. In addition, in-service training courses were developed involving three-day programmes for selected officers who would then return as local or regional trainers for their own staff. These 'Training for Trainers' courses were based on a package developed in the US and Canada (Bagshaw, 1988; Ramsay *et al.*, 1987), and were later backed up by further training in 'presentation skills', to enhance the quality of the training carried out locally.[3]

Establishments with the most pressing problems were the first to receive training courses, or were invited to send a staff member on the 'Training for Trainers' course at the training school. The male YOIs included in this research did both have a local trainer, who was in fact involved in local training (though often with very small numbers of staff) at the time of the research. This allowed the author to participate in training sessions, observe the reactions of the staff and seek their views concerning the usefulness of these programmes. Only a limited amount of training in suicide prevention had actually been carried out, at the time the research was being carried out. This was in part because few officers had joined the service recently enough to have received the New Entrants' training, and locally, staff were rarely available for training sessions, even if a 'Trainer' could organise courses. Staff shortages elsewhere meant that training – a 'non-essential task' – was frequently cancelled. In addition, at the time of the fieldwork, the concentration of effort on suicide prevention training had only recently begun.

Local training for hospital officers was fairly widespread (44 per cent), but less than 10 per cent of the uniformed staff had received what they saw as satisfactory local or national training. Almost half of the uniformed staff said that they had received 'some, but limited' local training, meaning that they had read the Circular (sometimes in groups), or they went through a short or introductory training session which did not altogether answer their questions:

> The only time we ever sort of skimmed over it was at college, and I can't remember anything about it. It was less than an afternoon. (BGO)

Governor grades and specialists were least likely to have received either local or national training in suicide prevention, and many commented that they had been rather 'left out' of things. Those who had received no training were slightly defensive in their response to the question:

> As you have probably picked up, there has been no local training here, and no national training ... things are moving painfully slow. I daresay a crisis would make it move faster. (Governor grade)

> The only training we've had is our experience of life. (PO)

Many staff had received other training, either in former jobs, or as related courses offered in psychiatric hospitals or other settings. Some prison service training evidently had taken place, however, and was continuing:

> I did the Training for Trainers' course. It was a three-day course designed to enable *us* to train hospital staff. It was interesting, but I came away convinced that if paperwork saved lives then we'd never have another suicide in prison! (PO)

> I say no – that is guardedly no. Even 18 years ago when I started as a prison officer there was a certain amount of input of advice on how to recognise the symptoms of depression and stress, the times when trainees are most at risk; and then again, when I did the two-year governors' training package, there was a lot of emphasis there, and quite rightly, too, on recognising the stress times and the difficult periods that inmates go through; and it's not only from the suicide prevention angle, it is also from the angle of when a person is likely to be able to respond better to motivation, when he needs constant support, and when is the time to encourage him to try and make a decision for himself. (PO)

Three-quarters of the staff thought that suicide prevention training was useful and necessary training for prison officers to have, but a quarter expressed reservations:

I mean, it's a relatively new thing for people to think almost in a binocular vision about suicide prevention as a complete and separate package. In my opinion I am not sure that it should even now be a separate package. (SO)

Yes I do, although I am not sure that learning how to fill in a form is the best way of doing it. (SO)

It's like fire prevention or first aid – it should be part and parcel of your job, not a separate issue. (PO)

Training was wanted, however, and felt to be necessary:

Yes I do, I think it should be reinforced that this is part of our normal work, it isn't just a specialist course that people go on. (SO)

Yes, it probably makes us a bit more aware of the sort of situation where we might have to watch out, where a suicide might arise. (BGO)

Again, senior and non-uniformed grades were the most likely to see the value of suicide prevention training:

Within a prison-setting, definitely. It enables virtually anyone to recognise someone undergoing periods of stress. It's not just the hospital staff, but say, the officer in the workshop who's got the advantage of seeing the inmate five days a week. It's also essential that people know the proper avenue to refer to members of the hospital staff. (Governor grade)

Many of the officers had seen others able to undergo training, and obviously wanted the training themselves, particularly where the response from the staff had been lively and participatory, sometimes continuing their discussions well after the training period and into the car park.

It's hard to say without having gone through the package myself. I believe it's quite a comprehensive package that the department has produced, and I think it increases awareness. I would very much like to go through it. (BGO)

Over three-quarters of the staff thought that this sort of training was relevant to the job of being a prison officer:

Yes, it reminds you that the people you are looking after are human, and it can lead you into the whole area of identifying human needs and responses – the whole social interaction field, if it's done properly. (BGO)

There was one other reason why it was important:

It can be useful to the staff for personal reasons, and not just for the benefit of the inmate population. (SO)

But the fact remained that unless it was isolated as an issue with its own priority, it would become just another routine task that may or may not be possible to carry out:

Yes, even though I say it should be part and parcel of the whole ethos, in reality it is not, because with the best will in the world, if something like suicide prevention is not constantly held up as something to watch for, something to deal with, something to incorporate in the system, the tendency is – with the speed the sausage machine tends to be forced into working these days – that if you are not very careful you can actually, I would not say forget about it, but it can take a back seat because of other pressured matters. (PO)

The word 'training' was often resisted; the notion of awareness was preferred:

I'd be careful about the word 'training', I prefer the word 'awareness'. You need training to identify the potential signs. It's easy to get complacent, but it's important to be aware that lurking beneath the surface are a huge number of extremely vulnerable inmates. (PO)

The word 'awareness' was substituted for 'prevention' in Prison Department training courses in 1990. Amongst the reservations and criticisms of training, and the equally evident expressed wish to receive it, there was some considerable scepticism about the whole purpose of the new procedures. This emerged as a theme throughout the fieldwork. The political climate in many prisons was rather tense at this time (Stern, 1989a), and this expression of suspicion about suicide prevention procedures emerged as a mixture of the 'general malaise', which was largely about other issues (working arrangements, lack of training, public criticism, lack of management support, feelings of alienation and so on; see Section IV, p.223), and a genuine feeling of confusion and vulnerability about suicide:

Staff don't always feel confident in handling the problem, but they do have the back-up – if in doubt, refer or admit it. They are always looking over their shoulders, because they feel should there be an inquest, it's an inquiry into *their* behaviour, and not the behaviour of the inmate. The person who's died takes no responsibility, and we've done nothing wrong – we've been asked to look after them but you can't afford to worry 24 hours a day. (PO)

Many thought that the procedures were introduced as a 'political sop', to alleviate media and public criticism, that the procedures were an 'umbrella': only that now the officer on the landing stood outside, and he was alone (see note 1, Chapter 4, p.249 regarding 'lack-of-care' verdicts).

It *is* embarrassing to have the press highlighting suicides in prison. We ought to be concerned, but not solely for that reason. It is difficult not to have a cynical view of policy actions, perhaps sometimes unfairly. You ask yourself, what are the *real* motives for introducing all these forms? (Governor grade)

If they want us to do the job properly then we need more time and we need more staff. We used to have much more flair and individuality as a service. Clerks could do what we do now; we're losing track of the real job, we're just adding up and rubbing out and altering. We're losing our skills. There's no initiative any more – it's all procedures ... it's all about trying to paint a rosy picture and when you look under the facade, nothing is happening. (PO)

Officers pointed out flaws in the procedures – whilst arguing that suicides in prison could never be prevented, because so many were simply unpredictable. One of the ironies, they argued, was that the instructions relied upon the 15-minute watch, as a method of prevention. Most suicides, as officers often knew, occurred in less than 15 minutes:

If someone is determined, they just time you. Once you've looked in, that's it, they've got 15 minutes – that's plenty long enough. (SO)

The Massachusetts Special Commission explicitly rejected the argument:

that if a person is determined to commit suicide, there is little anyone can do to prevent it ... The Commission's inquiries suggest that it is practically feasible to make enough improvements to cell conditions, and to methods of detainee surveillance and police training, to prevent almost all suicides.

(MSC, 1984:72)

Continuous watch, mentioned in the Circular as one method of managing seriously 'at risk' inmates, was simply not provided for in the regime, either in the hospital or on the wings. Hospital staff who had worked in National Health Service settings often compared the constraints of prison regimes with the constantly supervised open ward facilities in a hospital:

In a hospital, isolation in a strip cell is a last resort. In a prison, it's our only resort. (HO)

One of the major sources of criticism of these instructions was the fact that in the daily operation of prison life, practice inevitably fell short of policy, often as a result of permanent constraints, but also as a result of local features, such as staff sickness or other shortages, inadequate facilities, large numbers of receptions or failures of communication and agreement over practices. Suicide prevention, however, was also a new skill, a skill that prison staff wanted. Rather like 'welfare', however, it was also an old one that in some ways they already had. They needed recognition for those skills they held.

Awareness of procedures

Over three-quarters of the hospital staff, the governor grades and specialists said they were aware of how suicide prevention procedures were intended to work in their establishment. Uniformed officers were the least likely to understand the local procedures in full, just less than half being able to outline them during the interview. Most of the remainder, however (46 per cent of the uniformed staff), had at least a 'patchy' understanding of procedures, usually knowing what their own responsibilities were, even if they were unsure as to how the rest of the procedures fitted into the overall picture.

If an inmate on their wing or house was thought to be at risk, a third of the staff would refer them to the hospital; a quarter would deal with the problem themselves: as expected, more of the hospital and senior staff gave this response. Less than a quarter would refer the problem to their wing manager and the rest would do all of the above, referring the case to the hospital, informing the wing manager, and trying to resolve any immediate problems in the appropriate way:

> We refer to someone with a bit more expertise. Identifying the lad is the important part, the actual assessment is done by the hospital. We might take a bit more care when we're censoring his mail if we think he's a risk. (SO)

Training, and access to Circular Instructions, were obviously significant factors in the understanding of suicide prevention procedures. Many of the uniformed officers had come to understand procedures by their own efforts, or by having them explained by other officers during their working day. Many of the staff got the number of the forms wrong, gave the numbers the wrong way round, or were hesitant about the number. This was not included in the category of a 'patchy' understanding of how procedures worked, but was assumed to be a reasonable problem for staff to have to contend with!

Most of the signs of suicide risk suggested by the staff were related to a change in the person: either any change, or a withdrawal from others and activities. Forty-eight per cent of the staff said that some change in behaviour was, by itself, an important sign:

> If he's been with us a while, I'd look for changes in behaviour. If he's quiet, but becomes manic, or he's noisy and becomes quiet. (BGO)

A third of the staff said that withdrawal from others, or from activities was a major sign:

> Basically they might be withdrawn, or changing mood and manner; some of them get themselves in such a state, they might be dishevelled, unkempt or dirty ... these are the ones that are ready for a real depression. (BGO)

Some of the staff mentioned several different signs, and did not give more weight to any one sign in particular. A small number said they would not know what sign to look for. Other 'signs' mentioned included information contained in mail, other inmates coming to tell staff that they were concerned, hints given by the inmate him or herself and, again, less identifiable signs:

> Sometimes you can't pin-point the problem, but you can *sense* the anxiety. (BGO)

When asked an open-ended question about possible risk indicators, hospital staff gave a higher average number of factors, covering a wider range of the possible risk indicators identified in the literature (Home Office, 1986a; CI 3/87; CI 20/89), although uniformed officers obviously did know what to look for. Hospital officers often mentioned in response to this question, however, that they were not in the ideal position to detect early warning signs:

> These things are all risk indicators, but it's the discipline staff who have to look for these things on a regular basis. I can't do this, it's the officers who have regular, ongoing contact. (HSO)

This is an important aspect of suicide prevention: that the prison officers have a central role to play.

A third of the staff said that the suicide problem in prison should receive a lot or a great deal of attention:

> I think it should be given a high priority. It should be one of our corporate objectives. (Governor grade)

> Well, it has got to receive the highest priority because in the final analysis safety of life is our first priority. It is above security. (PO)

> As long as a person is in custody, we have got a moral responsibility to prevent them from harming themselves. (HSO)

Many felt that it should receive the amount of attention it was currently receiving (20 per cent), or that it should not receive any more attention than the many other prison problems (38 per cent):

> I think it's one of many problems the Prison Service has, and it should take its place alongside the rest of them. (SO)

Ten per cent of the staff thought that it should not receive much attention, or that it should receive less than was currently given:

> Not a lot. Because it's one of those things where, if it's ignored, it lessens. If it's made a major issue, it's one of the most infectious diseases I know. (PO)

> I'm not convinced, you see, that we're doing anything differently – clinically, to what we did before. What we are doing is filling in more forms, and I'm not sure that's a good thing. I think it's reducing the amount of time left available for contact with the individuals who need it. I think we get alerted to more guys as potential risks who turn out not to be suicidal ... that's no great imposition. (Specialist – psychiatrist)

How well procedures worked

Uniformed officers were the most likely to report problems concerning the operation of suicide prevention procedures in practice (37 per cent), with governor grades more likely to report few problems. Staff often responded to this question by drawing on their establishment's good record of few completed suicides to illustrate the apparent success of the way procedures worked.[4] Problems reported were often specific, and related to communication and agreement between departments, or the usefulness of the procedures themselves:

> When it works best is when it's avoided, by letting him have a cry on your shoulder, you defuse it. We've got three on special watch because we think they might cut themselves. It is good that we're all thinking about it, and are all knowledgeable about it. I've not seen any paperwork, mind. (SO)

> The identification process works, but the process of actually dealing with that person is a total failure. Staff are very cynical – there's a stock belief here that anyone who is ill, or who has been in trouble with the police, is not wanted by the hospital! (PO)

> The paperwork is fine, but I sometimes wonder what we're aiming at. Are we preventing a suicide, or covering ourselves in paperwork? Causation is not necessarily tackled. (PO)

Procedures did perhaps work better for the hospital staff, as their major concern was persuading the officers to use the referral forms at all (instead of passing informal messages to the hospital) or appropriately (that is, for suspected suicide risk alone, and not for a range of other problems). Other problems mentioned included lack of training, and the fears of the staff about the consequences of their observations:

> Yes, you're asking untrained people to commit themselves. (BGO)

Time was also a problem: for example, not having enough handing over time between shifts, or not being able to deal with urgent welfare problems. Other problems included staff shortages, the lack of continuity of staff on the wings, lack of information, inmate numbers, the lack of a personal officer system, problems of physical accommodation, staff co-operation, and the inflexibility of the procedures:

> The procedure itself, I do not think there is any problem. Not in it actually working, but I do not actually see the procedure itself as being particularly helpful. (Why is that?) To me, it has formalised the system into a paper transaction, which, because people are dealing with paperwork all day long, reams of it, the tendency is to think of it as part and parcel of yet another paper system. 'Oh, Joe Bloggins is at risk, we've heard that before, we send it to the Medical Officer, end of problem'. (SO)

> Well, it's important to remember that the paperwork system does not sweep away the need to actually talk to people, that is, the inmate. (HO)

Some hospital staff did feel that the new procedures had improved the identification and management of suicide risk:

> When it comes to referrals from staff – especially from discipline staff to the hospital – there has always been a reluctance to put pen to paper. Now that they've got to, that reluctance is slowly being eroded, and more staff are willing

to put down how they feel about the prisoner, which is to everyone's benefit.
(HSO)

The most popular aspect of the instructions was the referral form, 1997, which improved communication between discipline and hospital staff, encouraged feedback, and gave the discipline staff a resource to refer inmates to when they were seriously concerned.

When staff were asked how the procedures could be improved, most suggestions related directly to the problems mentioned above. Almost a third said that better communication would help; 15 per cent said they needed more time; 22 per cent wanted more training and 17 per cent mentioned several of these. Other suggestions included more staff, persuading the courts to remand and sentence fewer prisoners, better access to medical or psychiatric help, and more 'half-way' facilities, with hospital and discipline staff involved in specially organised units. More consultation with the inmate, better Hospital Officer cover, and learning more about the causes of such behaviour were all mentioned as ways of improving suicide prevention. One or two rather lengthy discussions raised the question of the role of Medical Officers, as their particular approach to the problem was felt to be a crucial determinant of the establishment's style of suicide prevention. The role of the medical (and hospital) staff are crucial issues, particularly in the light of current scrutiny and recent criticisms which are likely to pave the way for change (Home Office, 1990a; 1990e; Home Office Directorate of Prison Medical Services, 1990). It was mentioned on more than one occasion that staff felt uncertain about their own future in the prison service. Visiting psychiatrists bemoaned the perennial problem of how to deal with, or what to recommend for the 'borderline patient': is he really ill? Can we treat him? They were talking about the 'personality disordered' or the 'attention-seeker', neither of whom were really 'ill', nor were they 'clinically' depressed. These were the labels that self-injurers collected.

Communication and co-operation

Over half of all staff said that there were quite serious problems of communication and co-operation between the hospital and the discipline side of the institution. The contrast between uniformed- and hospital-staff perceptions of the nature and extent of this problem between the two departments is noteworthy (see Table 8.2). Governor grades and specialists saw plenty of problems, but not as many as the uniformed staff, who emerged as particularly frustrated with their apparent difficulties with the hospital both in the formal interviews, in informal discussions and during supplementary visits to other establishments.

The major problems given as examples were lack of feedback from the hospital, their unwillingness to accept inmates thought to be at risk onto the hospital, the lack of adequate instructions given to wing staff on the inmates' return, and the generally low level of consultation or information-sharing that went on. Hospital staff clearly had answers to most of these complaints, feeling that uniformed staff

Table 8.2   Co-operation and communication between hospital and discipline staff

	Officers		Hospital staff		Others	
	No.	%	No.	%	No.	%
Good	5	(14)	11	(46)	6	(29)
Some problems	5	(14)	5	(21)	6	(29)
Clear problems	25	(71)	8	(33)	9	(43)
Totals	35	(100)	24	(100)	21	(100)

$\chi^2=10.96$ d.f.$=4$ p<0.02

expected the hospital to provide a 'refuge' for discipline and control problems, and inmates not surviving on the wings. They felt that discipline officers often over-reacted to inmates' signs of distress, and were too keen to 'send their problems to us'. Wing staff usually ended up with 'the problem', in the long-term: hence their dim view of the co-operation they received.

I think the communication is quite reasonable. I am not sure that the *understanding* is quite the same. (BGO)

There are times when the units refer a young man who they consider to be at grave risk, and within 12 hours the medical personnel have seen him, interviewed him, and decided that he's not at immediate risk, and he will be sent back to the unit marked as 'risk category 2 – shared accommodation', end of problem. But of course that's not the end of the problem. (PO)

Number one, the inmate concerned has been talking to the medical officer who he doesn't know, rather than again under the old system, he would have been talking a lot more openly to his group officer, or his SO, or his PO, or even the Governor. He could have told the MO anything. (PO)

It used to be diabolical! I think it's much better than it was. I think there's a lot of confusion about territory and what sort of conditions and situations should be treated by the hospital and what should be treated as a discipline matter. So you get someone ringing the hospital saying, 'this guy's being a real pain, *do* something!', and the hospital will say, 'this guy's not ill – you deal with him!' There should be more overlap, somehow. (Specialist – chaplain)

Well, it's very difficult really, because – sometimes they say that they don't consider them to be a medical problem, they're more of a discipline problem. They say to us 'Oh, it's personality disorder, we can't do anything about it, because they're not medically ill, they're not mentally ill!' But if people are cutting themselves up and doing all sorts of weird and wonderful things, I mean we sometimes can feel completely out of our depth, don't we? Completely. (SO)

Accusations directed at the prison officers that they were behaving as 'pseudo-psychiatrists', were resented. At the same time, hospitals often complained that uniformed staff wanted to refer all their behaviour problems to the hospital, either for medication, or for 'cure'.

Relationships and communication were better where hospital staff appeared regularly on the wings, for example, to give out treatments. Otherwise, there was a distinct barrier detectable in all four establishments, materialising as a collective view expressed by uniformed officers that the hospital could 'pick and choose' their clients, that they kept themselves empty wherever possible, and that they received extra privileges (an allowance, and a pleasant working environment) for doing less work. Hospital staff, for their part, often argued that inmates could develop a better relationship with hospital officers, as their role was more 'therapeutic'. The consequences of communication and co-operation difficulties could be serious, and have been noted before:

> Other guards find their moves to help crisis-prone men blocked by the unresponsiveness of some treatment personel to their observations and referrals. Scenarios comprised of repeated unsuccessful attempts to secure mental health services for susceptible men culminate in despair and apathy. Such sequences can leave guards and human services personnel with the impression that they must each contend with non-cooperative allies, who function to undermine their helping efforts.
>
> (Johnson, 1977:269)

The problems between the two departments were somewhat reminiscent of the problems of throughcare and 'shared working' between the prison and probation services (Bottomley and Liebling, 1987; Jepson and Elliot, 1985). There were resentments, misunderstandings and unclear boundaries of responsibility. These particular misunderstandings between hospital and discipline staff did have a particularly vexed dimension: this was the question of whose problem suicide and self-injury really was: a medical or a discipline problem? Very few staff in any capacity argued that it might lie somewhere in between.

SECTION III: THE ROLE OF THE PRISON OFFICER

> Correctional staff, on recognizing the potential motivators, can make the single most important contribution in suicide prevention by discussing the inmate's problems, concerns, anxieties ... and referring for special medical or psychiatric services.
>
> (Scott-Denoon, 1984:72)

One of the major themes to emerge from the staff interviews was that prison officers did not easily see suicide *prevention* as being part of their primary role, only identification: they saw suicide as a medical problem, with suicide risk as a problem that medical staff were more properly qualified to assess.

The job of a modern prison officer

J.E. Thomas argued that in spite of assertions that the officer is associated with reformative goals, 'his role has always been to control' and 'his success or failure as an officer is measured against his ability to do that' (Thomas, 1972:xiv). It is for this reason that security and control are seen as the focus of a prison officer's job. It is in these areas that skills and pride are most obvious, that training is concentrated, and that status and respect are conferred. Welfare work, rehabilitation and counselling are less readily 'owned' without reservation or limitation – not because they are unpopular or unwanted, but because they are tasks which have never been 'given' to or uncritically accepted by prison officers. They are tasks which are more difficult to define, operationalise and perhaps, achieve; 'welfare' is increasingly seen as the vocation of specialists, such as probation officers, psychologists and psychiatrists (Jacobs, 1978; Toch and Klofas, 1982). Prison officers stand amidst confusion in our penal thinking: we are not even sure that welfare and rehabilitation comprise viable goals. Prison officers are the uncertain victims of this confusion, arguing as a group that they want to take on a more explicit welfare function, but arguing as individuals that they don't have the time, the skills, the training or the support required to achieve such a task. Within institutions, the range of effort, expertise and potential is extreme. How, then, do prison staff see themselves and their role? How do they see themselves in relation to suicide prevention, and the identification of 'risk' in inmates? Much of the uncertainty with which officers respond to explicit instructions regarding the management and prevention of suicide is an uncertainty about their 'role'. They are at once experts and laymen; specialists in the art of human management, without the qualifications to prove, or guarantee it. At times, they save or transform lives; at others, they do not or cannot respond to the human demands of their job.

The importance of welfare

In a survey carried out in 1982 (OPCS, 1985:53), 43 per cent of prison officers strongly agreed with the statement that 'Prison Officers are the best people to look after prisoners' welfare'. A further 31 per cent 'tended to agree'. Prison officers themselves were the most likely of a range of prison staff to agree with the notion that prison officers should be given more welfare responsibilities for inmates. The question of what exactly is meant by 'welfare', or whether suicide prevention is seen as a 'welfare issue' are not addressed, in this OPCS report or elsewhere.

Two-thirds of the uniformed staff interviewed in this research thought that their direct contact or work with the inmates was the most valuable part of their work:

> Not being soft, like – but they can relate to me. I think the contact with inmates is very important, and I feel I have a useful contribution to make. (PO)

Over half of the governor and specialist grades and collectively, 22 per cent of the other groups of staff thought that the paperwork involved in their job was the least valuable aspect of their work. In addition, a third of all staff thought that certain administrative procedures such as putting people on report for minor infringements, responding to duplicate requests for information from headquarters and region, daily detailing, and some of the 'inherited routines' were frustrating and lacking any clear value:

We push out too much paperwork, and as a result, things get missed. (SO)

Several of the staff commented that much of the current paperwork demanded of them could be completed by clerks, or should have been computerised long ago. Most frustrating of all was the fact that a lot of this work was being done by senior staff, 'whose time should really be spent on other things'. One of the objections to the recently introduced suicide prevention procedures was exactly this point: officers felt that the paperwork involved had taken precedence over the welfare and mental health of the inmate. As long as the right forms had been filled in, no complaints would be heard at inquests.

Almost two-thirds of the uniformed officers thought that welfare work was a very important part of a prison officer's job:

Yes. We do an awful lot that's not noticed, or categorised, or whatever, because we're the people who are here when it starts ... who they come and talk to. We might put them in contact with other people, but it's us who take the brunt of it all the time. We give advice out all day. (BGO)

It's not only important, it's rewarding as well. (SO)

Many of the staff (particularly the uniformed officers) added that it was particularly important in a young offenders' establishment:

Yes. This is the element of youth custody which has probably given me more satisfaction than any other ... after 19 years of not doing any of it. (PO)

The question of what welfare work included was difficult to assess. How far suicide attempts might be included within the realm of prison staff expertise emerged as a significant and related theme in the interviews:

I like to think that each and every prison officer, even though they might not like to admit it, is a psychiatrist in certain quarters, because we all assess and we all evaluate, even if they're just observing that 'this kid is a lot better than he was when he came in'. (Visiting Psychiatrist)

Where were the limits to this role?

Yes, it's important. As long as it doesn't take over the *primary* job, which is security. (PO)

Welfare was given less direct prominence when it was ranked amongst the rest of a prison officer's work. Almost two-thirds of the uniformed staff said that 'security' or control were the most important parts of a prison officer's job:

> The maintenance of good order, discipline and security. (BGO)

> There's a three-word phrase for it – custody, care, and control – but I think you've got to have custody and control before you can start on the care. (SO)

> I think it is threefold, and you can't say that any one is more important than any other, because of the interplay between all three areas. You have 'inmate care', which includes welfare aspects, but also care in its most basic aspects and entitlements; you have 'supervision and control', and you have 'security'. Those three aspects should be embodied in every prison officer, whatever the rank. At *times*, some of these are going to be more important than others. (Governor grade)

Smith argued in a discussion of prison officer stress that: 'A common source of conflict peculiar to prisoners and identified as early as 1959 is inherent in the ambiguous role of the penal system – treatment vs. custody' (Smith, 1984:11). This role conflict 'is the medium from which all other demands and conflicts arise' (Ibid.; see also Johnson, 1977). In these interviews with staff almost a quarter of the uniformed staff recognised that there was a direct conflict between the security and welfare aspects of their job:

> I think they feel a conflict, and I think there *is* often a conflict ... there should be a lot more discussion on those aspects. (BGO)

Non-uniformed staff were less likely to perceive a conflict:

> They may do, but they can *enhance* security. One of the best methods of control is that old cliché of staff–inmate relationships. They must give something of themselves, to get anything back from the inmates. (Specialist: Chaplain)

Many of the staff drew an analogy between the role of the family, where discipline and welfare were (happily, it was assumed) combined, and their own dual role. Prison probation officers expressed the view that it was difficult to have a trusting, working relationship with inmates when they, as probation officers, are drawn into the discipline and control arena. The tension between welfare and security was most clearly expressed and illustrated by the officers: those who are actually charged with the dual role. Smith illustrates the tendency for officers under stress to revert to their custodial role in order to avoid the 'double-bind' of the two functions (Smith, 1984:11). This conflict is central to the officers' doubts about their own ability to manage and prevent suicide attempts. The combination of poor training, poor communication and co-operation between departments, uncertainty about the nature of suicide and self-destructive behaviour and about the appropriate role of the prison officer in relation to its prevention, provide some serious obstacles to its achievement (see Johnson, 1977).

SECTION IV: UNDERSTANDING THE STAFF – HOPELESS AND ISOLATED?

Despite the limited amount of research available on prison staff problems, there is sufficient to confirm one of the consistent findings of this project: that staff are feeling vulnerable themselves (Thomas, 1972; Thomas and Pooley, 1981; OPCS, 1985; Stern, 1989a; in the US see Poole and Regoli, 1980). Despair, hopelessness and 'anomie' (Thomas, 1972) are themes emerging not just from the inmates, but amongst the staff:

> Staff are frightened – especially since Fresh Start. There is so much *uncertainty*, so many changes. (Governor grade)

The recent riots at Strangeways and elsewhere have made this more so (Staples, 1990; Woolf, 1991). Evidence of 'distrust, alienation and suspicion' between staff and management emerges throughout the literature (Stern, 1989a:63; Home Office, 1979: see also Poole and Regoli, 1980:225). Bagshaw and Baxter point out that it is: 'Failure to cope with (their) apparently conflicting functions (which) may lead to feelings of stress, helplessness, and eventually cynicism and feelings of hostility on the part of the Prison Officer' (Bagshaw and Baxter, 1987:168).

It is in the 'face-to-face' encounters with inmates that officers' various and conflicting duties are encapsulated. A recent study of anxiety levels in female prison officers in Scotland found that suicide attempts and self-injury incidents were amongst the most stressful aspects of the job (Liebling, 1990:36). Fear of violence and breaches of security are also major sources of anxiety for prison officers (Launay and Fielding, 1989). Security requirements and the need to form 'empathic relationships with inmates' have a tension between them that is difficult to resolve.

The notion of staff stress was definitely on the prison staff agenda; it was brought into the interviews again and again, as officers talked about their work. A 'stress package' had recently been issued by the Prison Department for assimilation into local training courses. Staff awareness of officer problems (depression, suicide, alcoholism, general levels of health and so on) was evident throughout the research. This concern was confirmed by recent literature: the causes of stress included staff–inmate confrontations, poor communication within the prison (Launay and Fielding, 1989), task pressures – under conditions of minimal training and supervision (Long et al., 1986:331) and the lack of any meaningful values with which to make sense of their work: 'They are in the anomic position of working for a goal which is negatively defined as the absence of punishment and is manifested by no acceptably measured results' (Duffee, 1974:157).

This complaint emerged consistently throughout the fieldwork. The psychological strain present in prison officers' work environment has been said to result in apathy, alienation, dissatisfaction, cynicism, and a lack of enthusiasm and concern for their charges (Gerstein et al., 1987; Poole and Regoli, 1980). Lack of support, feelings of 'burnout' and a lack of clarity about their role has been shown to contribute to anxiety, fatigue, tension and high levels of exhaustion (Cherniss, 1980; Gerstein *et al.*, 1987; Cheek and Miller, 1983; Posen, 1985; T. Smith, 1984; 1985; Toch and Klofas, 1982): 'A burnout sequence presupposes that the workers enter their careers full of idealism and of concern for clients, but that, after trials and failures, they end up feeling cynical and indifferent to human suffering' (Toch and Klofas, 1982:35).

Inmate or staff problems?

One of the findings that – far from being sought – emerged from the research was a pattern of parallels between staff and inmate problems. Three officer suicides were reported in Brixton and three in Risley; other recent cases were mentioned, almost invariably in establishments where inmate suicides had occurred. Many officers knew other officer colleagues who had attempted or committed suicide; they were concerned that their own mental and occupational health was not a concern of researchers or of management. Given the increasing size of the prison estate, it is perhaps not surprising that suicides and sick leave through depressive episodes occur in some number amongst staff, given the suicide rate and the (known) incidence of depression in the general community. Parallels emerged (often unnoticed in the telling) between explanations of staff and inmate problems: both groups of respondents were in need of a listening ear.

Officers talked of 'doing time' in establishments; they spoke of 'getting through my time, now', as they approached retirement; they 'coped', as establishments cope – barely, but continually, ever-challenged by the pressures of cuts, limited resources and dwindling contracted hours. *Time* was perhaps their most prominent concern, determining problems, solutions and disputes. Officers were often transferred, with little choice, to establishments all over the country. Northerners could not stay north – sooner or later, they had to uproot ('you're just a body to management – bodies in spaces'). Did anyone notice, I was asked, that 200 staff were redeployed countrywide in the aftermath of the Strangeways riot? ('Questions were asked about the location of the inmates – but no-one asked where the staff were!'). Officers occasionally lived in caravans outside prisons, or in lodgings upon transfer; sale of prison department quarters and differential house prices left them temporarily homeless. As a result, their families remained at home, and officers found themselves 'miles away from their loved ones' – just a number in the detail, to a 'faceless headquarters'. There was no one person to complain to ('you'd be complaining to a bureaucracy'). There are staff welfare officers, to whom staff make applications: they are Home Office appointees. Complaints and problems may have repercussions on promotion prospects. Parallels with Boards of Visitors, parole procedures and applications to 'welfare' for inmates were plain. Staff talked of mistrust; they felt alienated from management, undervalued (Stern, 1989a:63; Home Office, 1979:para.10.22). An OPCS survey (1985) concluded that prison officers' views of their job are rather jaundiced: 'It is a feeling that contains an odd mixture of bravado, cynicism, resentment and, it must be said, *fear*' (OPCS,

1985:56). Inquests illustrated the parallels between the predicament of the young inmate, and that of the officer 'in the dock' – a phrase used to describe the experience of giving evidence at an inquest. The Circular may be brought out during the inquest and worked through as though it were law:

> totally out of context in the daily life of an institution – they don't take account of the context, of the busy life of a wing, our *other* Circulars – on security and control. (SO)

More recently, staff have become afraid of litigation.[5] A newspaper report of an inquest on a prisoner suicide ended 'The trial continues today' (*Guardian* 25 October 1990:3). Officers commented that their position as a whole has become more vulnerable in several respects. Failure to carry out the tasks required by Circular Instructions (such as the completion of a 1997 when suspecting possible suicide risk) could result in serious consequences for the officer if the inmate should go on to harm himself. Police officers have been sued for large sums of money in recent suicide cases taken to the civil court by families (Kirkham v. Anderson; *The Times*, 4 January 1990). Stories are spreading to Britain from the US concerning inmates who deliberately throw themselves from a height, then sue the Prison Department for negligence for not noticing that they were feeling suicidal! The nature of the prison world, with its conflicting demands, staff shortages and lack of training in suicide prevention is not taken into account at the inquest. An individual prison officer may feel rather isolated when standing 'in the dock': '(The) isolation of the guard is supported by organisational role prescriptions that stress personal accountability rather than cooperation and collective responsibility' (Poole and Regoli, 1980:306).

Finally, in the collection of parallels connecting inmates' problems to those of the staff, they commented that educational and training aspirations they might have are overlooked in the struggle to run a prison (Stern, 1989a:64). Inmates, they pointed out, are given all these opportunities. Staff training is not given sufficient priority – either in suicide prevention, or many of the other skills that officers feel they could share with others, or claim as their own. As it is, unsure of their role, individual enthusiasms and contributions go largely unnoticed and unrewarded. According to Stern: 'Indeed the gradual erosion of the welfare role is often seen as one of the major factors in prison officers' loss of morale and growing discontent' (Stern, 1989:77). They are assessed on the basis of 'meaningless monitoring forms' – how many people do they unlock? – not, 'what is the quality of our work?' Much of their work is boring and repetitive – but such is the nature of prison life. For everyone.

Discussion

Staff perceptions and attitudes are an important determinant of approaches to the problem of suicide attempts in custody, and the conflicts involved in its management and prevention. It is clear from the responses to questions about the identification of risk that the level of contact between staff and inmates is felt to be a significant prerequisite for the success of any identification process. If change is a major sign of risk, then some knowledge of the inmates' usual behaviour and character is important. Continuity, time and involvement in routine welfare tasks are important facilitators of the identification of depression or despair. Personal Officer schemes were frequently mentioned as a useful system to have, as these schemes combined all aspects felt to be necessary to the task of detecting problems and providing support.

An emphasis amongst uniformed staff on the anticipation and prevention of discipline and 'manipulation' problems, so that potential infractions are as significant as actual infractions (Poole and Regoli, 1980:306), results in a conflict when self-injury is seen as *either* a discipline or a medical problem. The temptation was to see suicide as an almost exclusively medical or psychiatric problem, despite the eagerness of prison officers to be involved in all other aspects of 'welfare'.

Prison officers, more than any other group, are likely to see personal and individual causes such as depression and lack of communication as the main factors in prison suicide. Staff groups also differ to some extent in their ratings of other factors, more of the hospital staff seeing mental illness as an important factor, and few prison officers feeling that guilt is a large contributor to suicide. Most of the staff select or suggest factors which they see themselves as having little control over, despite the findings in Chapter 6 that practical and organisational factors can be of crucial significance in 'the onset of a suicidal crisis'. Some of these prison-related stressors are not in the hands of the prison officers, but lie with the larger world of managers and policy-makers, over whom the prison staff have little influence.

Few of the staff have escaped the potential trauma of an inmate suicide or suicide attempt. Most feel a combination of shock, guilt and frustration, although almost half of the uniformed grades felt they could cope with a suicide as they would any other part of their job.

Most of the staff see suicide and self-injury as separate problems, many stating that a 'genuine attempt' will always succeed. This view was held despite examples (freely related) of 'rescued' but genuine attempts they had encountered. The qualifiers, 'now, *that* was a close one ...', 'there are always exceptions ...', were heard many times. Despite the apparent consensus that the two behaviours were quite distinct, few of the staff could identify reliable ways of distinguishing between suicide attempts and other types of self-injury apart from factors relating to method and outcome. Given the restricted means of attempted suicide in prison, it is even less likely in the prison setting than outside that severity and type of injury is related directly to intent (see Morgan, 1979:9). Situational pressures such as bullying, threats and the destruction of relationships were seen as likely to provoke suicide attempts, although many of the staff believed that successful suicides could be a result of 'cries for help' that 'went wrong'.

Prison officers liked to see staff–inmate relationships as good. The experience of imprisonment was described as rather pointless, as even where opportunities existed, inmates did not generally make use of them. The major problems of imprisonment were lack of contact with outside and the loss of freedom. Weaker inmates were known to suffer more immediate problems of taxing, teasing and violence.

Training for staff in suicide prevention procedures was in the midst of its execution during the fieldwork period. At this early stage, officers felt that the training they had received was limited in several respects. It was thought to be superficial, infrequent and, in some ways, inappropriate. Staff felt on the one hand that they had 'managed without' for many years, but they also expressed the view that this training package did not resolve their own fears and anxieties about potential suicides, the inquest and the inevitable publicity to follow. Their own skills were being neglected, and their suspicions about the real purpose of the Circular and the training package were pertinent. They still felt 'out of their depth', despite an elaborate system of referral. The crucial role played by prison staff in suicide prevention was not reflected in the extent of training reported. Their knowledge of signs of risk to look for was as likely to be informed by experience and hearsay as by training. Officers perceived the most problems with suicide prevention procedures as they were understood to operate in principle. They saw failure of communication (particularly with the hospital) as being a major obstacle. They also saw the institutional response to suicidal inmates as a limited and bureaucratic response, without sufficient resources, time or training to be effective. Dispute as to the appropriate location for potentially suicidal inmates was clear.

Methods of improving suicide prevention procedures suggested by staff included more staff and hospital officers, fewer prisoners, better access to medical and psychiatric help, more 'inter-disciplinary' units involving officers and specialists, better consultation with inmates and hospital staff, and learning about the causes of suicide in prison. Staff forced their own feelings of vulnerability on to the research agenda, showing that their own problems were often a mirror image of those suffered by inmates. Unsupported themselves, they asked why prison officer suicides were not of interest to outsiders and managers.[6]

The major difficulties expressed by staff shared a common theme: a theme of separation and conflict: of role, department, location, responsibility and label. Whose responsibility is the problem: medical or discipline staff? Where should the inmate be located: the hospital, or on the wing? Can prison officers have a view about suicide risk, or not? Is the inmate 'genuinely suicidal', or not? Is he or she 'clinically depressed', or not? *Is* it a psychiatric problem, or not? *Is* suicide related to self-injury, or not? Some of these divisions are enshrined in a Circular Instruction which holds the medical officer ultimately responsible for the detection of risk, and the prevention of suicide, but has little to say about the overlapping problems and needs of the vulnerable. Throughout the research, but particularly at this point, there was a major theme absent from all discussions and interviews: the notion of integration.

Part III

Conclusions

Chapter 9

Understanding suicides in prison

Vulnerable prisoners in high-risk situations

Self-mutilation is the culmination of a process, influenced by the environment of penal confinement and the prison as a social system, rather than a discrete event. However, the inmate is not the helpless pawn of this environment. Rather he contributes to this process through his interpretations of his experiences and his capacity to tolerate stress. His contributions, in turn, are products of this social and psychological conditioning previous to his current confinement. It is important to investigate why individuals initiate this process.

It is equally important, however, to investigate the intervention of the environment in affecting outcome ... The magnitude and appearance of suicide rates ... are profoundly affected by the social context and response to suicide attempts ... (In this study) the very existence of the response demonstrated that the human environment was concerned over the survival of the inmate. This assurance, minimal as it may be, may have been sufficient to terminate suicidal behaviour.

(Johnson, 1973:240–41)

SECTION I: EXPLAINING SUICIDES IN PRISON

Prison suicide research has remained isolated from advances made in other areas of prison research and from sociological critiques. The role of individual factors has been prominent: psychiatric explanations are assumed to play a major role in accounts of suicides both in and out of prison. Research in prison sociology has indicated the importance of environmental variables in understanding issues such as absconding, riots and disturbances. The role of environmental variables and of interactive explanations for prison suicide have been slow to appear, but may be of equal significance in this field. Prison suicide research needs to be brought into the broader world of prison sociology. This book represents an attempt to do this.

There are several methodological and theoretical limitations inherent in research to date on prison suicides, attempted suicides and self-injury. The figures on which such studies are based are inadequate, as are the records from which much of the data is extracted. Control groups are rarely used, and studies are aimed almost exclusively at the prediction of the suicidal inmate. Just as the search for the causes of crime has been abandoned in many criminological circles in favour of situational crime prevention, the search for the causes of suicide in prison has never been at the forefront of research. Studies aimed at the identification of the inmate at risk of suicide have been based on inadequate or small samples, and the range of variables they consider is small and inconsistent. Those risk factors which have been identified may only describe a proportion of those completed suicides occurring in prison. It may be the case that different types of prison suicide occur (for example, amongst the psychiatrically ill, lifers and the young), each having a different 'profile'. 'What goes on' in prison may be unavailable in any form of documentation, however carefully collected, and despite the increasing volume and availability of this kind of recorded information. It is clear that there are serious difficulties inherent in relying upon statistical information alone when trying to establish the incidence and nature, and develop explanations for, suicides in prison.

This concluding chapter will discuss the methodological approach adopted as a result of the limitations found in previous research. The implications of the research presented in Chapters 6 to 8, and their theoretical significance will be then be considered.

Understanding the problem

There are three issues in prison suicide research which must be understood, and which this study aims to clarify. These are:

1   the notion of vulnerability
2   the relevance of situational factors
3   the management and prevention of suicide and attempted suicides in prison

Psychiatric illness factors have been overstated in prison suicide research. This may also be true of studies carried out in the community (Kelleher, 1988). A general theory should be formulated which is capable of addressing both individual and situational dimensions of the problem. The notion of vulnerability has been explored here, both in terms of contributory background factors and current identifying features. Previous research has omitted to investigate whether the experience of imprisonment may be different for the potentially suicidal inmate. It is shown here that the 'vulnerable' group have different experiences, and also perceive their situation differently, often finding themselves worse off than others in terms of their contacts with outside, and many aspects of their daily life inside. Relationships with other inmates can be difficult and frightening, the suicide attempt group being more likely to be isolated and friendless throughout the sentence. A culture of exploitation and victimisation (Irwin and Cressey's 'convict culture', 1962), leaves those with the fewest resources and strengths at the bottom of a powerful hierarchy. Self-injury may sometimes be the only way in which it is possible to manipulate a hostile environment. Unlike all other efforts to manipulate, this technique is considered to be weak and negative: no status is conferred on those who declare their bankruptcy. The 'inmate code': 'don't weaken' and 'play it cool'

(Sykes and Messinger, 1960:8; Johnson, 1976) is broken. There is a sub-culture of self-injury in young offender institutions: it is the culture of the weak; it is both imported and situationally induced. With the thieves and convicts (cf. Irwin and Cressey, 1962) there are victims, or the vulnerable. The 'argot' used by staff and inmates alike is a language of contempt: 'slashers' and 'cutters', with their 'tram-lines' and 'scratches', are 'inadequate', 'manipulative' and 'attention-seeking'. If they 'top themselves', they have made 'attention-seeking gestures' that 'went wrong'. The function of the words used most commonly to describe suicide attempts and/or self-injury in prison is not to maintain secrecy or to evoke barriers to communication between inmates and staff (cf. Bondeson, 1989:122–23), but to allow both parties to avoid confronting the realities of pain and desperation: suicide attempts are thereby dismissed. The language denies their validity, and the distress they express.

Inmates may make these 'gestures' as a last-ditch effort to provoke a solution, or to draw attention to their plight. Despite worn statements by staff that this was 'a cry for help', help is rarely forthcoming. The 'gesture' is a declaration of resourcelessness: the bravest plea the inmate can muster. Without rescue or support, their determination to escape from misery is likely to take a different and more dangerous course.

Alternatively, the inmate may omit any 'cry for help' and proceed directly down a pathway to suicide. Not even daring to manipulate their own rescue, these inmates simply give up. The signs may have been perceptible to the astute: how did they spend those hours alone in their cells? How were they mixing with other inmates? What sort of contact did they have with the outside? How well were they coping with the experience of imprisonment – were they making any use of their sentence? Had they shown poor coping strategies in other ways?

There is a third possibility: that the threat of suicide never becomes real; that adopting a method of escape which provides some short-term relief becomes a coping mechanism in itself for some inmates. Such young prisoners are nevertheless declaring a type of bankruptcy which places them in a high-risk category. Their recourse to repeated self-injury exposes their lack of resourcefulness. It may indicate poor relationships with others, low self-esteem and a low threshold for prison-induced stress. One of their few coping skills may be the art of escape by avoidance, not the most useful or realistic skill with which to face a term of imprisonment.

Suicidal behaviour, and intent, may each be viewed as a continuum along which the vulnerable may quickly progress (O'Mahony, 1990). Self-injury, once accomplished, increases the risk of suicide by a factor of between ten and one hundred (Kreitman, 1988; Pallis, 1988:35). It is clear that inquiring into the reasons for self-injury (particularly where the stated intention is suicide) is a valid route towards understanding the pathway to suicide. Looking at the overlap between these traditionally distinct concepts provides a clearer understanding of suicide risk than looking at either behaviour alone, or at the distinctions between them.

Contributory factors may include the disruption of relationships, lack of communication and support, bullying, threats, fear and violence, uncertainty, isolation, boredom, 'enforced idleness', insomnia and the prospect of a long or meaningless sentence devoid of future hopes or plans. Inmates who do nothing during the day, or sleep through hours of inactivity, become restless and anxious at night. This is not the sleeplessness of depression but the restive preparations of despair (see Chapter 6). It is essential to understand the onset of a suicidal crisis in the inmates' own words. Common feelings of hopelessness, loneliness, isolation, depression and boredom are expressed by those who come close to the suicidal act. Many unseen features of the prison experience have a direct bearing on the build-up of suicidal feelings. For young prisoners, aspects of the prison situation may be particularly important. The young are at least as prone to suicide in prison as any other age group. This finding remains largely unexplored. Young-prisoner suicides may be less likely to resemble suicides in the community and are less likely to show evidence of psychiatric illness than other prison suicides. The roles of imitation, boredom and bullying may be of particular concern in young offender institutions and remand centres or wings. It may also be that the threshold at which suicide is reached is lowered by the presence of others who make suicide attempts. Prison pressures for young offenders may include physical, economic and psychological victimisation (cf. Bowker, 1980). With no escape route, legitimate or illegitimate, suicide becomes a very real option. Tumim's review identified the young prisoner as an especially vulnerable group: 'The young are particularly vulnerable. They are more likely than adults to lack the inner resources to deal with being held in a local prison or remand centre' (Home Office, 1990d:22).

The impulsivity of young prisoner suicide attempts may persuade staff that they are not 'serious and genuine' attempts. Such an assumption is wrong. Young offenders are taking their own lives in custody at a rate which is increasing more rapidly than amongst any other group. The most common motivation for these attempts was a mixture of escape and communication. As Hawton and Catalan found in their study of suicide attempts amongst adolescents, what is being communicated is the declaration that 'things got so unbearable, I didn't know what else to do' (Hawton and Catalan, 1987). Those who are most at risk are those who cannot generate their own problem-solutions. Figure 9.1 draws together some of the factors which may contribute to the onset of a suicidal crisis.

It is the combined effects of feelings of hopelessness, their histories, their current situation, and the fact that they cannot generate solutions to that situation that propel the young prisoner towards suicide. Situational triggers or provoking agents may be decisive in a suicide attempt at different thresholds, depending on both the inmate's vulnerability, and the level of stress he or she experiences. Different sets of circumstances can produce many outcomes. As shown in Chapter 6, those inmates who are most vulnerable often find themselves subject to the worst stresses in prison. They are more likely to be isolated, to be without activity, and to be without contact from home. Those inmates who are least resourceful are also exposed to the most severe provoking agents. These constellations of variables are interacting: poor family support may act as both a predisposing factor, rendering

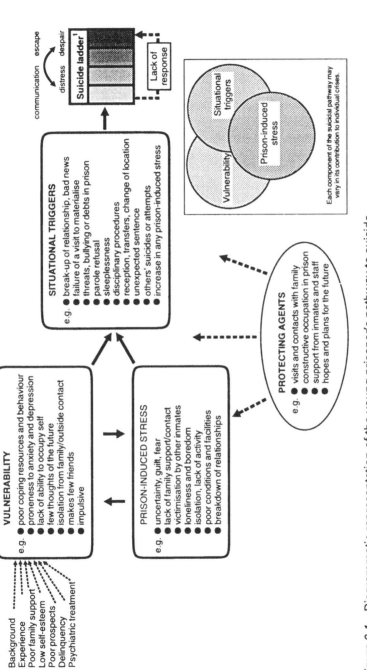

Figure 9.1 Diagrammatic representation of the young prisoner's pathway to suicide

Note: 1. The 'Suicide Ladder' (Eldrid, 1988) indicates a pathway from feelings and thoughts of suicide, through self-injury and failed suicide attempts to completed suicide. The inmate may be propelled along the continuum of suicidal action by the (lack of) institutional response.

The following labels appear in the figure:

VULNERABILITY
e.g.
● poor coping resources and behaviour
● proneness to anxiety and depression
● lack of ability to occupy self
● few thoughts of the future
● isolation from family/outside contact
● makes few friends
● impulsive

Background
Experience
Poor family support
Low self-esteem
Poor prospects
Delinquency
Psychiatric treatment

PRISON-INDUCED STRESS
e.g.
● uncertainty, guilt, fear
● lack of family support/contact
● victimisation by other inmates
● loneliness and boredom
● isolation, lack of activity
● poor conditions and facilities
● breakdown of relationships

SITUATIONAL TRIGGERS
e.g.
● break-up of relationship, bad news
● failure of a visit to materialise
● threats, bullying or debts in prison
● parole refusal
● sleeplessness
● disciplinary procedures
● reception, transfers, change of location
● unexpected sentence
● others' suicides or attempts
● increase in any prison-induced stress

PROTECTING AGENTS
e.g.
● visits and contacts with family
● constructive occupation in prison
● support from inmates and staff
● hopes and plans for the future

communication escape
distress despair
Suicide ladder[1]
Lack of response

Vulnerability
Situational triggers
Prison-induced stress

Each component of the suicidal pathway may vary in its contribution to individual crises.

the inmate vulnerable to feelings of anxiety and low self-esteem; it may also provide a situational stress, as promised visits fail to materialise. Likewise, fear may act as a prison-induced stress, increasing at particular times, perhaps ultimately providing the final catalyst to suicidal action once a particular threshold is reached. The ability to cope with imprisonment varies between inmates and is amenable to simple investigation, by prison officers.

The aforementioned account calls into question any conception of young prisoner suicide as an exclusively or predominantly psychiatric problem. These are people in psychological distress, not necessarily amounting to mental disorder. Suicide in prison – at least amongst young prisoners – is to a large extent a problem of coping. The only solution currently offered by medical resources for being unable to cope is the option of temporary sanctuary in a hospital. It is important to recognise that non-medical solutions must be put forward in any effective suicide prevention strategy: some of these will be considered below. Remaining with the notion of understanding the problem for the moment, a second key issue can now be addressed. What are the methodological implications of the research reported here, and how has the methodological approach adopted in this book contributed to understanding young prisoner suicide and suicide attempts?

Methodological implications

Few previous studies of suicides and suicide attempts in custody have looked beyond the records of prisoners and into the subjective world of both inmates and staff. The originality of the present research project, guided by one or two exceptional studies, and by research in other areas of prison life (or in other areas of criminology), lies in its commitment to listening to its subjects and encouraging them to take the role of informers and teachers. In an address to the 1989 Prison Chaplains' Conference, Reverend Keith Pound, the Chaplain General, said that the role of the prison chaplain is to practise the art of listening, and to ask questions no-one else is asking. These are the principles of good prison-suicide research. Jack Dominion argued at the same conference that our prisons are full of the psychologically wounded, in whom love and hope have never been given a chance to grow. They lack self-esteem, they are hungry for recognition; they experience the world as hostile. The role of empathy: the ability to feel the inner world of the person, the ability to listen and the effort to avoid judging him or her, are important routes towards the restoration of those qualities that are missing in their lives: 'If the person we are listening to is to have confidence in us, he or she must feel that their inner world is reached and penetrated accurately ... Many people have never been properly heard in all their lives' (Dominion, 1988).

The long, semi-structured interview comprises the core of this research. One of its most important conclusions is that the experience of imprisonment cannot be fully apprehended by psychological scales and measurements alone (cf. Bukstel and Kilmann, 1980; Banister, 1973; Walker, 1983; Walker, 1987). Of more value is a detailed discussion with inmates of their experiences of custody, including possible thoughts of suicide precipitated by their current situation.

An exploration of the nature of suicide attempts in prison, as understood and managed by the staff, has not been undertaken in previous studies.

This book did not proceed from the premise that suicide attempts should be understood from a predominantly psychiatric perspective. It was this approach that led to the heart of staff fears expressed during the research fieldwork that they were not qualified to deal with the identification of suicide risk at all. It is of crucial importance to appreciate the problems faced by staff in the management and prevention of suicides in prison. Quite apart from feeling inadequately prepared to deal with the problem in the way they are asked to (by identifying risk factors and referring the inmate to the hospital), prison staff also perceive major problems of co-operation and communication between departments. They feel inadequately trained, and yet see themselves as held accountable for decisions they make about potential suicide risks. They have no say in decisions to return an inmate thought to be at risk of suicide from the hospital back to the wing. Completed suicides occurring on wings may be bitterly resented by those who discover the body, particularly amongst staff members who had been seeking some support for the inmate. If there are non-medical aspects to suicide in custody, non-medical staff should be involved in prevention policy.

Explanation and understanding risk

It is possible, based on the results of this research, to begin to formulate a new conception of risk which may be seen as more satisfactory and supplementary to the 'profile' approach to suicide prevention outlined in Chapter 2. The conventional profile suffers from several limitations, the most important of which is its failure to identify inmates who may go on to make a suicide attempt. Based as it is on limited statistical probabilities, many of those inmates who are especially vulnerable to suicidal thoughts in prison will not be identified by its narrow parameters. Nor will these 'typical characteristics' necessarily distinguish individuals at high risk of suicide from the rest of the prison population, many of whom share those characteristics found to be associated with suicide on the outside.

A new understanding of risk should be based on the notion of vulnerability to suicide. Staff with current training in 'the identification of risk' see it as a specialist skill which they learn to carry out as a separate and distinct part of their work. This rather limited and unsuccessful notion of risk identification should be reconceptualised: inmates can and will participate in their own risk assessment; they will indicate their own vulnerability, admit their current problems and even attempt to avoid some of the stresses leading to suicidal feelings in custody. 'Suicide risk' may be reframed in terms of inmates' coping ability; it is indicated in indirect ways by evidence of poor coping in other areas of prison life. In order to assess this ability, or its absence, staff should be engaged in the process of listening and communicating. As indicated in Chapter 8, the questions, 'What do you do when you're locked in your cell?' and 'What sort of plans do you have for when you get out?' may be better questions, and may be more accurately answered, than 'Are you feeling suicidal?'.

The process of identifying risk is not enough. The assessment of risk poses a question: what then to do with the vulnerable prisoner, or the poorest copers? Identifying vulnerability does not comprise a solution in itself, any more than isolation in stripped conditions addresses the problem of suicidal feelings. At present, at worst, inmates at risk of suicide are shuffled between the hospital and the wing, or between different prisons, with neither doctors nor prison officers feeling that the problem belongs in their hands. The practical implications of this state of affairs have been seen in 'lack of care' verdicts returned by inquest juries (R v. Birmingham and Solihull Coroner). A view of suicide risk as either present or absent, as either the psychiatrist's problem or 'one for the discipline staff', is wholly inadequate.

It has been argued in previous studies that the prison population is a particularly 'suicide prone' group. This argument receives a substantial amount of support from the present research, not just as a result of inmates' propensity to show those risk characteristics associated with suicide outside, but importantly, because of the poor coping skills and the limited future prospects shown by many inmates. The evidence for this can be seen throughout: in their lack of any constructive use made of either enforced-idle or occupied time. Opportunities are missed, nothing is planned and consequently the sentence is lived in the present. For most inmates, it serves no purpose and provides no support.

Debates about the aims of imprisonment have fluctuated between future-oriented goals (Rule 1: A good and useful life; positive custody) and present-oriented goals ('humane containment') (Bottoms, 1990:3–8). The recent mission statement issued by the Prison Service (cited in the Introduction, this volume) has been criticised on the grounds that it 'omits some crucial dimensions of the aims of imprisonment' (Bottoms, 1990:17); it has been characterised as a 'humane containment plus' formula (Ibid. :16), lacking any real and practical moral commitment to prisoners' rights, standards, opportunities or to their future. The need for some conceptual dimension of future hope in the articulation of aims has been identified and justified on practical, humanitarian and ethical grounds (Dunbar, 1985; Bottoms, 1990; Stern, 1989a). The lack of any ideals or aspirations for the future leaves prison staff to 'operate in a moral vacuum' (Dunbar, 1985; Stern, 1989a:229). Many have argued that the 'sense of futility' in the prison service should be avoided through simple messages and practical details (Dunbar, 1985; Bottoms, 1990). The three principles of relationship, individualism and activity were identified by Dunbar (1985:35) as holding the key to good regimes. The dimensions of hope and possibility ('even in the most unlikely individuals', Bottoms, 1990:23) hold the key to the minimisation of suicidal thoughts and feelings amongst prisoners. We do not have to predict the suicidal individual in order to be aware that hopelessness, enforced idleness, fear, inactivity and despair comprise the pathway to suicide. It is a matter for the public and for policy-makers to decide whether some notion of social, economic or even 'spiritual' rehabilitation might point the way to a better future. The concept of 'care' has an explicit meaning: it must incorporate respect, nurturing and hope for the future. These concepts are as important for the short-term prisoner (and the remand prisoner) as they are for the long-termer. Without care and without hope, there is nothing. A better link between stated aims and practice would be a welcome development:

> Many of you will share the view that suicide prevention cannot be seen primarily as a matter of procedures and precautions. In its widest sense it must be about creating a climate in which suicidal thoughts and feelings are less likely to take root. Inmates will normally be less prone to resort to suicidal behaviour in the establishment where regimes are full, varied and relevant; where staff morale is high and relationships with inmates are positive; where inmates are treated fairly and as individuals; where good basic living conditions are provided; where every effort is made to encourage contacts with family and the community. In short, the problem of suicide can never be separated from the Service's over-arching duty to treat prisoners with humanity and prepare them for release.
> (Addendum to CI 20/1989, issued 12 December, 1990:1–2)

Moving forward in research

Prison suicide research and research on suicides in the community should inform each other, whilst recognising important differences of context. The notion of 'resourcelessness' applies to vulnerable people in the community as well as to those in prison. Understanding the aetiology of such phenomena in the community might contribute to our understanding of the effects of a prison sentence, or of long stretches of time spent in idleness and isolation. On the other hand, the problem of prison suicide should also be considered as a distinct phenomenon, with a unique context: extrapolating directly from research results found in community samples is ill-advised. The range of methods available, the timing and the motivation of such attempts in prison need to be understood within the particular environment in which they occur. We can enter the field informed by community studies, but should appreciate the different character of this context. Research on prison suicides should also be increasingly informed by the methodology and concepts of sociological research into other areas of prison life.

This book has not considered suicide attempts amongst young people in other institutions, such as hospitals, educational or army establishments. It has not included suicide attempts occurring after release from prison. The research field-work was restricted to inmates serving sentences in young offender institutions. It excluded remand centres, police cells and the courts, despite reports of young suicides in these settings. It has not attempted to analyse groups of suicide attempters according to their perceived degree of risk, nor has it followed up any of the cases involved in the research in order to monitor long-term outcomes. It has not considered the effects of medication nor the significance of physical ailments in suicide risk.

Future research is required on inmates who recover from suicidal crises, on those who go on to repeat their attempts, and on differences between males and females in the development and expression of suicidal feelings. A study of suicide verdicts, and of possible differences between inquests held in cases of unnatural deaths in custody and those in the community would be most informative. A study of suicide attempts in local and remand centres and amongst adult prisoners will follow the project reported in this book. It should be supplemented by further research on treatment methods, an evaluation of staff training and by comparative studies in National Health Service hospitals, youth treatment centres and other types of environment.

SECTION II: POLICY INTO PRACTICE

Evaluating policy and practice

Most of the establishments visited during the course of the fieldwork were young offender institutions for sentenced inmates, with little overcrowding, relatively stable populations and good facilities. Circumstances in which Circular Instructions on Suicide Prevention were being implemented were favourable. In addition, the advance notice of impending research doubtless encouraged establishments to ensure that their suicide prevention procedures were in reasonable working order at the time of – or throughout – any expected visit. In this context, problems that were encountered or reported were more fundamental than organisational.

The limitations of suicide prevention policy raised by prison staff during the research fell into two groups. First, operational difficulties relating to the proper implementation of the Circular on suicide prevention (for example, the problem of communication). Secondly, limitations relating to the scope of the Circulars themselves were raised. The identification and assessment of suicide risk had been made more systematic by the new Instructions, but notions of treatment and support were not adequately articulated in the Instructions, nor implemented in practice. The emphasis placed on risk assessment left staff feeling helpless: they were faced with a task they felt unqualified to carry out, the outcome of which they felt accountable for. Inmates were not the only group to be troubled by fear.

Briefly, four limitations in current policy and its implementation were reported by the staff: poor communication and co-operation between departments within establishments, particularly between the hospital and the discipline staff on the wings; staff suspicions about the purposes and usefulness of instructions which were clearly intended to 'protect the Department at inquests'; the application of a blanket set of procedures to widely differing types of establishment; and the lack of resources such as training and staff.

The problem of communication and co-operation was clear: three-quarters of the uniformed staff reported serious difficulties between the wings and the hospital.

Prison staff were thought by hospital staff to be making inappropriate referrals to the hospital, occasionally inundating them with 'non-medical' problems. Staff on wings reported inadequate feedback once referrals had been made. Disagreements inevitably arose as to whether or not the inmate was a 'suicide' or medical problem. Temporary respite in the hospital, followed by a swift return to the wing was seen as an inadequate response to wing staff's fears about the inmate's safety. Prison officers felt that the hospital did not share information or opinions with the wing on the inmate's return.

Secondly, doubts were expressed about the purposes of a set of instructions which were appearing with increasing prominence at inquests. Observation at 15-minute intervals, for example, does not prevent the determined suicide, and is intrusive and unhelpful for the potentially suicidal. Fifteen minutes allows more than enough time to accomplish a self-inflicted death. It is this aspect of the suicide prevention procedures which received the most cynical remarks from the staff. It was assumed that complying with these procedures ensured that they had acted properly in the event of a successful suicide. Only continuous observation on a ward could provide realistic prevention. For the suicidal inmate, observation was useless, not even an effective situational deterrent. What they needed was treatment, counselling, support and the resolution of particular problems. Staff felt they did not have the time, nor the training to provide such support.

Thirdly, staff (and occasionally, inmates) at the four centres studied often mentioned that the identification and assessment system introduced by CI 3/1987 and CI 20/1989 may have been more appropriate to local and remand centres, where high turnovers, staff shortages and little activity or interaction between staff and inmates precluded all but the 'bare bones' of a suicide prevention system. In young offender institutions, where operational pressures were fewer, a wholly different approach to the detection of risk and the management of the suicidal would be possible.

Fourthly, the issue of training: at the time of the research few of the staff had received either local or national training in suicide prevention. Those that had felt that it had not answered their own queries about suicide attempts, nor had it allayed their fears that some of the responsibility for suicide prevention inevitably rested with the officers, and yet they had no influence over decisions about the inmate's risk categorisation or location.

Officers felt defensive. They recognised that they had extensive knowledge of the inmates and their suicide attempts, yet lacked the confidence to query decisions made by the hospital – decisions that might be based on minimal contact with the prisoner concerned. In order to fulfil the spirit of the suicide prevention Circulars, as enshrined in the above Addendum (Home Office, 1990b), conflictual relationships between staff and between departments should also be resolved.

Finally, we can look briefly at the practical implications of the arguments outlined in this study, and at future directions for policy and practice.

New directions for policy

In 1990, the Chief Inspector of Prisons, Judge Stephen Tumim published his review of prison suicide prevention procedures (Home Office, 1990d) and 123 recommendations were made. He concluded that only an integrated and proactive approach by all staff (and where appropriate, inmates) would improve the prison service strategy in preventing suicides. Confinement in prison, he argued, under conditions of inactivity and with the lack of any purpose, can only serve to emphasise extremes of human feeling, such as boredom and despair. Substantial evidence for the recommendations made in Tumim's detailed report can be found in this book. Extensive and exploratory interviews with inmates expressing suicidal feelings, with those 'at risk' and with inmates from the general population illustrate the essentially psychological or cognitive (rather than exclusively medical) problem of prison suicide. Vulnerability can be recognised and alleviated in simple ways. Education, activity, contact and concern might avert many crises.

In the light of the research presented in the previous chapters, certain procedural conclusions can be drawn. First, a Circular Instruction cannot, on its own, constitute a satisfactory response to the increasing numbers of suicide attempts taking place in prison. Staff training, continuity, good communication between departments, time and resources, and a commitment to a suicide prevention strategy, are all essential components. One of the major problems that has to be addressed in order to reduce the likelihood of recourse to both self-injury and suicide attempts is the issue of bullying (see McGurk and McDougal, 1986; Shine *et al.*, 1990). Reducing both the opportunities and the conditions which facilitate such behaviour would have favourable effects, not the least of which may be the curtailment of epidemics of suicide attempts.

Prison Department policy on suicide prevention is informed largely by studies of those risk factors found to be associated with suicide risk on the outside (such as previous psychiatric treatment, depression, alcohol abuse, and social isolation). In prison, many of these characteristics are shown by a large proportion of the inmate population, thus detracting from the relevance of such factors in providing an indication of suicide risk. There may be other important factors in the prison situation, for particular groups of prisoners, and as argued above, a different conception of risk is required.

Distinctions should also be drawn between sentenced and remand prisoners, whose populations may be distinct in their levels of psychiatric morbidity. The adult male remand population has a high prevalence of psychiatric disorder, including schizophrenia, alcoholism, depression and other problems which are related to suicide (Gunn, 1991, pers. comm.). Many may be in prison for the preparation of medical reports for the courts because of suspected psychiatric disturbance. The sentenced population, on the other hand, shows relatively low levels of depressive illness and schizophrenia – conditions known to be associated with increased suicide risk – whilst problems such as drug abuse, personality disorder and sexual disorders are high (Gunn, 1991, pers. comm.). Psychiatric explanations may contribute to the suicide figures amongst remand prisoners to a greater degree than amongst the sentenced population. A psychiatric assessment may be more relevant for remand prisoners thought to be at risk of suicide than for sentenced prisoners showing evidence of psychological distress rather than psychiatric illness.

It may be that distinctions should be drawn between remand and sentenced prisoners, and between young prisoners and adults, in the formulation of policy. Procedures which stress interaction and support should supplement the 'bare bones' of an identification and assessment system which prevents by physical restraint. In addition to pre-release courses, sentenced inmates should be offered 'coping skills' courses, which address both sentence and post-release survival. Legitimate alternatives to self-injury should be provided and made obvious to inmates experiencing difficulties during the sentence. Under no circumstances should the response to a suicide attempt be punitive: isolation in stripped conditions is sometimes assumed by inmates to be a punishment for their behaviour. Staff training should supplement its current emphasis on the identification of risk factors with a thorough discussion of the meaning of a suicide attempt and the reframing of the concept of risk. To attribute a unitary meaning to these acts (i.e. attention-seeking) is potentially dangerous and misleading. Training should be aimed at encouraging all staff to appreciate the complexity of such behaviour and its possible causes and motivations, which are multiple. It should be stressed that 'attention-seeking behaviour' often precedes suicide.

Most evaluation studies of treatment and training in suicide prevention in the prison context (of which there are none in the UK) show that therapeutic intervention is both possible and effective (Sperbeck and Parlour, 1986; Hopes and Shaull, 1986; Jenkins *et al.*, 1982; Wicks, 1972; Ramsay *et al.*, 1987). The authors of these studies also agree that more systematic research is needed on suicide attempters in the prison setting before advances can be made. The use of behavioural contracts, psychological counselling and support and a change of environment, including movement to a different wing, or to shared accommodation, have all been shown to contribute to recovery from a suicidal crisis (Sperbeck and Parlour, 1986; Ramsay *et al.*, 1987). There is a case for developing innovative methods of psychological support. As we might expect from the results of studies in the community (e.g. Hawton and Catalan, 1987), different groups of prisoners are found to respond to different types of treatment. The young and first-time offenders should not not be isolated in response to suicide threats as they do not cope well in single cells (Sperbeck and Parlour, 1986). Good morale amongst staff is essential to successful treatment (Langlay and Bayatti, 1984; Bluglass, 1990; Scottish Home and Health Department, 1985; Sainsbury, 1988).

In the search for constructive solutions, we have much to learn from community studies: that proper assessment takes time (Hawton and Catalan, 1987), that negative attitudes from staff interfere with recovery (Morgan, 1979; Hawton and Catalan, 1987); that non-medically qualified staff can assess the state of the patient as adequately as medical staff (Gardner *et al.*, 1982), and that the patient will report his or her own problems and may participate in the definition of appropriate treatment. Cognitive or group therapy is found to be an effective method of treatment with adolescents (Sainsbury, 1988). Trained prison staff can be very effective agents of therapy as they are in daily contact with inmates. Staff should be encouraged 'to engage in casual and frequent conversations with inmates, since these may often reveal cognitive and affective suicidal clues' (Sperbeck and Parlour, 1986:97).

Finally, it is apparent from recent reports (Home Office, 1990d; Woolf, 1991) that the Prison Department and other relevant agents are in many respects committed to the alleviation of 'prison-induced distress' in both inmates and, increasingly, amongst staff. This book aims to contribute to the understanding of that distress and of the young prisoners who are susceptible to it.

Notes

INTRODUCTION

1 *Parasuicide* is a term first used by Kreitmen (Kreitman, 1969; 1977) in order to distinguish between 'suicidal acts' and acts which simulate or mimic suicide, but which may not be oriented primarily towards death. The use of this term is problematic and has not been adopted by the author for reasons outlined in Chapter 2. A *'suicidal act'* has been defined as 'any act of deliberate self-damage, which the person committing the act could not be sure of surviving' (Stengel, 1970). *'Suicide'* has been defined as 'self-inflicted death', usually with the intention of dying (Stengel, 1970; Eldrid, 1988; Schneidman, 1985). See Kreitman (1969) and Stengel (1970), and also Schneidman (1985) for a discussion of the many difficulties pertaining to these definitions, about which there is little agreement.

2 Suicides and self-inflicted deaths in prison 1985–1989

Year	1985		1986		1987		1988		1989	
Local/remand	25	(21)	16	(13)	35	(33)	24	(22)	34	(23)
Dispersal	–	–	2	(1)	3	(2)	3	(1)	2	(2)
Cat. B	2	(2)	2	(2)	4	(3)	4	(4)	2	(1)
Cat. C	–	–	1	(1)	1	(1)	4	(3)	5	(4)
Open	–	–	–	–	–	–	–	–	–	–
Female	1	(–)	–	–	–	–	–	–	–	–
YOI*	1	(–)	–	–	3	(3)	2	(1)	5	(3)
Totals	29	(23)	21	(17)	46	(42)	37	(31)	48	(33)

Source: Adapted from Home Office, 1990d:50–51
Note: * The self-inflicted deaths in YOIs do not include all young-prisoner deaths; many occur in local and remand centres. The figures in brackets are deaths confirmed as suicide by Coroners' inquests. The figures for young-offender prison suicides are included in Chapter 3.

3 In R v. Southwark Coroner, Ex-parte Hicks [1987] 1 WLR 1624 it was held that a verdict of lack of care was appropriate where the death was caused by neglect of the inmate's physical or medical condition (in this case, epilepsy), and other persons had a real opportunity of doing something which could have prevented the death. Lack of care was not thought to be appropriate in this prison suicide case, where care was simply the common-law duty of care, and it was plain that the deceased had intended to kill himself. He had been depressed and low, but there was no evidence that he was not responsible for his actions. The verdict 'lack of care' could only be appropriate where the deceased's physical and/or mental condition were the *true cause of death*. An example of such a case would be where a deranged man, incapable of forming any intention and known to be in such a condition that he required constant care, was neglected and jumped through

a window to his death (R v. Birmingham and Solihull Coroner, Ex-parte Secretary of State for the Home Department. July 1990). Whether the death had been aggravated by lack of care was an issue for the new inquest jury. The second inquest was held on 24–25 October 1990. The jury decided that the suicide had occurred 'in circumstances aggravated by lack of care' (*Guardian* 25 October 1990:3). In Knight and others v. the Home Office and Governor of HMP Brixton, Mr Justice Pill held that the 'duty of care' owed by the Prison Medical Service to prisoners was not comparable with that owed by NHS psychiatric hospitals to its patients (see British Medical Association, 1990; also Smith, 1984; Home Office, 1990a; Sim, 1990; and Kappeler *et al.*, 1991).

4 Fresh Start: New staffing structures and working practices brought into the prison service in the late 1980s, intended to improve efficiency and match tasks to the hours available in the working day. Overtime bans, and the unification of governor and officer grades were major changes designed to secure a more organised and better managed service with a well-paid basic salary and a career structure. The recruitment of more prison staff and the enhancement of regimes were promised to follow from its implementation.

5 A personal or group officer 'will play an important and continuing part in the preparation of sentence plans'. He:

> should be the first point of contact for the offenders assigned to him. While retaining the right of access to specialists without enquiry as to the nature and content of the interview, offenders should be encouraged to approach their personal officer on any problems which may arise during the course of the sentence. Personal officers should be given opportunities to talk to the offenders assigned to them about their offending behaviour and its consequences for others as well as themselves. They should help them to adjust to custody, assess their reactions to it and identify any welfare problems.
>
> (CI 40/88: Regimes in Young Offender Institutions, para. 19)

1   SUICIDES IN PRISON: RATES AND EXPLANATIONS

1 Smalley noted that 'the number of females, nine, is too small for statistical analysis'; they were therefore excluded from the rest of the study (Smalley, 1911:41).

2 'Between 1868 and 1877 more than 2,000 people accused of the criminal offence of attempted suicide were committed to the House of Detention at Clerkenwell' (Priestly, 1985:70).

3 Goring also commented:

> From the statistical point of view, a very real difficulty contained in this question is fortunately removed by the fact that the special immunity from accidental death, afforded to prisoners, happens to be nicely balanced by their increased liability to die from suicide.
>
> (Goring, 1913:153)

4 This is an unfortunate choice of base rate, as suicides as a proportion of *deaths* are not an indication of suicide *rates*.

5 Williams has suggested (MRC, University of Cambridge) that since the removal of the offence of attempted suicide from the criminal statutes, suicide has ceased to be the preserve of the police. In 1961, the beginning of psychiatric interest in the nature and causes of suicide was encouraged (Williams, 1989, pers. comm.).

6 Most of the figures given below (for Europe and Canada) are taken or translated from Bernheim's detailed study of prison suicide rates in Canada and 11 different European countries (Bernheim, 1987).

7 This figure is reached by calculating 46 per cent of the prison death rates, 1980–1985, of which 46 per cent were suicides.

8 The rate for children in Juvenile Detention facilities, on the other hand, was 1.6 per 100,000 ADP – much lower than the rate for children in the community, at 3.5 per 100,000 (Flaherty, 1983:89).

9 UK ratio of receptions to ADP is 5:1; in the US the ratio is 11:1. For remand inmates only the ratio is 6:1 in the UK and 36:1 in the US (Criminal Justice Statistics, 1988:605–7; 614–15; Prison Department Statistics, 1988; US Department of Justice, Criminal Statistics, 1988).

10 Information about the proportion of suicides amongst these deaths is not given. It is known that suicides constitute a higher proportion of all deaths in prison than in the community (Winfree, 1985; Tuskan and Thase, 1983).

2   THE PRISON SUICIDE PROFILE

1 In Japan and Israel the ratio is equal (Bernheim, 1987:118).

2 Whether this accurately reflects 'the facts' or reflects stereotypes relating to male and female behaviour is a matter for speculation. The assumptions may be that women commit suicide as a result of mental illness, or internal factors, whereas men commit suicide as a result of external 'rational' factors (cf. Allen, 1987 by analogy).

3 It is likely that female prison suicides do differ from their male counterparts, not least because the female prison population differs in significant respects (age, offence-type, family and employment history, psychiatric history, etc.) from the male population (Zamble and Porporino, 1988; Heffernan, 1972). It is also apparent from a small number of studies that female prison suicides may be achieved by different methods and for different reasons than male prison suicides (Hatty and Walker, 1986; see discussion in Chapter 7).

4 Charter 87, a campaigning organisation in the UK concerned about suicide and at-tempted suicide by asylum seekers held in detention without charge or trial, and ordered to be deported, provided detailed information about several cases of suicide and attempted suicides: 'Such people do not need to be protected from themselves ... but from their circumstances' (Charter 87 *Newsletter*, Oct./Nov. 1990). The anxiety and uncertainty of their situation, and exacerbated by language and cultural difficulties, may 'lead to attempted suicide' (Ibid.). Since their campaign, new procedures have been introduced for most political asylum-seekers arriving in the UK. Many fear imprison-ment and torture if they return to their own countries.

5 Many of the disorders found to be relatively more common in prison than outside (e.g. drug abuse, sexual and personality disorders) are marginal issues in psychiatry, despite being classified as psychiatric disorders by International Classification of Diseases and Disorders (ICD). In a forthcoming study by Gunn et al., 38 per cent of sentenced adult males were given a psychiatric diagnosis. Of this group, 10 per cent of men (22 per cent of women) were drug dependent, 8 per cent were alcohol dependent, 5–6 per cent were found to have anxiety neuroses (many of these groups could also be diagnosed as personality disordered). A further 7–8 per cent had a diagnosis of personality disorder alone. Outside, it is thought that 10–12 per cent of the general population suffer from minor neurotic or depressive illnesses (Gunn, 1990; 1991, pers. comm.).

6 Under observation: this term describes the special procedures whereby inmates are isolated, normally on a hospital wing, and checked during 15-minute intervals. Different degrees if special watch procedures are employed, from less frequent checks to continual observation and the removal of all dangerous objects (such as cell contents and clothes).

7 The same might be said of Instructions issued to prison department establishments on

the management and prevention of suicide. The notions of 'treatment' or support, once the inmate potentially at risk has been identified, are absent from these Circulars.

8 Hunger-strikers are not technically included amongst suicide attempt figures. The feelings expressed and the circumstances leading to food refusal amongst prison inmates may be similar to those associated with other types of self-harm. Inmates may refuse food for several days or on several occasions before making a suicide attempt. The association of hunger-strike with political protest is misleading. No discussion of food refusal in the literature on suicide attempts in prison was found.

9 This finding is taken to suggest a clear lack of 'social integration' amongst prison suicides, it is worth bearing in mind that three of the four widowers in this group were charged with killing their wives.

10 No conclusive evidence for this assertion, or for the assumption that inmates know which methods are likely to be more effective, is available. In the community, the young show very little understanding of the dangerousness of different types and amounts of drugs used in overdoses (Hawton *et al.*, 1982a).

11 Sparks has suggested that the word 'strategic' may be less invidious than the term 'manipulative' (Sparks, 1990, pers. comm.). This would be consistent with the notion of the appeal function of a suicide attempt, and avoids some of the temptation for staff (and others) to dismiss the behaviour or, worse, to punish it.

3   YOUNG PRISONER SUICIDES AND SUICIDE ATTEMPTS: A SPECIAL CASE?

1 Young Offenders in custody (or 'young prisoners') are defined by the Prison Department as:

> Those sentenced to imprisonment when under 21 (replaced, along with borstal, by youth custody from 24 May 1983) or detention in a young offenders institution from October 1988, who have not subsequently been reclassified as adults; it therefore encompasses inmates reaching 21 or more without being reclassified.
>
> (Home Office, 1988a)

The term 'young offender' may also include juveniles, aged between 14 and 16. The term 'young adult offender' would exclude this group.

2 The analysis of these figures is my own, but would not have been possible without the kind assistance of Dr Enda Dooley in extracting this data from his study of all prison suicides, 1972–1987. The comparison is limited by the fact that significant differences between the adult and young offender suicides could not be explored without separating them from the original total figures given in Dooley's paper.

3 These figures do not take into account the increase in young prisoner suicides between 1987 and 1990 (see below).

Self-inflicted deaths of young prisoners 1987–1990*

1987	7
1988	9
1989	11
1990	8

Note: *Up-dated from Home Office, 1990d:22; Prison Reform Trust, 1990:5. In 1990, 16 per cent of self-inflicted deaths were by young prisoners, reflecting their proportion in the prison population.

4 Baroning: a mode of economic gain whereby tobacco or canteen goods are loaned and borrowed, with high rates of 'interest' expected in return. Inmates may be threatened

with violence if they default on payments. 'Taxing' involves the forcible removal of inmates' goods. (Shine *et al.*, 1990:119–20).

5 The Werther Effect aquires its name from J. W. von Goethe's novel, *The Sorrows of Young Werther*, which had a tremendous impact on many young men, inciting several to suicide, it is believed (Schmidte and Hafner, 1988).

4 A CHANGE OF DIRECTION

1 In 1991 six verdicts of lack of care were brought at the inquests of suicides in custody (Inquest, 1991). The case cited in the Introduction (R v. Birmingham and Solihul Coroner, July 1990) and its subsequent appeal which failed to overturn the lack-of-care verdict brought, has apparently set a precedent. This case has become a watershed in prison suicide history. The effects of such a verdict on suicide prevention in practice are mixed. Fear of such verdicts within establishments can lead to a defensiveness and a withdrawal of involvement from potentially 'at risk' cases. The Circular Instructions are not legal documents and should not be used as such. Condemnation may not be as effective as support. On the other hand, the exposure of poor practice, lack of communication and organisational difficulties has helped to transform practice in some establishments. The campaign to achieve such damning verdicts at inquests should be met by an equally fierce campaign by the prison department and by individual establishments to exclude such a possibility, despite the odds.

2 A new version of the F213 was introduced into establishments in March 1990. This is a longer form, with more details required (place of injury, time and date of examination, circumstances in which injury sustained), and more room for comment.

3 The information included on the Major Incident form is time and date of incident, time and date last seen alive, whether suicide took place in public view, whether next of kin and coroner have been informed, were there any apparent lapses in security, vigilance or failure to comply with MO's directions or Standing Orders, whether the family are critical of the department, method, date and verdict of inquest and whether the inquest inferred lack of care. An attempt at suicide requires four of these questions to be answered: did the suicide (sic) take place in public view; were there any apparent lapses in security, vigilance or failure to comply with MO's directions or Standing Orders; is the inmate's family critical of the department, and method used in attempt. All information on Minor Reports is sent to Regional Offices (monthly); Major Incidents are sent immediately to Regional Office and to the Deputy Director's Office, using British Telecom Gold electronic mail. This recording system is out of date since the introduction of Incident Management Support Units as part of the prison service reorganisation in September 1991.

5 INVESTIGATING SUICIDES IN PRISON

1 During the small number of reception interviews observed, this question has been asked with eyes down on a desk, in the presence of other inmates, or in reverse: 'not feeling suicidal at all?'.

2 The issue of whether or not to ask for and use keys during prison research is a vexed one. Staff in young offender establishments are far more willing to agree to keys being issued than those in adult prisons. The major arguments against the use of keys are (1) personal safety (risk of being taken hostage) and (2) one's image *vis-à-vis* the inmates. Regarding (1), if I had felt at risk at any stage throughout the research, I would have returned the keys and managed without. As for (2), chaplains carry keys, and this does

not seem to interfere with their counselling and pastoral role. As a chaplain once said to me, 'my keys are to open doors, not just to shut them'.

3   It is possible given the number and variety of variables included in the questionnnaire that some of the apparently significant results (those reaching a level of p<0.05) are in fact spurious. However, as those responses which have shown appreciable differences between the two inmate groups are in a consistent direction, and are compatible with the theory of vulnerability and poor coping supported throughout this book, all the results are presented in the text. See also the comment in Chapter 6 about this data refinement process (see note 1 below).

4   At this stage in the writing process the choice of material to be included in an account of the research process is consistent with (but was not determined by) feminist writing: 'a feminist approach to research or a feminist methodology usually involves a focus on socially significant problems; feminist researchers typically become involved with the research subjects; they also aim to record the impact of the research on themselves' (Gelsthorpe, 1990:94).

5   The wish to build up a relationship of trust, and to provide an atmosphere that facilitated honesty and an open discussion of difficult questions required a stance which expressed to the inmate that I would believe and value his words, suspending 'suspicion'. As Jack Dominion pointed out at the Prison Chaplaincy Conference (1989), adopting this stance may provide the young offender with the first opportunity he or she has ever had to be believed. Many inmates expressed surprise that the interview had no other purpose besides recording their own version of events.

6   UNDERSTANDING YOUNG PRISONER SUICIDES AND SUICIDE ATTEMPTS: IN THEIR OWN WORDS

1   *A Note on Statistics.* As indicated in a note in Chapter 5, too much faith in statistical methods of data presentation can ignore complexities in the data obscured by the neatness of categorisation. In this chapter, indicators of the level of statistical significance are given as a guide to the reader who may prefer a signpost to the more important trends emerging from the interviews. Any p value lower than 0.05 shows that the table contains differences between the groups well over those that might have been expected by chance. The smaller the p value, the greater these differences are. In some cases, the numbers in the tables are so small that these statistical tests become less reliable. Bourke, Daly and McGilvray argue that only when more than 20 per cent of the cells in a table are below 5 is there any reason to doubt the reliability of this statistical test (Bourke *et al.*, 1985:115). Robson (1983) argues that the significance values may still be a guide to the reader, providing that some indication of the small numbers is given.

2   The measure of previous convictions used in the research was the number of previous convictions, not the number of court appearances. Although the number of court appearances has been found to be significantly associated with future reoffending (Phillpots and Lancucki, 1979), it is the extent of (known) previous offending behaviour that is known to be associated with suicidal behaviour in prison (Griffiths, 1990a and 1990b).

3   In 63 per cent of these cases there was evidence from both the interview and the record. In a further 18 per cent of cases, the information was found in the record. In a last 18 per cent of cases the information came from the interview only.

4   Rule 43: The term 'Rule 43' is used in Young Offender Establishments, even though the equivalent of the adult 'Rule 43' for young offenders is Rule 46. The definition of Rule 46 is as follows:

Young Offender Institution Rule 46: Removal from association

(1)   Where it appears desirable, for the maintenance of good order or discipline or in his own interests, that a prisoner should not associate with other prisoners, either generally or for particular purposes, the governor may arrange for the prisoner's removal from association accordingly.

(2)   An inmate shall not be removed under this Rule for a period of more than 24 hours without the authority of a member of the board of visitors, or the Secretary of State. An authority given under this paragraph shall in the case of a female inmate aged 21 years or over, be for a period not exceeding one month and, in the case of any other inmate, be for a period not exceeding 14 days, but may be renewed from time to time for a like period.

(3)   The governor may arrange at his discretion for such a prisoner as aforesaid to resume association with other prisoners, and shall do so if in any case the medical officer so advises on medical grounds.

(Prison Department (1989), *The Management of Vulnerable Prisoners*, Report of a Prison Department Working Group:63)

The Working Group were established in 1988 in order to review policy and practice in relation to inmates segregated on Rule 43(6), including their treatment and access to activity. Use of the term 'own request' to describe those inmates who are 'voluntarily' segregated for their own protection is incorrect, according to the Working Party Report. The measure is a management option available to the Governor and is not subject to the prisoners' discretion.

The Report argues that Rule 43 is not a desirable situation for prisoners, whether convicted or unconvicted, having various detrimental consequences from the prisoners' point of view:

it deprives the prisoner of normal association; it can prevent access to facilities for work, recreation and education; it has a stigma which can label a prisoner for the whole of his sentence; it overrides other considerations for appropriate allocation (including proximity to home); it keeps the prisoner's offence in the forefront of the minds of those who have to make assessments of him.

The only benefit is the provision of physical protection from assault or intimidation from other inmates.

5   Possible inverse links between absconding and suicide are not raised in the literature, but it is clear from several sources that absconding provides an 'escape route' which is chosen in preference to self-injury or suicide attempts where possible (see CI 40/88:59). Research on absconding behaviour and its associated causes (Laycock, 1977, Banks *et al.*, 1975) and observation of adjudication procedures following absconds from YOIs confirm this impressionistic link between the two types of incident.

6   There is a widely held assumption explicit in suicide prevention procedures that suicides can be predicted and action taken to avert them. This assumption is of crucial importance at inquests and may influence the verdict. The extent to which individual suicides are in fact predictable remains a complex and somewhat confused issue. Prison staff tend to assume that 'genuine suicides will never be predicted'. Both extremes are flawed. It is likely that certain types of suicide are more 'predictable' and 'preventable' than others.

7   The prison officer could, with little extra training, enquire about areas 3–5 as a lead into ordinary 'welfare' concerns, *and* as a possible probe into vulnerability or risk. If he was seriously worried by any of the responses given, he could investigate areas 1 and 2 in the inmate's file, perhaps alerting other staff (probation, Chaplain, psychologist) about the *particular* area of concern (rather than subsuming the whole picture under *suicide*

risk), such as the lack of visits, difficulties with other inmates, or problems sleeping. Keeping all inmates active, and helping them to make more constructive use of their time/sentence would be obvious ways of minimising risk. The importance of encouraging constructive occupation is clear from these results.

8 A long-term research project (which included remand prisoners) on suicide attempts in male prisons has been carried out by the Institute of Criminology as a follow-up to the study reported in this book. It is due for completion in May 1992 and publication will be forthcoming.

8   MANAGING TO PREVENT SUICIDE: STAFF ATTITUDES AND PERSPECTIVES

1 Senior Officer (see Abbreviations at the front of the book).

2 Taxing: See example, in Chapter 6 (p. 147).

3 Much of the recent training carried out on suicide prevention had been criticised on the grounds of poor presentation, or poor choice of trainer. Staff were resistant to instruction that was felt to be unhelpful or inappropriate, particularly if the officer chosen to present the short course was significantly younger and less experienced than the 'old hands' he was trying to teach.

4 At one establishment there were three suicides in the year following the completion of the fieldwork. On a return visit after the first (and subsequent discussions with staff), it was clear that these tragedies made a great deal of difference to the atmosphere in the hospital and on the wings, and to the confidence of the staff. Many of the staff reported feeling 'devastated', and two were tempted to leave the service.

5 In the US there have been more than 10,000 civil suits filed against local jails (Winfree, 1985:14). In the UK a recent judicial review failed to overturn a 'lack of care' verdict in the case of a prisoner suicide. A new inquest was ordered, but a new jury also returned a verdict of 'suicide in circumstances brought about by lack of care' (*Independent* 27 October 1990:2). See also Kappeler *et al.*, 1991.

6 A new strategy for staff care and support, especially following incidents, has been launched by the Prison Department. Local 'care teams' are being established. Awareness of staff needs is increasing, and probably constitutes one of the major avenues towards better suicide prevention strategies within individual establishments.

Bibliography

Albanese, J S (1983) Preventing Inmate Suicides, *Federal Probation* 47:65–69.

Allebeck, P, Allgulander, C and Fisher, L D (1988) Predictors of Completed Suicide in A Cohort of 50, 465 Young Men: Role of Personality and Deviant Behaviour, *British Medical Journal* 297:176–178.

Allen, H (1987) *Justice Unbalanced: Gender, Psychiatry and Judicial Decisions.* Open University Press: Milton Keynes.

Anderson, O (1987) *Suicide in Victorian and Edwardian England.* Clarendon: Oxford.

Anthony, H S (1973) *Depression, Psychopathic Personality and Attempted Suicide in a Borstal Sample.* HORU Report No. 19, HMSO: London.

Atkinson, J M (1982 edn) *Discovering Suicide: Studies in the Social Organisation of Sudden Death.* Macmillan: London.

Australian Office of Corrections (1985) Suicide and Other Deaths in Prison Including Victorian Results from the National Deaths in Corrections Study. Unpublished Report, Research Unit, Office of Corrections: Victoria, Australia.

Backett, S (1987) Suicides in Scottish Prisons, *British Journal of Psychiatry* 151:218–221.

Backett, S (1988) Suicide and Stress in Prison, in Backett, S, McNeil, J and Yellowlees, A (eds) *Imprisonment Today.* Macmillan: London: 70–84.

Bagshaw, M (1988) Suicide Prevention Training: Lessons From the Corrections Service of Canada, *Prison Service Journal* 70:5–6.

Bagshaw, M and Baxter, K (1987) Interactive Skills Training for Prison Officers, in McGurk, B J, Thornton, D M and Williams, M *Applying Psychology to Imprisonment.* HMSO: London.

Baldwin, P (1988) Women in Prison, in Backett, S, McNeil, J, and Yellowlees, A (eds) *Imprisonment Today.* Macmillan: London: 53–70.

Bancroft, J and Hawton, K (1983) Why People Take Overdoses: A Study of Psychiatrists' Judgements, *British Journal of Medical Psychology* 56:197–204.

Banks, C, Mayhew, P and Sapsford, R (1975) *Absconding From Open Prisons.* Home Office Research Studies, 26 HMSO: London.

Banister, P A (1973) Psychological Correlates of Long-term Imprisonment: 1 Cognitive Variables, *British Journal Of Criminology* 13:312–322.

Barraclough, B M and Hughes, J (1987) *Suicide: Clinical and Epidemiological Studies.* Croom Helm: London.

Barraclough, B M, Bunch, J, Nelson, B and Sainsbury, P (1974) A Hundred Cases of Suicide: Clinical Aspects, *British Journal of Psychiatry* 125:355–73.

Beck, A T (1976) *Cognitive Therapy and the Emotional Disorders.* International Universities Press: New York.

Beck, A T, Brown, G and Steer, R A (1989) Prediction of Eventual Suicide in Psychiatric Inpatients by Clinical Ratings of Hopelessness, *Journal of Clinical and Consulting Psychology* 57(2):309–310.

Beck, A T, Weissman, A, Lester, D and Trexler, L (1974) The Measurement of Pessimism: The Hopelessness Scale, *Journal of Clinical and Consulting Psychology* 42:861–865.

Bernheim, J C (1987) *Les Suicides en Prison*. Editions du Meridian: Canada.

Biles, D (1988) Draft Guidelines For The Prevention of Aboriginal Deaths in Custody, *Royal Commission into Aboriginal Deaths in Custody* Research Paper No.2. Australian Institute of Criminology: Canberra.

Biles, D (1989a) Australian Deaths in Custody 1980–1988: An Analysis of Aboriginal and Non-Aboriginal Deaths in Prison and Police Custody, *Royal Commission into Aboriginal Deaths in Custody* Research Paper No.7. Australian Institute of Criminology: Canberra.

Biles, D (1989b) Australian Deaths in Prisons 1980–1988: An Analysis of Aboriginal and Non-Aboriginal Deaths, *Royal Commission into Aboriginal Deaths in Custody* Research Paper No.11. Australian Institute of Criminology: Canberra.

Biles, D (1990) *International Review of Deaths in Custody* Criminology Research Unit Paper No. 15. Australian Institute of Criminology: Canberra.

Biles, D (1991) Deaths in Custody in Britain and Australia, *Howard Journal* 30(2): 110–120.

Birtchnell, J and Alacron, J (1971) The Motivation and Emotional State of 91 Cases of Attempted Suicide, *British Journal of Medical Psychology* 44:45–52.

Bluglass, R (1990) Recruitment and Training of Prison Doctors, *British Medical Journal* 301:249–250.

Bondeson, U V (1989) *Prisoners in Prison Societies*. Transaction: New Jersey.

Bottomley, A K (1979) *Criminology in Focus: Past Trends and Future Prospects*. Martin Robertson: Oxford.

Bottomley, A K (1990) Lord Justice Woolf's Inquiry into Prison Disturbances, unpublished submission.

Bottomley, A K and Liebling, A (1987) Young Offender Throughcare, unpublished report submitted to Home Office.

Bottomley, A K and Liebling, A (1988) Throughcare For Young Offenders in Custody, *Prison Service Journal* 74:9–13.

Bottoms, A E (1990) The Aims of Imprisonment, in Garland, D (ed.) (1990) *Justice, Guilt and Forgiveness in the Penal System* Occasional Paper No. 18. Centre for Theology and Public Issues, University of Edinburgh, pp. 3–37.

Bourke, G J, Daly, L E and McGilvray, J (1985) *Interpretation and Uses of Medical Statistics* (3rd edn). Blackwell: Oxford.

Bowker, L H (1977) *Prison Subcultures*. Lexington: Massachusetts.

Bowker, L H (1980) *Prison Victimization*. Elsevier: New York.

Bowker, L H (1982) *Corrections: the Science and the Art*. Macmillan: New York.

Bowlby, J (1965, 1st edn 1953) *Child Care and the Growth of Love*. Penguin: Middlesex.

British Medical Associaton (1990) *Working Party Report on the Health Care of Remand Prisoners*. BMA: London.

Broadhurst, L G and Maller, R A (1990) White Man's Magic Makes Black Deaths in Custody Disappear, *American Journal of Social Issues* 25(4):279–89.

Broderick Report (1971) *Death and Certification of Coroners*. Cmnd. 4810. HMSO: London.

Brown, G W and Harris, T (1978) *Social Origins of Depression: A Study of Psychiatric Disorder in Women*. Tavistock: London.

Bukstel, L H and Kilmann, P R (1980), Psychological Effects of Imprisonment on Confined Individuals, *Psychological Bulletin* 88(2):469–493.

Bulmer, M (1977) *Sociological Research Methods: An Introduction*. Macmillan: London.

Bulmer, M (1980) Comment on 'The Ethics of Covert Methods', *British Journal of Sociology* 31 (1): 59–65

Burgess, R G (1982) *Field Research: A Sourcebook and Field Manual*. Allen and Unwin: London.

Burtch, B E (1979) Prisoner Suicides Reconsidered, *International Journal of Law and Psychiatry* 2:407–413.

Burtch, B E and Ericson, R V (1979) *The Silent System: An Inquiry into Prisoners who Suicide and Annotated Bibliography.* Centre of Criminology: University of Toronto.

Burtch, B E and Ericson, R V (1985) The Silent System: Official Responses to Suicidal Prisoners, in Fleming, T (ed.) *The New Criminologies in Canada: State, Crime and Control.* Oxford University Press, Toronto: 313–326.

Carlen, P (1983) *Women's Imprisonment: A Study in Social Control.* Routledge: London.

Carroll, L (1974) *Hacks, Blacks and Cons: Race Relations in a Maximum Security Prison.* Heath: Massachusetts.

Casale, S (1989) *Women Inside: The Experience of Women Remand Prisoners in Holloway.* The Civil Liberties Trust: London.

Chambers, D R (1989) The Coroner, the Inquest and the Verdict of Suicide (Editorial), *Medicine, Science and the Law* 29(3):181.

Chambers, D R and Harvey, J C (1989) Inner Urban and National Suicide Rates, a Simple Comparative Study, *Medicine, Science and the Law* 29 (3):182–185.

Cheek, F and Miller, M D S (1983) The Experience of Stress for Prison Officers: A Double-bind Theory of Correctional Stress, *Journal of Criminal Justice* 11 105–120.

Cherniss, C (1980) *Staff Burnout: Job Stress in the Human Services.* Sage: Newbury Park.

Chiles, J A, Strosahl, K, Cowden, L, Graham, R and Lineham, M. (1986) The 24 Hours Before Hospitalization: Factors Related to Suicide Attempting, *Suicide and Life-Threatening Behaviour* 16 (3):335–342.

Christie, N (1981) *Limits to Pain.* Martin Robertson: Oxford.

Clarke, R V G and Cornish, D B (1983) *Crime Control in Britain: A Review of Policy Research.* State University of New York Press: Albany.

Clarke, R V G and Martin, D N (1971) *Absconding From Approved Schools* Home Office Research Studies 12. HMSO: London.

Clarke, R V G and Mayhew, P (eds) (1980) *Designing Out Crime.* HMSO: London.

Clemmer, D (1940) *The Prison Community.* Holt, Rinehart & Winston: New York.

Cohen, S and Taylor, L (1972) *Psychological Survival: The Experience of Long-term Imprisonment.* Harmonic, Penguin: London.

Coid, J (1984) How Many Psychiatric Patients in Prison? *British Journal of Psychiatry* 145: 78–86.

Coid, J, Wilkins, J, Chitkara, B and Everitt, B (1990a) Self-mutilation in Female Remanded Prisoners : II A Cluster Analytic Approach to Identification of a Behavioural Syndrome, unpublished paper.

Coid, J, Wilkins, J and Chitkara, B (1990b) Self-mutilation in Female Remanded Prisoners: III The Association with Firesetting and Pyromania, unpublished paper.

Consumers of Mental Health Services (1988) unpublished proceedings of conference, London.

Cookson, H M (1977) A Survey of Self-Injury in a Closed Prison for Women, *British Journal of Criminology* 17(4):332–347.

Cookson, H and Williams, M (1990) Assessing the Statistical Significance of Rare Events, unpublished paper (restricted circulation) DPS Report Series 1:33.

Cooper, H H A (1971) Self-Mutilation by Peruvian Prisoners, *International Journal of Offender Therapy and Comparative Criminology* 15(3):180–188.

Correctional Service of Canada (1981) *Self-inflicted Injuries and Suicides.* Bureau of Management Consulting: Canada.

Coroners Rules (1984) SI 552. HMSO: London.

Cressey, D R (Ed) (1961) *The Prison: Studies in Institutional Organization and Changes.* Holt, Rinehart and Winston: New York.

Cullen, J E (1981) *The Prediction and Treatment of Self-injury by Female Young Offenders* DPS Report, Series 1 No.17. Home Office: London.

Danto, B L (1973) *Jail House Blues: Studies of Suicidal Behaviour in Jail and Prison.* Epic Publications: Michigan.

Danto, B L (1978) Suicide Among Murderers, *International Journal of Offender Therapy and Comparative Criminology* 22(2):140–148.

Davies, B (1990) Report From Suicide Prevention Working Party, unpublished confidential report, Swansea.

Davis, J A (1971) *Elementary Survey Analysis.* Prentice Hall: New Jersey.

Denzin, N (1978) (ed.) *Sociological Methods: A Sourcebook* (2nd edn) McGraw-Hill: London.

Diekstra, R F W (1987) Renee: Chronicle of A Misspent Life, and Renee or the Complex Dynamics of Adolescent Suicide, in Diekstra, R F W and Hawton, K (eds) (1987) *Suicide in Adolescence.* Martinus Nijhoff Publishers: Dordrecht, pp. 25–77.

Diekstra, R F W and Hawton, K (eds) (1987) *Suicide in Adolescence.* Martinus Nijhoff Publishers: Dordrecht.

Dobash, R P, Dobash, R E and Gutteridge, S (1986) *The Imprisonment of Women.* Basil Blackwell: Oxford.

Dominion, J (1988) Address to Prison Chaplaincy Conference: Nottingham.

Dooley, E (1990a) Prison Suicide in England and Wales 1972–1987, *British Journal of Psychiatry* 156:40–45.

Dooley, E (1990b) Non-natural Deaths in Prison, *British Journal of Criminology* 30(2):229–234.

Dooley, E (1990c) Seminar given to Institute of Criminology, February, 1990.

Douglas, J (1967) *The Social Meanings of Suicide.* Routledge: London.

Douglas, J (1970) *The Relevance of Sociology.* Appleton-Century Crofts: New York.

Duffee, D (1974) The Correctional Officer and Organizational Change, *Journal of Research in Crime and Delinquency* 11(2) :155–179.

Dunbar, I (1985) A Sense of Direction, unpublished report to the Prison Department.

Durkheim, E (1964) *The Rules of Sociological Method.* The Free Press: New York.

Dyer, J A T and Kreitman, N (1984) Hopelessness, Depression and Suicidal Intent in Parasuicide, *British Journal of Psychiatry* 144:127–133.

Education, Science and Arts Committee (ESA) (1990) *Prison Education* Third Report. HMSO: London.

Eldrid, J (1988) *Caring for the Suicidal.* Constable: London

Elpern, S and Kemp, S (1984) Sex-role Orientation and Depressive Symptomatology, *Sex Roles* 10 (11/12):987–992.

Erikson, R V (1975) *Young Offenders and their Social Work.* Heath: Massachusetts.

Esparza, R (1973) Attempted and Committed Suicide in County Jails, in Danto, B L (ed.) *Jail House Blues.* Epic Publications: Michigan.

Farmer, R D T (1988) Assessing the Epidemiology of Suicide and Parasuicide, *British Journal of Psychiatry* 153:16–20.

Fawcett, J and Mars, B (1973) Suicide at the County Jail, in Danto, B L (ed.) *Jail House Blues.* Epic Publications: Michigan.

Feather, N T (1985) Masculinity, Femininity, Self-esteem, and Subclinical Depression, *Sex Roles* 12 (5/6):491–499.

Feld, B C (1977) *Neutralizing Inmate Violence: Juvenile Offenders in Institutions.* Ballinger: Massachusetts.

Fenwick, F (1984) Accounting for Sudden Death: A Sociological Study of the Coroner System, unpublished doctoral thesis, University of Hull.

Flaherty, M G (1983) *The National Incidence of Juvenile Suicide in Adult Jails and Juvenile Detention Centres,* University of Illinois: Urbana-Champaign.

Foster, J (1990) Having a Field Day, *New Society* 15 June 1990, p.28.

Fromm, E (1962) *Beyond the Chains of Illusion*. Abacus edn. (1986): London.

Gaes, G G (1985) The Effects of Overcrowding in Prison, in Tonry, M and Morris, N (1985) *Crime and Justice: An Annual Review of Research* Vol. 6. University of Chicago Press: Chicago.

Gardner, R, Hanka, R, Roberts, S J, Allon Smith, J M, Kings, A A and Nicholson, R (1982) Psychological and Social Evaluation in Cases of Deliberate Self-poisoning Seen in an Accident Department, *British Medical Journal* 284:491–493.

Gaston, A W (1979) Prisoners, in Hankoff, L D and Einsidler B (eds) *Suicide: Theory and Clinical Aspects*. PSG: USA.

Geary, R (1980) *Deaths in Prison*. NCCL Briefing Paper. National Council for Civil Liberties: London.

Gelsthorpe, L (1990) Feminist Methodologies in Criminology: a New Approach or Old Wine in New Bottles?, in Gelsthorpe, L and Morris, A (eds) *Feminist Perspectives in Criminology*. Open University Press: Milton Keynes.

Gelsthorpe, L and Morris, A (1988) Feminism and Criminology in Britain, in Rock, P (ed.) *A History of British Criminology*. Oxford University Press: Oxford.

Genders, E and Player, E (1989) *Race Relations in Prison*. Clarendon Press: Oxford.

Gerstein, L, Topp, C and Correll, G (1987) The Role of the Environment and Person When Predicting Burnout Among Correctional Personnel, *Criminal Justice and Behaviour* 14(3):352–369.

Gibbons, D (1990) The Ultimate Price: Women's Deaths in Prison, unpublished CQSW thesis, Hatfield Polytechnic.

Gilligan, C (1982) *In a Different Voice: Psychological Theory and Women's Development*. Harvard University Press: Massachusetts.

Gillilend, D (1990) Research Note: Attempted Suicide Among Adolescents, *British Journal of Social Work* 20:365–371.

Goffman, E (1968) *Asylums*. Penguin: London.

Goldney, R D and Burvil, P W (1980) Trends in Suicidal Behaviour and its Management, *Australian and New Zealand Journal of Psychiatry* 14:1–15.

Golombak, H and Garfinkle, B D (1983) *The Adolescent and Mood Disturbance*. International Universities Press: New York.

Goring, C (1913) *The English Convict*. HMSO: London

Gould, M S (1988) Suicide Clusters and Media Exposure, paper published in Blumenthal, S J and Kupfer, D J (eds) *Suicide Over the Life Cycle*. American Psychiatric Press: Washington D. C.

Gould, M S and Shaffer, D (1986) The Impact of Suicide in Television Movies, *New England Journal of Medicine* 315:690–694.

Gould, M S, Wallenstein, S and Kleinman, M (1987) Time Space Clustering of Teenage Suicides, unpublished paper, Division of Child Psychiatry: University of Columbia.

Gouldner, A W (1973) *For Sociology: Renewal and Critique in Sociology Today*. Allen Lane: London.

Gover, R M (1880) Notes by the Medical Inspector, in Appendix No. 19, *Prison Commission Annual Report*, 1880. HMSO: London

Griffiths, A W and Rundle, A T (1976) A Survey of Male Prisoners, *British Journal of Criminology* 16(4):352–366.

Griffiths, A W (1990a) High and Low Offenders Compared, *Medicine, Science and the Law* 30(3):214–216.

Griffiths, A W (1990b) Correlates of Suicidal History in Male Prisoners, *Medicine, Science and the Law* 30(3):217–218.

Grindrod, H and Black, G (1989) *Suicides at Leeds Prison: An Enquiry into the Deaths of Five Teenagers During 1988/89*. Howard League for Penal Reform: London

Gudjonnson, G H (1988) Interrogative Suggestibility: its Relationship with Assertiveness, Social Evaluative Anxiety, State Anxiety and Method of Coping, *British Journal of Clinical Psychology* 27:159–166.

Gunn, J, Robertson, G, Dell, S and Way, C (1978) *Psychiatric Aspects of Imprisonment.* Academic Press: London.

Gunn, J (1990) Meeting the Need, unpublished paper, Institute of Psychiatry: London.

Hammersley, M and Atkinson, P (1983) *Ethnography: Principles in Practice.* Tavistock: London.

Hammerlin, Y and Bodal, K (1988) *Suicide and Life-threatening Activities in Norwegian Prisons During the Period 1956 through 1987.* Ministry of Justice, Prison Department, Norway.

Hankoff, Leon D (1980) Prisoner Suicide, *International Journal of Offender Therapy and Comparative Criminology* 24(2):162–166.

Harding, S (ed.) (1987) *Feminism and Methodology.* Open University Press: Milton Keynes.

Harding-Pink, D (1990) Mortality Following Release From Prison, *Medicine, Science and the Law* 30(1):12–16.

Hatty, S E and Walker, J R (1986) *A National Study of Deaths in Australian Prisons,* Australian Centre of Criminology: Canberra.

Hawton, K (1978) Deliberate Self-poisoning and Self-injury in the Psychiatric Hospital, *British Journal of Medical Psychology* 51:253–259.

Hawton, K (1986) *Suicide and Attempted Suicide Amongst Children and Adolescents.* Sage: London.

Hawton, K (1987a) Assessment of Suicide Risk, *British Journal of Psychiatry* 150:145–153.

Hawton, K (Update) (1987b) Attempted Suicide in Adolescents, *Association for Child Psychology and Psychiatry Newsletter* 9(1):5–9.

Hawton, K and Catalan, J (1987) *Attempted Suicide: A Practical Guide to Its Nature and Management* (2nd edn). Oxford University Press: Oxford.

Hawton, K, Cole, D, O'Grady, J and Osborn, M (1982a) Motivational Aspects of Deliberate Self-poisoning in Adolescents, *British Journal of Psychiatry* 141:286–291.

Hawton, K, Osborn, M, O'Grady, J and Cole, D (1982b) Classification of Adolescents who take Overdoses, *British Journal of Psychiatry* 140:124–131.

Hawton, K, O'Grady, J, Osborn, M and Cole, D (1982c) Adolescents Who Take Overdoses: Problems and Contacts With Helping Agencies, *British Journal of Psychiatry* 140:118–123.

Hayes, Lindsay M (1983) And Darkness Closes In ... A National Study of Jail Suicides, *Criminal Justice and Behaviour* 10(4):461–484.

Heffernan, E (1972) *Making it in Prison: The Square, The Cool, and the Life.* Wiley and Sons Inc: London.

Heilig, S (1973) Suicide in jails: A Preliminary Study in Los Angeles, in Danto, B L (ed.) *Jail House Blues.* Epic Publications: Michigan.

Hempel, C G (1966) Explanation in Science and History, in Dray, W H (1966) *Philosophical Analysis and History.* Harper and Row: New York.

Holding, T A and Barraclough, B M (1975) Psychiatric Morbidity in a Sample of a London Coroner's Open Verdicts, *British Journal of Psychiatry* 127:97.

Home Office (1978) *A Survey of the South East Prison Population* Research Bulletin No.5:12–24. HORPU: London.

Home Office (1979) *May Committee Inquiry into The United Kingdom Prison Services.* HMSO: London.

Home Office (1984) *Suicides in Prison.* Report by HM Chief Inspector of Prisons. HMSO: London.

Home Office (1985) HM YCC and Remand Centre Glen Parva. *Report by HM Chief Inspector of Prisons.* HMSO: London.

Home Office (1986a) *Report of the Working Group on Suicide Prevention*. HMSO: London.
Home Office (1986b) *Report on the Work of the Prison Department*. 1985/6 Cm.11 HMSO: London.
Home Office (1987) Circular Instruction 3/1987: *Suicide Prevention*. HMSO: London.
Home Office (1988a) *Report on the Work of the Prison Service 1987–8*. HMSO: London.
Home Office (1988b) H. M. Remand Centre Risley. *Report by H. M. Chief Inspector of Prisons*. HMSO: London.
Home Office (1988c) H. M. Prison Hull. *Report by H. M. Chief Inspector of Prisons*. HMSO: London.
Home Office (1988d) Circular Instruction 40/1988: *Regimes in YOIs*. HMSO: London.
Home Office (1989a) Circular Instruction 20/1989: *Suicide Prevention*. HMSO: London.
Home Office (1989b) *Briefing* No.11, 24 July:2.
Home Office (1990a) *Report on the Work of the Prison Service 1988–1989*. HMSO: London.
Home Office (1990b) Suicide Prevention and Follow-up to Deaths in Custody, Addendum to CI 20/89.
Home Office (1990c) H. M. Prison Leeds. *Report by H. M. Chief Inspector of Prisons*. HMSO: London.
Home Office (1990d) *Report of a Review by Her Majesty's Chief Inspector of Prisons For England and Wales of Suicide and Self-harm in Prison Service Establishments in England and Wales*. HMSO: London.
Home Office (1990e) Scrutiny Team on Prison Medical Services, *Report of an Efficiency Scrutiny of the Prison Medical Service Vols I and II*. Home Office: London.
Home Office Directorate of Prison Medical Services (1990) *Guidelines for Prison Medical Officers on the Use of Protective and Unfurnished Rooms as a Clinical Intervention*. Prison Medical Directorate: London.
Home Office Statistical Bulletin (1990) 12/90: *The Prison Population in 1989*. Government Statistical Service: London
Hopes, B and Shaull, R (1986) Jail Suicide Prevention: Effective Programmes Can Save Lives, *Corrections Today* 48(8):64–70.
Howard League (1990) *Criminal Justice* Vol. 8, No.2 – Parliamentary Questions.
Hull Prison Board of Visitors' *Annual Report* (1988) Hull Prison.
Inquest (1991) *Annual Report*: London.
Irwin, J (1970) *The Felon*. Prentice-Hall: New Jersey.
Irwin, J and Cressey, D R (1962) Thieves, Convicts and the Inmate Culture, *Social Problems* 10(1):142–155.
Jacobs, J (1978) What Prison Guards Think: A Profile of the Illinois Force, *Crime Delinquency* (24):185.
James, E (1989) The Prison Chaplaincy: A Mission to an Urban Priority Area, unpublished Conference Paper, Prison Chaplaincy Conference 1989.
Jenkins, R L, Heidemann, P H and Powell, S (1982) The Risk and Prevention of Suicide in Residential Treatment of Adolescents, *Juvenile and Family Court Journal* 33(2):11–16.
Jepson, N and Elliot, K (1985) Shared Working between Prison and Probation Officers, unpublished Home Office Report: University of Leeds.
Johnson, E (1973) Felon Self-mutilation: Correlates of Stress in Prison, in Danto B L(ed.) (1973) *Jail House Blues*. Epic: Michigan.
Johnson, R (1976) *Culture and Crisis in Confinement*. Heath: Massachusetts.
Johnson, R (1977) Ameliorating Prison Stress: Some Helping Roles for Custodial Personnel, *International Journal of Criminology and Penology* 5:263–273.
Johnson, R (1978) Youth in Crisis: Dimensions of Self-destructive Conduct Among Adolescent Prisoners, *Adolescence* 13 (51): 461–482.
Johnson, R and Toch, H (1982) *The Pains of Imprisonment*. Sage: California.

Jones, A (1986) Self-mutilation in Prison: A Comparison of Mutilators and Non-mutilators, *Criminal Justice and Behaviour* 13(3):286–296.

Jones, H, Cornes, P and Stackford, R (1977) *Open Prisons*. Routledge and Kegan Paul: London.

Kappeler, V E, Vaughn, M S and Del Carmen, R V (1991) Death in Detention: an Analysis of Police Liability for Negligent Failure to Prevent Suicide, *Journal of Criminal Justice* 19:381–393.

Kelleher, M (1988) Question to Professor Kreitman, in *The Clinical Management of Suicide Risk*, Proceedings of a Conference held at The Royal Society of Medicine: London.

Kelly, L (1988) *Surviving Sexual Violence*. Blackwell: Oxford.

Kennedy, D B (1984) A Theory of Suicide While in Police Custody, *Journal of Police Science and Administration* 12(2):191–200.

Kitsuse, J I and Cicourel, A V (1963) A Note on the Uses of Official Statistics, *Social Problems* 11:131–139.

Knapman, P and Powers, M J (1985) Quashing the Inquisition, *The Law and Practice on Coroners*. Barry Rose: Chichester, pp.167–174.

Kreitman, N (1969) Parasuicide (Letter), *British Journal of Psychiatry* 115:746–747.

Kreitman, N (1977) (ed.) *Parasuicide*. Wiley and Sons: London.

Kreitman, N (1988) Some General Observations on Suicide in Psychiatric Patients, in *Proceedings of a Conference on The Clinical Management of Suicide Risk*. Royal Society of Medicine, London.

Kreitman, N, Carstairs V and Duffy J (1991) Association of Age and Social Class with Suicide among Men in Great Britain, *Journal of Epidemiology and Community Health* 45:195–202.

Langlay, G E and Bayatti, N N (1984) Suicide in Exe Vale Hospital, 1972–1981, *British Journal of Psychiatry* 145:463–467.

Launay, G and Fielding, P (1989) Stress Among Prison Officers: Some Empirical Evidence Based on Self-report, *The Howard Journal* 28(2): 138–148.

Laycock, G K (1977) *Absconding From Borstals* Home Office Research Study, 41. HMSO: London.

Lester, D and Gatto, J (1989) Self-destructive Tendencies and Depression as Predictors of Suicidal Ideation in Teenagers, *Journal of Adolescence* 12:221–223.

Liebling, A (1991) Suicide and Self-Injury Amongst Young Offenders in Custody, PhD thesis submitted to University of Cambridge.

Liebling, H (1990) A Study of Anxiety Levels in Female Prison Officers Working in Different Conditions of Security and Female Hostel Staff, unpublished MPhil Thesis, University of Edinburgh.

Lloyd, C (1990) *Suicide in Prison: A Literature Review* Home Office Research Study 115. HORPU: London.

Lofland, J (1971) *Analysing Social Settings*. Wadsworth: New York.

Long, N, Shouksmith, G, Voges, K and Roache, S (1986) Stress in Prison Staff: An Occupational Study, *Criminology* 24(2):331–345.

MacAllister, D (1990) Youth Custody Throughcare: The Role of the Community Based Probation Officer, unpublished PhD thesis: University of Hull.

McCain, G, Cox, V C and Paulus, P (1980) The Effect of Prison Crowding on Inmate Behaviour, unpublished Final Report: University of Texas.

McCloone, P and Crombie, I K (1987) Trends in Suicide in Scotland 1974–84: An Increasing Problem, *British Medical Journal* 295:629–631.

McClure, G M G (1984a) Trends in Suicide Rate for England and Wales 1975–80, *British Journal of Psychiatry* 144: 119–126.

McClure, G M G (1984b) Recent Trends in Suicide Amongst the Young, *British Journal of Psychiatry* 144: 134–138.

McClure, G M G (1987) Suicide in England and Wales, 1975–1984, *British Journal of Psychiatry* 150: 309–314.

McClure, G M G (1988) Suicide in Children in England and Wales, *Journal of Child Psychology and Psychiatry* 29(3):345–349.

McDermott, K and King, R (1988) Mind Games, *British Journal of Criminology* 28(3):357–378.

McGurk, B J and Fludger, N L (1987) The Selection of Prison Officers, in McGurk, B J, Thornton, D M and Williams, M *Applying Psychology to Imprisonment.* HMSO: London.

McGurk, B J and McDougal, C (1986) *The Prevention of Bullying Among Incarcerated Delinquents* DPS Report, Series II, no.114 (restricted circulation): London.

McMurran, M (1986) *Drinking Less.* Glen Parva: Leicester.

McMurran, M and Hollin, C (1989) Drinking and Delinquency: Another Look at Young Offenders and Alcohol, *British Journal of Criminology* 29:386–394.

McNeill, P (1989) *Research Methods* (2nd edn). Routledge: London.

Maltsberger, J T (1986) *Suicide Risk: The Formulation of Clinical Judgment.* New York University Press: New York.

Mandaraka-Sheppherd, A (1986) *The Dynamics of Aggression in Women's Prisons in England and Wales.* Gower: Aldershot.

Mann, P (1985) *Methods of Social Investigation.* Basil Blackwell: Oxford.

Maris, R W (1981) *Pathways to Suicide: A Survey of Self-destructive Behaviours.* Johns Hopkins University Press: Baltimore.

Mathieson, T (1965) *The Defences of the Weak: A Sociological Study of a Norwegian Correctional Institution.* Tavistock: London.

Matza, D (1964) *Delinquency and Drift.* Wiley: New York.

Massachusetts Special Commission (1984) Suicide in Massachusetts Lock-Ups 1973–1984, unpublished Final Report Submitted to the General Court: Massachusetts.

Merton, R K, Fiske, M and Kendall, P L (1956) *The Focussed Interview; A Manual of Problems and Procedures.* Bureau of Applied Social Research: Columbia University.

Mezey, G and King, M (1987) Male Victims of Sexual Assault, *Medicine, Science and the Law* 27(2):122–124.

Mezey, G and King, M (1989) The Effects of Sexual Assault on Men: a Survey of 22 Victims, *Psychological Medicine* 19:205–209.

Modestin, J and Wurmle, O (1989) Role of Modelling in In-patient Suicide: a Lack of Supporting Evidence, *British Journal of Psychiatry* 155:511–514.

Monat, A and Lazarus, R S (1985) *Stress and Coping: An Anthology.* Columbia University Press: New York.

Moore, R G, Watts, F N and Williams, J M G (1988) The Specificity of Personal Memories in Depression, *British Journal of Clinical Psychology* 27:275–276.

Morgan, H G (1979) *Death Wishes: The Understanding and Management of Deliberate Self-harm.* Wiley: Chichester.

Morris, A (1987) *Women, Crime and Criminal Justice.* Basil Blackwell: Oxford.

Moser, C and Kalton, G (1971) *Survey Methods of Social Investigation* (2nd edn). Heinemann: London.

NACRO (1985) *Black People in the Criminal Justice System.* NACRO Briefing Paper: London.

NACRO (1990) *News Digest No. 62* Parliamentary Questions. NACRO: London.

New South Wales Bureau of Crime Statistics and Research (1990) *Crime and Justice Bulletin* (8) NSW.

Nie, N H, Klecka, W R and Hull, C H (1989) *Statistical Package for the Social Sciences Primer.* McGraw-Hill: New York.

Oakley, A (1981) *Subject Woman.* Robertson: Oxford.

O'Connor, M (1984) Probation: The Outside Connection, *Prison Service Journal* 55:2–3.

Office of Corrections Resource Centre (1988) *Suicide and Other Deaths in Prisons includ- ing Victorian Results from the National Deaths in Corrections Study*. Research Unit Office of Corrections: Canada.

Office of Population Censuses and Surveys (1985) *Prison Staff Attitudes*. HMSO: London.

Office of Population Censuses and Surveys (1988) *Morbidity Statistics*. HMSO: London.

Office of Population Censuses and Surveys (1990) *Mortality Statistics*. HMSO: London.

O'Mahony, P (1990) A Review of the Problem of Prison Suicide, unpublished (restricted circulation) report: Dublin.

O'Mahony, P (1991) Prison Suicide Rates: What Do They Mean? Paper presented at Deaths in Custody Conference, Canterbury (proceedings forthcoming).

Orlowski, R J (1986) Suicide and Self-Injury, unpublished paper presented to Michigan Department of Corrections.

Ovenstone, I M K and Kreitman, N (1974) Two Syndromes of Suicide, *British Journal of Psychiatry* 124:36–45.

Paerregaard, G (1975) Suicide Among Attempted Suicide: A 10-year Follow-up, *Suicide* 5(3):140–144.

Pahl, R (1977) 'Playing the Rationality Game: the Sociologist as a Hired Expert' in Bell, C and Newby, H (eds) *Doing Sociological Research*. Allen and Unwin: London.

Pallis, D J (1988) Open Forum Discussion, in *The Clinical Management of Suicide Risk*, Proceedings of a Conference held at The Royal Society of Medicine: London.

Pallis, D J, Gibbons, J S and Pierce, D W (1984) Estimating Suicide Risk among Attempted Suicides II: Efficiency of Predictive Scales after the Attempt, *British Journal of Psychiatry* 144:139–148.

Park, R E (1925) *The City*, Reprinted as Park, R E and Burgess E W (1967) University of Chicago Press: Chicago.

Parker, H J (1974) *A View From The Boys*. David and Charles: Newton Abbot.

Pescosolido, B A and Mendelsohn, R (1986) Social Causation or Social Construction of Suicide? An Investigation into the Social Organisation of Official Rates, *American Sociological Review* 51:80–101.

Phillips, M (1986) *Suicide and Attempted Suicide in Brixton Prison*. DPS Report: London.

Phillpots, G J O and Lancucki, L B (1979) *Previous Convictions, Sentence and Reconviction*, Home Office Research Study 53.

Polsky, H (1962) *Cottage Six*. Wiley: New York.

Poole, E and Regoli, R (1980) Work Relations and Cynicism among Prison Guards, *Criminal Justice and Behaviour* 7(3) 303–314.

Porporino, F (1983) Coping Behaviour in Prison Inmates: Description and Correlates, PhD Dissertation, University of Ontario, Canada.

Porporino, F J and Zamble, E (1984) Coping with Imprisonment, *Canadian Journal of Criminology*, 26:403–421.

Posen, I (1985) Survey of Work-Stress at Holloway, in Williams, M and Bateman, V (eds) (1985) *Proceedings of the Prison Psychologists' Conference 1985* DPS Report Series II No. 149. HMSO: London.

Power, K G and Spencer, A P (1987) Parasuicidal Behaviour of Detained Scottish Young Offenders, *International Journal of Offender Therapy and Comparative Criminology* 31(3):227–235.

Priestly, P (1985) *Victorian Prison Lives 1830–1914*. Methuen: London.

Prison Commission *Annual Report 1897*. HMSO: London.

Prison Commission *Annual Report 1880*. HMSO: London.

Prison Commission *Annual Report 1911*. HMSO: London.

Prison Department (1989) *The Management of Vulnerable Prisoners*, Report of the Prison Department Working Group. PRT: London.

Prison Reform Trust (1983) *Arrangements for the Prevention of Suicide in Prison*, Submission by the Prison Reform Trust to HM Chief Inspector of Prisons. PRT: London.

Prison Reform Trust (1990) *Prison Report 13*. PRT: London.

Prison Statistics England and Wales 1972–1988. HMSO: London.

Ramsay, R F, Tanney, B L and Searle, C A (1987) Suicide Prevention in High-risk Prison Populations, *Canadian Journal of Criminology* 29(3):295–307.

Rich, C L, Ricketts, J E, Fowler, R C and Young, D (1988) Some Differences Between Men and Women Who Commit Suicide, *American Journal of Psychiatry* 145(6):718–722.

Robins, E, Murphy, G E, Wilkinson, R H, Gassner, S and Kaynes, J (1959) Some Clinical Considerations in the Prevention of Suicide, Based on a Study of 134 Successful Suicides, *American Journal of Public Health* 49:888–898.

Robson, C (1983) *Experiment, Design and Statistics in Psychology* (2nd edn). Penguin: Middlesex.

Rood de Boer, M (1978) Children's Suicide, in Eekelaar, JM and Katz, SM *Family Violence: An International and Interdisciplinary Study*. Butterworths: Toronto, pp. 441–459.

Ross, R R, McKay, H B, Palmer, W R T, Kenny, C J (1978) Self-mutilation in Adolescent Female Offenders, *Canadian Journal of Criminology* 20(4) 375–392.

Roy, A and Linnoila, M (1986) Alcoholism and Suicide, *Suicide and Life-threatening Behaviour* 16(2):162–188.

Royal Commission into Aboriginal Deaths in Custody (1988) *Interim Report*. Australian Government Publishing Service: Canberra.

Sainsbury, P (1988) Suicide Prevention – An Overview, in Morgan, H G (ed.) *The Clinical Management of Suicide Risk*, Proceedings of a Conference held at The Royal Society of Medicine: London.

Samaritans (1990) *Who Cares if I Live or Die? : Suicide in Great Britain*. The Samaritans: London.

Sapsford, R (1983) *Life Sentence Prisoners*. Open University Press: Milton Keynes.

Schmidte, A and Hafner, H (1988) The Werther Effect after Television Films: New Evidence for an Old Hypothesis, *Psychological Medicine* 18:665–676.

Schneidman, E (1973) *Deaths of Man*. Quadrangle: New York.

Schneidman, E (1985) *Definition of Suicide*. Wiley: New York.

Scott-Denoon, K (1984) *B.C. Corrections: A Study of Suicides 1970–1980*. Corrections Branch: British Columbia.

Scottish Home and Health Department (1985) *Report of the Review of Suicide Precautions at H. M. Detention Centre and Young Offenders Institution, Glenochil*. HMSO: Edinburgh.

Scraton, P and Chadwick, K (1986) *In the Arms of the Law: Coroners' Inquests and Deaths in Custody*. Pluto Press: London.

Scraton, P and Chadwick, K (1987) Speaking Ill of the Dead: Institutionalized Responses to Deaths in Custody, in Scraton, P. (ed.) *Law, Order and the Authoritarian State*. Open University Press: Milton Keynes.

Seager, C P and Flood, R A (1965) Suicide in Bristol, *British Journal of Psychiatry* 111:919–932.

Seeley, J R (1970) The Making and Taking of Problems: Toward an Ethical Stance, in Douglas, J *The Relevance of Sociology*. Appleton-Century Crofts: New York.

Shaffer, D (1974) Suicide in Childhood and Early Adolescence, *Journal of Child Psychology and Psychiatry* 15:275–291.

Shils, E A (1959) Social Inquiry and the Autonomy of the Individual, in Lerner, D (ed.) (1959) *The Human Meaning of the Social Sciences*. Meridan: New York, pp.114–157.

Shine, J, Wilson, P and Hammond, D (1990) Understanding and Controlling Violence in a Long-term Young Offender Institution, in Fludger, N L and Simmons, I P *Proceedings*

From Psychologists Conference 1989. DPS Report Series I No. 34:115–132 Directorate of Psychological Services: London.

Sim, J (1990) *Medical Power in Prisons: The Prison Medical Service in England: 1774–1989.* Open University Press: Milton Keynes.

Sinclair, I (1971) *Hostels for Probationers,* Home Office Research Studies No. 6. HMSO: London.

Smalley, H (1911) Report by the Medical Inspector, in *Report by the Prison Commissioners.* HMSO: London.

Smart, C (1977) *Women, Crime and Criminology: A Feminist Critique.* Routledge: London.

Smith, R (1984) Ample Scope for Improving the Health of Prisoners, *British Medical Journal* 288: 1939–1940.

Smith, R (1985) Report on Seven Deaths at Glenochil, *British Medical Journal* 291: 353.

Smith, R (1986) The State of the Prisons, *British Medical Journal* 287–288 (serialised).

Smith, T (1984) Stress in the Prison Service, *Prison Service Journal* 56:10–11.

Smith, T (1985) Stress in Prison Officers, in William, M and Bateman, V (eds) (1986) *Proceedings of the Prison Psychologists' Conference* 1985. DPS Report Series II No. 149. HMSO: London.

Sparks, R (1989) Problems of Order in Dispersal Prisons: Notes on a Research Process, unpublished paper.

Sperbeck, D J and Parlour, R R (1986) Screening and Managing Suicidal Prisoners, *Corrective and Social Psychiatry* 32(3): 95–98.

Staples, J (1990) (Editorial), *Prison Service Journal* (79):1.

Stengel, E (1964, 1980 edn) *Suicide and Attempted Suicide.* Penguin: London.

Stengel, E (1970) Attempted Suicide (Letter), *British Journal of Psychiatry* 116:237–238.

Stengel, E (1971) Suicide in Prison: The Gesture and the Risk, *Prison Service Journal* 2: 13–14.

Stengel, E and Cook, N (1958) *Attempted Suicide: Its Social Significance and Effects.* Chapman and Hall:London.

Stern, V (1989a) *Bricks of Shame* (2nd edn). Penguin: London.

Stern, V (1989b) *Imprisoned by our Prisons.* Penguin: London.

Stephens, J (1987) Cheap Thrills and Humble Pie: The Adolescence of Female Suicide Attempters, *Suicide and Life-threatening Behaviour* 17 (2):107–118.

Stoppard, J M and Paisley, K J (1987) Masculinity, Femininity, Life Stress and Depression, *Sex Roles* 16 (9/10):489–495.

Sutherland, E H (1937) The Professional Thief, *Journal of Crime, Law and Criminology* 28:161–163.

Sykes, G (1958) *The Society of Captives.* Princeton University Press: Princeton.

Sykes, G and Messinger, S (1960) The Inmate Social System, in Cloward, R (ed.) (1960) *Theoretical Studies in Social Organization of the Prison.* Social Sciences Research Council: USA.

Taylor, P and Gunn, J C (1984) Violence and Psychosis II: Effect of Psychiatric Diagnosis on Conviction and Sentencing of Offenders, *British Medical Journal* 289:9–11.

Taylor, S (1982) *Durkheim and the Study of Suicide.* Macmillan: London.

Thomas, J E (1972) *The English Prison Officer Since 1850.* Routledge: London.

Thomas, J E and Pooley, R (1981) *The Exploding Prison: Prison Riots and the Case of Hull.* Junction: London.

Thornton, D (1990) *Depression, Self-Injury and Attempted Suicide Amongst the YOI Population* in Fludger, NL and Simmons, IP (eds) *Proceedings of the Prison Psychologists' Conference,* DPS Report Series 1: 34: 47–55.

Toch, H (1975) *Men in Crisis: Human Breakdowns in Prison.* Aldine: New York.

Toch, H and Klofas, J (1982) Alienation and Desire for Job Enrichment Among Correctional Officers, *Federal Probation* 46 (1):35–47.

Toch, H, Adams, K and Grant, D (1989) *Coping: Maladaptation in Prisons*. Transaction: New Brunswick.

Topp, D O (1979) Suicide in Prison, *British Journal of Psychiatry* 134:24–27.

Turner, T H and Tofler, D S (1986) Indications of Psychiatric Disorder amongst Women admitted to Prison, *British Medical Journal* 292:651–653.

Tuskan, J J and Thase, M E (1983) Suicides in Jails and Prisons. *Journal of Psychosocial Nursing and Mental Health* 21(5):29–33.

US Department of Justice (1988) *Criminal Statistics*.

Vinson, T (1982) *Wilful Obstruction: The Frustration of Prison Reform*. Methuen: North Ryde.

Vrandenberg, K, Krames, L and Flett, G (1986) Sex Differences in the Clinical Expression of Depression, *Sex Roles* 14(1/2):37–49.

Walker, M, Jefferson, T and Senerivante, M (1990) *Ethnic Minorities, Young People and the Criminal Justice System*. ESRC Project No. E06250020: Main Report. Centre for Criminological and Socio-Legal Studies: Sheffield.

Walker, N D (1977) *Behaviour and Misbehaviour: Explanations and Non-explanations*. Blackwell: Oxford.

Walker, N D (1983) Side-Effects of Incarceration, *British Journal of Criminology*, 23:61–71.

Walker, N D (1987) The Unwanted Effects of Long-term Imprisonment, in Bottoms, A E and Light, R (eds) *Problems of Long-Term Imprisonment*. Gower: Aldershot.

West, D J (1965) *Murder Followed by Suicide*. Cambridge Studies in Criminology XXI, Heinemann: London.

Wicks, R J (1972) Suicide Prevention: A Brief for Corrections Officers, *Federal Probation* 36:29–31.

Wicks, R J (1974) Suicidal Manipulators in the Penal Setting, *Chitty's Law Journal* 22(7):249–250.

Widom, C S (1989) Child Abuse, Neglect, and Violent Criminal Behaviour, *Criminology* 27(2):251–271.

Wilkins, J and Coid, J (1990) Self-mutilation in Female Remand Prisoners: 1. An Indicator of Severe Psychopathology, unpublished paper.

Williams, M (1986) Differences in Reasons for Taking Overdoses in High and Low Hopelessness Groups, *British Journal of Medical Psychology* 59:269–277.

Williams, M and Hassanyeh, F (1983) Deliberate Self-Harm, Clinical History and Extreme Scoring on the EPQ, *Personality and Individual Difference* 4(3):347–350.

Williams, J M G and Scott, J (1988) Autobiographical Memory in Depression, *Psychological Medicine* 18:689–695.

Winfree, L T (1985) American Jail Death-Rates: A Comparison of the 1978 and 1983 Jail Census Data, paper presented at the Annual Meeting of the American Society of Criminology, San Diego, California.

Women's Equality Group (1987) *Breaking The Silence: Women's Imprisonment*. Strategic Policy Unit: London.

Wool, R and Dooley, E (1987) A Study of Attempted Suicides in Prisons, *Medicine, Science and the Law* 27(4):297–301.

Wool, R (1991) Prison Suicides, unpublished paper presented at Deaths in Custody Conference, Canterbury.

Woolf, Lord Justice (1991) Report of an Inquiry into the Prison Disturbance April 1992. HMSO: London.

Wormith, J S (1984) The Controversy Over the Effects of Long-term Incarceration, *Canadian Journal of Criminology* 26(4):423–438.

Zamble, E and Porporino, F J (1988) *Coping, Behaviour and Adaptation in Prison Inmates*. New York: Springer-Verlag.

Zingraff, M T (1980) Inmate Assimilation: A Comparison of Male and Female Delinquents, *Criminal Justice and Behaviour* 7(3):275–292.

CASES CITED

Kirkham v. Anderson (appeal) reported in *The Times* 4 January 1990.
Knight and others v. Home Office and Governor of Brixton Prison, reported in *The Independent* 24 January 1990.
R v. Southwark Coroner, Ex-parte Hicks [1987] 1 W. L. R. 1624.
R v. Birmingham and Solihull Coroner, Ex-parte Secretary of State for the Home Department. (Appeal, unreported, 31 July 1990.)

Name index

Subject index